Dear WebMD Member,

Welcome to WebMD!

WebMD is offering you this book – **Women's Moods** by Deborah Sichel, MD, and Jeanne Watson Driscoll, MS, RN, CS – as a special thank-you for electing to become a WebMD member. Now that WebMD has merged with OnHealth, coming to WebMD is like walking into your favorite bookstore and finding that it's merged with another favorite across town. We've moved a lot of the great content, features, and tools from OnHealth to WebMD – creating a combined site that has the best of both! At the combined site, **http://my.webmd.com**, you can get same great advice from OnHealth experts like infertility expert Amos Grunebaum, MD, Dan Savage and Judy Sobiesk of Savage Family Matters, and Louanne Cole Weston of Sex Matters®. And you'll also recognize some of your favorite OnHealth tools like the Diet and Fitness Journal, Pregnancy Calendar, and Ovulation Calendar.

I would like to invite you to take advantage of WebMD's high-quality, original content and up-to-date health news created by the WebMD news team of doctors and medical journalists. At WebMD you can participate in online communities, manage your health with our Health-E-Tools, join an interactive chat session, even find a specialist physician in your area or request advice from one of WebMD's experts – and get instant support and feedback. Quite simply, WebMD is the online destination that puts a wealth of health information and resources at your fingertips.

So don't wait any longer, log onto **http://my.webmd.com** and let your fingers find your way to good health and wellness.

Again, thank you for choosing WebMD. We're delighted you've made the decision to join one of the Web's leaders in health information.

Sincerely,

Marjorie Martin

Marjorie Martin
Editor-in-Chief, WebMD
http://my.webmd.com

WOMEN'S MOODS

WHAT EVERY WOMAN MUST KNOW
ABOUT HORMONES, THE BRAIN,
AND EMOTIONAL HEALTH

Deborah Sichel, M.D.,
and
Jeanne Watson Driscoll, M.S., R.N., C.S.

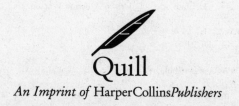

Quill
An Imprint of HarperCollinsPublishers

A hardcover edition of this book was published in 1999 by William Morrow and Company.

HarperCollins books may be purchased for educational, business, or sales promotional use. For information please write: Special Markets Department, HarperCollins Publishers Inc., 10 East 53rd Street, New York, NY 10022.

First Quill edition published 2000.

Illustrations by Karen Merrill

The Library of Congress has catalogued the hardcover edition as follows:

Sichel, Deborah.
    Women's moods : what every woman must know about hormones, the brain, and emotional health / Deborah Sichel and Jeanne Watson Driscoll.
      p.   cm.
Includes bibliographical references and index.
ISBN 0-688-14898-0
   1. Women—Mental health. 2. Women—Psychology. 3. Mood (Psychology). 4. Emotions. I. Driscoll, Jeanne Watson.

RC451.4.W6S57 1999
616.89'0082—DC21
                                       99-25412
                                         CIP

ISBN 0-380-72852-4 (pbk.)

01 02 03 04 WB / RRD 10 9 8 7 6 5 4 3 2 1

This book is dedicated to our daughters,
Lorrie and Katie Driscoll
and
Megan and Lauren Schiff.
They are our pride and joy.

Contents

Part III. Pregnancy

Part IV. Postpartum: A Vulnerable Time

Part V. Negotiating Menopause

ACKNOWLEDGMENTS

We would like to acknowledge the women whom we have cared for and who have invited us into their lives to share their journey.

We acknowledge Kathleen O' Meara, Hal Cash, and Cassandra Morabito, our colleagues at Hestia Institute: Center for Women and Families. They have supported us through the gestational period of this book and have wondered for years both silently and aloud, "How's the book, and when is it going to be done?" Thanks for your love and patience.

We would like to acknowledge Nancy Berchtold, founder of Depression After Delivery, National. Nancy introduced us to Beth Vesel, our agent, who enabled us to fulfill this vision.

Thanks to Toni Sciarra, our editor at William Morrow, whose skill and integrity are much appreciated. We also thank her for her continuing vision and belief in our message.

We acknowledge Susan Golant, a skilled word sculptress, who helped us to refine our manuscript, maintaining the heart and soul of the information. She has been a joy to work with. Thank you.

Thank you to Karen Merrill, our illustrator, who persevered to create visuals to clarify the models, and to Marie Snyder for her ever-present availability and support.

Specifically from Deborah: "My grateful thanks to my husband, Dr. Harold Schiff, for his assistance and editing of the neurological content and for his and my daughters' patience and love. To Dr. Ronald Marcus, who taught me to love obstetrics and to care for women. To Dr. Katherine Wisner, Dr. Meg Spinelli, Dr. Andrew Nierenberg, Dr. Selwyn Oskowitz, and Dr. Phyllis Scherr, sincere appreciation for their continued and invaluable support to me."

Specifically from Jeanne: "I thank my daughters, parents, and family, who are always there for me. I thank my dear friends and colleagues, who have provided much love, support, and guidance on the personal level, specifically Sheila Mansfield, Eloise Clawson, Diane Semprevivo, Barbara Rosenthal, and Cheryl Beck. I thank my nurse colleagues around the North American continent, who have been so supportive of our work and share our passion for the care of women and their families. Saving the best for last, I want to thank my husband, David, a continuous source of strength, love, and support."

PREFACE

The writing of this book began four years ago when we submitted a proposal on a work about how women's reproductive hormones affect their emotional lives and how this aspect of women's mental health is peculiarly invisible to most psychiatrists, obstetricians, gynecologists, and the medical establishment in general. Having to collect and process the many components of this book took longer than we originally anticipated, because at first it all seemed so complicated.

Along the way, however, we realized that the concepts underlying the book were really much simpler than we had previously believed. We would be teaching women about their extraordinary brains; about how their genetic heritage and difficult life events, coupled with the reproductive phases of their lives, could usher in emotional disturbances; and about how their various hormones might affect specific areas of their brains to produce symptoms.

While at first glance this may not seem all that simple, we believe that we have distilled all of these interacting components to their essence. They are now rendered in understandable terms and embrace all the information you need to know in order to care for your amazing brains and move toward better emotional health in the future. In the process we have drawn on our combined forty years of clinical experience with women. As we have struggled to understand the stories of our patients' lives, they have become our best teachers, and they will be yours, too.

This is a whole new way to conceptualize women's health and to treat women! We have arrived at this new way of caring for women and promoting their emotional well-being through contemplation and questioning, correlating what we were hearing from our patients with available and emerging research in both the basic and clinical sciences. This approach takes into account life experiences, genetics, neurobiochemistry, reproductive biology, and psychology. Each part is equally important.

In addition we have evolved a model for understanding that has worked well for our patients. Using the metaphor of an earthquake, with its ominous precursors—tremors—we have been able to anticipate the impact of life experiences, stress, and reproductive hormones on the biochemical processes of the brain. The brain is the major organ of the body, yet it is sadly mistreated and ignored in the area of well-being and health. With the latest research we can demonstrate metaphorically that living life has a biochemical effect on the brain.

In the following pages we will describe our assessment model, which takes into account the various fault lines that can lead to an earthquake. We will teach you about the biochemistry of your brain, and the toll that unremitting stress takes on your brain's biochemistry. You will understand how the female reproductive hormones affect your mood and well-being. You will read about how mood and anxiety disorders can emerge throughout the female reproductive years, from your first menstrual period to menopause.

Working closely with our patients, we have also developed a plan of care (the NURSE Program) that tells them, "Your brain matters." Without paying attention to your brain, all aspects of life—emotional, physical, and spiritual—will suffer. The NURSE Program encompasses mind, body, and soul. As the synthesizers of women's stories, we have had the privilege and honor of accompanying many on their personal journeys of healing as they reclaimed their mental health using this valuable tool.

For too long women have been expected to fit into the model of male physiology and neurochemistry. For most of our lives many of us have felt that we didn't conform to that model, but we've had no other choice, since none other was forthcoming. Consequently, until very recently, we have felt invisible in the area of health care. But today we have found our voices and are speaking up.

Female biochemistry, neurology, and psychological development are quite different from those of men. In evolutionary terms the genders have been designed differently to carry out distinct tasks. This doesn't mean that women's tasks are less important than men's are, only that they're different. We talk about these differences as a *given,* not a moral or ethical issue.

Countless new patients have looked at us as tears streamed down their faces, saying, "Do you know you're the first person who has heard what I'm saying without trying to tell me how to feel or invalidating my feelings? I feel better just knowing that you understand." A woman's unique reality must be taken into account in order for true healing to occur.

That is what this book is about: understanding and healing. Our approach is eclectic, although its essence is very simple—caring. We care enough to sit with someone in pain. We support, facilitate, and promote our patients' journeys toward health, while concurrently providing them with guidance, information, resources, and interventions, as needed. We believe that women are entitled to health: physical, emotional, and spiritual.

In the end we hope that this book enlightens you, empowers you, and heals you. We aim to change the politics of women's health by providing you with knowledge of your brain, biology, neurochemistry, and psychology. Since knowledge is power, this will enable you to be empowered, to speak your truth, and to be heard.

A few stylistic notes. Unless we received their permission, we have changed the names and identifying characteristics of all the women whose stories we tell. Indeed, most of the case histories you will read are composites of the many accounts we hear daily in our clinical practice and in the seminars and workshops on women's mood and anxiety disorders that we present in North America. It has been fascinating, albeit sad, to realize how universal these stories are. Many tell of victimization, marginalization, and silencing.

And for the purposes of clarity and readability, we have decided to write this book using Deborah's voice. This in no way implies that Jeanne's contribution is anything less than equal. We each bring to this book our individual ways of looking at the same puzzle. We have discussed, pondered, researched, laughed, cried, yelled, and resolved conflicts to get at the essence of our message. It could not have been written without both sides of each of our brains.

The writing of this book has strengthened our relationship as friends and colleagues and our respect for each other's humanness. Somehow we found the resources to mobilize ourselves through the difficulties, putting aside our egos in favor of a spiritual process. In truth, the message transcends both of us.

We wish you peace and healing on your journey.

In the end, I find I can't separate brain from body. Consciousness isn't just in the head. Nor is it a question of mind over body. If one takes into account the DNA directing the dance of the peptides, [the] body is the outward manifestation of the mind.

—Dr. Candace Pert, *former chief brain biochemist at the National Institute of Mental Health*

Part I

A NEW WAY TO
UNDERSTAND YOUR
EMOTIONAL WELL-BEING

Chapter 1

BREAKING THE SILENCE

Jeanne's Story

My passion for the topic of this book began on a very personal level. I graduated from the University of Delaware in 1971 with a Bachelor of Science in nursing and began my career as an intensive- and cardiac-care nurse, with a special interest in death and dying. After I got married, I went on to get my master's degree in psychiatric nursing, hoping someday to open a hospice to care for the dying. Little did I know that after the birth of my first baby I would be helping myself recover from a "deathlike" experience that redirected my whole life, personally and professionally.

My transformative experience began on April 11, 1976, with the birth of our first daughter, Lorraine. I had been given a spinal anesthesia for the birth. Afterward, the nurse came to help me go to the bathroom. As a medical-surgical nurse, I knew that after spinal anesthesia the patient needs to remain flat to prevent spinal headaches. I asked the nurse if I should stay in bed. "No," she replied, "you don't need to. The needles are so small that headaches rarely happen."

That was the beginning, the experience that taught me that as a patient I needed to take care of myself and trust my intuition. Twenty-four hours later I felt as though someone were trying to suck my brain out through my ear. The headache did not go away for three weeks postpartum. Breast-feeding was a nightmare; my nipples were cracked and sore. I thought that all new mothers breast-fed while curling their toes, seeing stars, panting, and crying. I felt so strange— like a robot—pretending I was fine while all the time the anticipated joys and pleasures of having a new baby were turning into painful, confusing realities.

One night Lorraine was crying, and I couldn't get her to stop. I tried everything. Finally I placed her—more like flung her—into her bassinet. She wailed even harder at first, but then stopped. Although she had fallen asleep, I panicked, terrified that I had killed her. I put a mirror under her nose to be sure she was alive. She was fine, but I wasn't. Thoughts of her potential death began to reverberate in my head, swelling my anxiety and terror.

I couldn't get these horrible images out of my mind. Soon after, when I was nursing her, I imagined that my husband, David, was going to come home from work and find us both dead, covered in blood. In response to these thoughts and images, my heart would pound and race, my pulse became irregular, and I couldn't breathe. I thought I was losing my mind and was going to die. Welcome to motherhood!

I was so ashamed and scared, I couldn't share any of this with David. I was terrified that social services or the police would remove me from my home for abusing my daughter. If anyone knew what was in my mind! It was horrible.

Finally, when I divulged my physical symptoms to a friend (not telling her about the thoughts that accompanied the feelings), she set up an appointment with a cardiologist. After two hours of cardiac monitoring, the doctor told me that he had no idea what I had, and that his wife had breast-fed and *she* never had any of these symptoms. I was sent home. In the parking lot the symptoms returned, but I was not going back inside that ER!

Although my electrocardiogram (EKG) was normal, I was convinced that something was wrong with my heart. The sensations were all physical. Who would think that they stemmed from anxiety? I had a master's degree in psychiatric nursing, yet I didn't connect the thoughts and the physical symptoms at all, nor did any of my care providers.

Over the next few months the physical symptoms and the violent thoughts slowly abated. When, after fourteen months, I discovered that I was pregnant with our second child, my worst fear was that the thoughts would return.

Unfortunately, they did, and more quickly this time. Katie was born in April 1978. By the second postpartum day, I imagined that if I kissed either of my daughters, I would suck their cheeks off their faces and they would bleed to death. The mysterious irregular heartbeat, light-headedness, shortness of breath, and the concomitant fear of death resumed, too.

This time the doctors checked my thyroid functions and did complete blood counts and other hormone tests, to no avail. All were normal. They had no idea about what was causing the symptoms and didn't once link them to the fact that I had just had another baby.

For the next year every day was an ordeal. Finally, about ten months postpartum, the thoughts went away.

I was very angry that this had happened to me and that no one knew what it was. As is my usual style, I began to study and investigate the area of postpartum mental health, reading the research on labor, delivery, breast-feeding, and postpartum. Something had happened to me after my babies were born, but I couldn't find a word about my experience in any books or journals. Both the psychiatry and the obstetric texts made reference to maternity or "baby blues" and psychosis. All the books dispatched with these disturbances in only one paragraph.

I knew I was not psychotic. The word "psychosis" refers to a mental state in which an individual's perception of reality is impaired—she may hallucinate, become incoherent and delusional, and can display bizarre behavior. I had no hallucinations and stayed in close touch with reality. I knew I would not act on my thoughts, but I was terrified nonetheless. My symptoms had persisted too long to be considered baby blues. That usually lasts a few weeks, and crying, which is a hallmark of the blues, had not been one of my major symptoms. What I had experienced was a mystery, but it changed my life and my career.

I was now on a mission. I was going to direct my "creative rage" into positive action. I diverted all my interest in death and dying into the area of the psychosocial aspects of postpartum and lactation. I was going to use my experience to help others. I became a childbirth educator, lactation consultant, and parent educator. I was motivated and passionate.

In 1981, when my children were three and five, I began my career as a psychiatric clinical nurse specialist in the obstetrical-gynecological-neonatal nursing division of Brigham and Women's

Hospital. I was determined to change the paradigm—that a new mother's experience is always joyful and ecstatic, that after giving birth you simply adjust and cope. I was going to turn my horrific experience into a positive force. I was going to tell the truth about these not-so-nice feelings and help women feel empowered and mentally strong.

It was during that first year at the hospital that I met Deborah. I knew right away that we were kindred spirits. I would tell Deborah that she practiced psychiatry like a nurse, which in my mind was the highest of compliments. She cared for the whole woman: mind, body, and soul. Our relationship continued after her fellowship ended and she left the hospital to begin her private practice. I would refer patients to her, as none of the psychiatrists in the hospital concentrated on this type of work at that time.

Eight years after we met, I left my position at the hospital and started my private practice as a nurse psychotherapist/consultant. Our collective journey as colleagues and friends had begun. This book is based on those experiences.

Deborah's Story

When I met Jeanne, I was working on a fellowship in obstetrical and gynecological psychiatry at the hospital. I had attended medical school in South Africa, where I was born. Because of that country's emphasis on family practice, training of physicians there includes significantly more obstetric and gynecologic preparation than in the United States. Indeed, my love of obstetrics and gynecology had blossomed in South Africa under the teaching of a few outstanding professors who had deeply influenced how I understood and cared for women patients.

I came to Boston University for psychiatric training and there became interested in the psychiatric illnesses of women during their reproductive lives—the places where medicine, psychiatry, and gynecology intersect. In fact, today I'm as comfortable in the labor and delivery rooms and the neonatal intensive-care units as I am in my psychiatry practice. Due to my personality, I resist accepting anything just because it is espoused as current medical or psychiatric doctrine. Undaunted by traditional attitudes and bureaucratic systems, I like to make my own observations and adjust my care to my patients' needs.

In fact, in twenty years of practice I have found that I can provide the best care by looking at the larger picture, never seeing my patients from just one perspective but rather as a whole, as I integrate their obstetrical, medical, and psychiatric concerns. So perhaps it wasn't surprising that in the early stages of my training I became fascinated with how postpartum mental illnesses develop.

Based on what I had encountered in my patients, I began to explore and rethink traditional assumptions about postpartum illness. I was intrigued by the rapid onset of depression or psychosis that some women experienced—sometimes within days of delivery. My supervisors usually attributed these symptoms to a woman's ambivalence about motherhood, her grief for the loss of the pregnancy experience, or her unresolved hostility from previous conflicts. But I believed there was much more to the picture than psychoanalytic interpretations.

Going Down the Wrong Road

In the United States mental illnesses as they relate to female hormones were and still are barely acknowledged. For instance, in the early 1980s, the most frequent treatment for women with postpartum depression was counseling to help resolve their hypothetical conflicts and losses. Counseling revolved around talk about their distress and their inability to care for their infants. It was expected that if a woman did her work in the counseling relationship, she would recover. However, even with this type of help many women continued to have depressive symptoms well into their second postpartum year. Those experiencing postpartum psychosis were treated with antipsychotic medication and "tincture of time."

In my mind these explanations and approaches missed the mark. I could not accept that emotional conflict or ambivalence about motherhood in previously healthy women who had been completely well during pregnancy and through delivery would so quickly result in such a high degree of distress. I found few explanations for many of the physical symptoms that predominate in these illnesses, including agitation, increased heart rate, breathing difficulties, diarrhea, nausea, and appetite and sleep changes. It seemed to me that these distressing symptoms alone would be enough to prevent mothers from caring adequately for their babies, regardless of any inner conflict.

In addition, some of these new mothers were just basically very ill, and talking to them during counseling sessions achieved little. Over time I came to believe that many aspects of women's moods were seriously misunderstood. Indeed, I have found that the old interpretations of women's emotional symptoms during and after pregnancy and at other stages of their reproductive lives (such as bouts of PMS or at menopause) often blame and victimize them and do little to help them.

Although a woman's biology is the cornerstone of her mental health, it remains an invisible dimension to most health-care providers. The unique biology of female reproductive events can have a profound impact on women's mental health, yet *we have not incorporated this biology into the diagnostic picture.* For instance, mood and anxiety disorders can worsen under different hormonal circumstances. When these patterns go unrecognized, symptoms are frequently misinterpreted and treatment is inadequate, allowing these symptoms to remain or escalate.

Researchers have found that the areas of the brain in which female reproductive hormones act are the very same areas that regulate mood stability and behavior. In any situation in which a woman experiences emotional and behavioral symptoms, her hormonal status should be taken into account. Yet when a woman consults a clinician for any type of emotional difficulties, I have found it rare for the professional to ask her about her menstrual cycle or any other hormonal aspects of her life, even though this knowledge not only helps with the diagnosis but may also indicate how best to manage the problem.

This issue is exacerbated by the fact that women rarely obtain proper evaluation and treatment for their emotional needs. When they're feeling down or distressed, most don't go to mental-health clinicians for help. Instead they first visit a primary-care provider such as a family practitioner, internist, nurse practitioner, or obstetrician/gynecologist. This may be because of a preponderance of physical symptoms or because they want to investigate purely physical reasons for how they feel before they are willing to consider the emotional explanation. If they have some form of depression or anxiety disturbance, they are likely to be referred to a psychologist or a social worker. Still others will seek help from a religious counselor.

Invariably, where a woman goes for help will determine the kind of help she gets. If she consults a primary-care physician, she will receive a full medical workup for physical symptoms such as headaches, stomachaches, or chest tightness, although these symptoms may well indicate anxiety emanating from her brain. If she goes to a psychologist, she will receive a recommendation for psychotherapy or counseling, without an appraisal of her medical situation or how her symptoms may relate to her reproductive events and hormonal fluctuations. No matter whom she consults, however, it is unlikely that anyone will tell her how her symptoms may be originating from a brain that is in distress.

In fact, I've found that in most situations clinicians never make the effort to delineate exactly why these symptoms emerge. They don't evaluate women as whole beings, taking into account all the elements that contribute to their mental health. Consequently they misunderstand the interplay of the psyche, brain chemistry, and reproductive state that cause these problems.

Unfortunately, going to the wrong kind of clinician can create considerable delay in getting the right kind of help—help that recognizes that the individual is suffering from a mood or anxiety disorder and that her fluctuating hormones may be contributing to it. Furthermore, women often receive little information about how the different phases of their reproductive lives are likely to affect their moods. As a result, if they suffer from mood disturbances such as severe PMS or postpartum depression, they may find that these issues persist for much of their childbearing years, until well into menopause.

A More Enlightened View

New research in brain biology has begun to demonstrate that specific brain structures and chemicals are directly involved in the emotional symptoms some women experience during their reproductive lives. One such chemical that facilitates communication between nerve cells in the brain (also known as neurotransmitters) is *serotonin*. A serotonin imbalance has been implicated in depression.

While I was working on my fellowship at Brigham and Women's Hospital, scattered scientific investigations began to report that estrogen, the main hormone released by the ovaries (it is responsible for supporting all of the reproductive events in a woman's life from puberty to menopause) has a profound effect on serotonin in the brain. More research followed, demonstrating the numerous ways that estrogen acts on nerve cells communicating in the brain.

These findings led me to suspect that the impact of changing hormone levels on serotonin and other brain chemicals might have an enormous (but as yet unexplored) influence on women's psychiatric symptoms in their childbearing years. I was sure that most of the symptoms I was seeing in new mothers at the hospital reflected their heightened sensitivity to particular brain chemicals following the profound hormonal changes that occur after childbirth.

In 1986 Jeanne attended a meeting of a newly formed group, Depression After Delivery (DAD), where she met Dr. James A. Hamilton of San Francisco. Dr. Hamilton had been involved for many years in the treatment of women with postpartum depression. Jeanne returned from that meeting thrilled and excited with his explanations that these disorders are biochemically driven. She shared his unique approach with me and urged me to meet with him and discuss our shared views.

The following year we attended the Depression After Delivery meeting together. I found in Dr. Hamilton a meeting of the minds. I felt inspired by the work that this fine man had done and the care that he had tirelessly given to women. There was a humanity here. I spoke with him at length about how he believed postpartum illnesses emerged. He felt implicitly that these problems were biologically driven and that women were victims of severe illnesses, usually mistreated and certainly misunderstood. Mainstream medicine and psychiatry in the United States paid little attention to these problems, resulting in woefully inadequate recognition and treatment.

I was intrigued by Dr. Hamilton's view that estrogen and other hormones were in some way responsible for the onset of these problems. He had also been the first physician to explore the use of estrogen to prevent these disorders. In his search for a common mechanism that triggered these illnesses, he had grouped different types into several subcategories.

As I saw more and more women in the postpartum period, I, too, realized that I was actually observing different illnesses that had been formerly lumped together under the diagnosis of "postpartum depression." Depending on when the symptoms began and on their specific characteristics, it became clear to me that we were in fact, looking at something new.

Discovering a New Syndrome

One particular group of postpartum women intrigued Jeanne and me. Though their initial complaints had to do with anxiety and over-concern about their babies, it puzzled us that the dread these women described on the phone did not match the emotional state we observed once they came into the office.

On the phone they seemed overwrought with distress. "It's urgent," they would tell us. "I have to come in." Then they made frantic statements such as "I'm afraid to be alone with my baby," "I need other adults at home," "I don't want to bathe my baby," " I'm frightened of dropping or falling with the baby."

Yet their urgency to be seen did not match the demeanor they displayed when they sat in front of us. In our offices they seemed calm, as if holding themselves together. They made vague, tearful references about what was bothering them but couldn't tell us what was so compelling about it. It didn't make sense. We felt that they were holding back, hiding something, but what? They wouldn't let on.

As the women came to trust us, the issues became clearer. They began to disclose that they were having violent thoughts, sometimes involving harm toward their infants. Because these obsessions were alien and abhorrent to them, the women were ashamed and had remained silent, unable to reveal these thoughts even to their husbands or partners. As we learned to gently uncover the repetitive nature of their fantasies and fears, we realized that these women did not fit the usual picture of postpartum depressive or psychotic disorder.

Although we were unsure what their symptoms meant, we felt that our patients would benefit from meeting and sharing with others who had similar experiences. Given the numbers of new cases we were seeing (sometimes one new woman a week), we decided to begin treating them in a group. One particular group included a judge, a stay-at-home mom, a Wall Street banker, a physician, a social worker, and a kindergarten teacher—all well-adjusted, highly functioning individuals prior to the eruption of these symptoms. They talked and cried as they shared their outlandish fears.

As you will see in Chapter 15, when we began treating these women's symptoms with newly available antidepressant medications such as Prozac and Anafranil, their thoughts miraculously resolved, their anxieties disappeared, and they recovered their former caring selves. In a subsequent surprising development, some women experienced a recurrence of the alarming thoughts premenstrually, despite the fact that they were on therapeutic dosages of medication and in group therapy. Once their periods started, however, these thoughts disappeared once more.

Our results showed us that these symptoms had nothing at all to do with rage or latent psychological hostility—the women had all been too well for their entire lives to be at risk for such problems. Rather, the disturbing psychiatric symptoms had much to do with hormones and brain chemistry. Some type of temporary chemical dysregulation—most likely involving serotonin—had occurred in their brains after delivery. After this incidence it appeared that a temporary relapse occurred in the days preceding menstruation.

Remembering Dr. Hamilton's observations as he worked with estrogen, I wondered whether the precipitous drop in estrogen levels after delivery disturbed the delicate balance of serotonin in the brain, initiating a cascade of biochemical events that might account for the rapid onset of thoughts about harming the babies. The symptoms we had observed—the sudden appearance of a distinctive form of anxiety characterized by obsessional thoughts without any corresponding compulsive behavior—was entirely new to clinicians. We called the newly defined syndrome *postpartum obsessive-compulsive disorder* or *postpartum OCD*.

The new mothers we studied experienced a heightened vigilance about the possibility of harm to their baby. They worried, for instance, about how easily their infant could slip into the bathwater and drown. But rather than mobilizing them to exercise more caution in performing this task, the worry persisted, much like a phonograph needle becoming stuck in a groove of an old, scratched record, causing their thoughts to become locked in a biochemical groove.

In the case of postpartum OCD this "groove" happens as follows: The women move from the identification of a potentially dangerous situation (a normal occurrence) to the active thought of the event's actually happening, with the mother imagining herself as the instrument of harm. From then on, every potential danger translates into a real possibility, because they fear their thoughts might become actions: "If I think it, I might do it."

When a new mother in the throes of postpartum OCD worries about dropping her baby, she visualizes the consequence and her thoughts fix on that image, unable to move on to a normal resolution—mobilizing to protect her infant. Even objects in the home like knives, scissors, and microwave ovens pose a potential danger. In postpartum obsessive-compulsive disorder the normal protective instinct goes into overdrive, interfering with a mother's performance rather than enhancing it.

When we eventually published a paper on this disorder, numerous clinicians told us they had seen the same syndrome in thousands of women. This new postpartum disorder turned out to be quite common, and if misunderstood or untreated, it could devastate women's lives.

So profoundly were we affected by these new moms' revelations and the desperation with which they sought treatment and solace, we determined to break the silence of suffering and victimization that women during the childbearing years had experienced for so long. We began to discuss and describe this syndrome in many of the workshops and seminars that we gave together and individually around the United States.

Moving Forward

During this time, in addition to my private practice, I was employed part-time at Massachusetts General's psychiatry program. While there, I experienced a life-altering event that quickly put everything into perspective, as such things do. I was diagnosed with malignant melanoma—a skin cancer that, if left untreated in its earliest stages, is almost always deadly. After three surgeries to remove all traces of malignant cells, I was given a fairly optimistic prognosis. However, there was no way of knowing that a cell or two had not escaped into my circulation to appear later as a metastatic cancer. If that occurred, I knew that my condition would be fatal.

I remember the day Jeanne accompanied me to one surgery. I was reflecting on where we were in this journey to help women. Although areas of women's mental health were marginally improved, I fretted that there was a long way to go before these issues became mainstream knowledge, taught to all physicians- and nurses-in-training. Within my dark hour my thoughts were about how we had to do better.

"Do you remember how we used to fantasize that we could establish a place within the community where we could provide more comprehensive care for women?" I asked Jeanne. "Maybe now is the time to do this. Perhaps this is the reason that we met in the neonatal intensive-care unit all those years ago. In Yiddish there is a word for this—*besheert*—which means intended or preordained. Well, our relationship is the epitome of *besheert*. We are each so passionate about this work that we can't ignore this energy."

Following this powerful realization, I decided to leave my position at the hospital to follow what my heart told me to do—establish a community-based women's mental-health center and widen the net of education and increase the number of women we reached.

With renewed vigor to follow our dream, we searched for appropriate space in which to start our community project and begin the most important phase of our work with women. By December 1995 we were ensconced in our new offices in Wellesley, Massachusetts, with three other experienced clinicians who felt the same way we did about treating and informing women and their families. With a close collaborative practice, there was plenty of opportunity for talking and processing thoughts. We agreed to call our center Hestia Institute: Center for Women and Families.

Why Hestia? Three thousand years ago Hestia was the Greek goddess of home and hearth, protector of the family and the temple. Representing warmth, comfort, and a spiritual presence, Hestia was the center of the home and represented illumination and the soul of the family. Women, in their role as nurturers, turned to Hestia as their source of inspiration, protection, and beauty. It is this essence that we offered our patients and ourselves.

We had come a long way.

Emerging Patterns

In the early years of our practice, we predominantly saw women who experienced mood and anxiety disorders after the births of their babies, but as our understanding of the connections between all the reproductive phases increased, we began treating patients whose emotional problems correlated with PMS, pregnancy, infertility treatments, and menopause. Along with puberty, these are the times when significant hormonal shifts occur.

At each visit we carefully noted our patients' menstrual-cycle phase, because this so vitally affects how they feel. A woman who is experiencing PMS, for instance, may seem downhearted and sluggish the week before her period begins but energized and cheery shortly thereafter.

As we worked with our patients, we began to see predictable correlations between menstrual-cycle phases, reproductive events such as childbirth or menopause, and mood disturbances. In time we could anticipate when a woman might enter a risk period for the emergence or worsening of mental disturbance. For instance:

- Ten percent of all women will have an episode of depression during pregnancy, and we found that many of those who suffer from depression during pregnancy will undergo a worsening of their condition after delivery.
- Fifty percent of women who use birth-control pills experience depression due to the effects of the hormones in the Pill. Oral contraceptives can also induce anxiety episodes and can worsen depression in a woman who has a propensity for it.
- In the United States, 15 percent of women of childbearing age and their partners experience problems conceiving. Most of these couples will consult gynecologists who specialize in fertility treatments. They receive powerful medications like Pergonal, Clomid, and Metrodin that stimulate the ovaries to produce many eggs. But fertility medications can produce significant mood and anxiety problems, because they act on chemical pathways in the brain involved in the expression of these symptoms. These problems may or may not disappear after the woman discontinues the medication. Moreover, such a reaction suggests a biochemical vulnerability to mood and anxiety changes at a later hormonal event.
- Women who suffer from severe mood disorders such as manic depression (see Chapter 4) frequently experience a worsening of symptoms premenstrually. It is not uncommon for these women to become psychotic before their periods, often requiring hospitalization. Yet when they are admitted, no clinician connects the last week of the menstrual cycle with the deterioration of their mental state.
- Women who have PMS will often experience depression and anxiety after the birth of their babies. Yet rarely do their health-care providers give them anticipatory guidance and education during their pregnancies.
- Menopause can be preceded by mood and anxiety disorders for many women, as this is a time of irregular hormonal fluctuations. Unfortunately, not all hormone-replacement therapy is the same, and gynecologists rarely assess their patients' unique life histories and biochemical brain vulnerabilities.

- Menopause can be associated with a first-time onset of depression due to the decline in estrogen.

In treating so many women for psychological disorders, we also learned that unless one takes into account a patient's menstrual cycle and how her brain is affected by other hormonal shifts—be they puberty, the premenstrual period, use of birth-control pills, infertility treatments, pregnancy, miscarriage, postpartum, or menopause—it is difficult to assess accurately why she is feeling the way she does. As a result of our many observations, we realized that mapping a woman's emotional life over time, incorporating all of these events, affords her the best way to understand how mood disturbances arise.

Beyond Hormones

It would be easy to point to your fluctuating hormones as the sole reason for emotional symptoms. However, in so doing, we would overlook several other essential elements that we can't ignore. Because all of these symptoms emanate from the brain, it is vital for you to understand how your brain works and what this organ needs to maintain balance. In Chapter 3 we explain the workings of the brain, especially as they relate to your moods and hormones.

As you will see, your genetic heritage also plays an important role. Illnesses like depression and manic depression often run in families, so a careful family history can help determine whether you are at risk for one of these conditions.

Moreover, life events can make a profound impression on your brain. *The brain is an organ just like any other in your body, and like all other organs, it can be hurt by a variety of situations.* When your brain is hurting, emotional and physical symptoms occur. It is therefore important to correlate reproductive events in your life with the impact of highly stressful life situations. In order to fully appreciate mood problems, you need to pay attention to your life story.

In our office we have developed a unique way to map the evolution of a woman's emotional life, integrating her brain chemistry, the impact of her hormones on that chemical balance, her genetic history, and stressful life events. This helps us to develop a comprehensive picture of a patient's emotional life, showing her quite concretely how she arrived at the point of requiring mental-health care and what she might expect for the future. We will be sharing this mapping device with you in Chapter 6.

Throughout this book we will show you how to integrate the essential components of life events, genetics, reproductive events, and brain chemistry, so that you understand how mood and anxiety symptoms have emerged across your lifetime. We hope to empower you with this knowledge.

The Task Before Us

In increasing numbers a silent epidemic of mental disorders is occurring in the lives of women during their reproductive years. This book fills the informational gaps, explaining the profound effects the female sex hormones can have on your emotional life. It chronicles the years from the beginning of menstruation through menopause, exploring the potential causes, treatments, and prevention of mood and anxiety problems at each phase. We will show you how hormonal changes and stressful life events can interact to alter brain chemistry and how an experience at one point in your reproductive life may predict the outcome at another. In the chapters that follow, you will learn not only where you have come from emotionally but also what you can expect in the future.

As in our clinical practice, women are their own storytellers in this book. From them you will learn how to appraise what your vulnerabilities may be and how to get help if you are or have been experiencing problems. As you read, we hope that the old stereotypes of emotional illness will fall away, and blame and stigma will transform into hope and empowerment. We aim to end the epidemic of silence.

Chapter 2

THE INVISIBLE WOMAN

Some months ago a colleague consulted me about one of his female patients. Although the woman had been hospitalized for two weeks, her depressive condition had not improved. My colleague wondered what other medications might be more effective. He had even considered electroconvulsive therapy—a treatment that can be successful when all else fails.

My colleague began to recount the history of Anna's problems. But after fifteen minutes of talking, I realized that he had told me little that would help me come to a conclusion about what type of illness she had. Of course, he had already told me that she had a depressive disorder, but since there are several types of depression, identifying the type that she had was an important first step in determining the treatment.

I learned that Anna's father had died three years earlier, which was, my colleague believed, the cause of her current difficulties. I was curious to know what had happened since her father's death, particularly the extent of Anna's grief reaction. Although it is normal for bereavement to induce emotional distress for a while, grief can evolve into depression if it persists for months at a time. Pivotal life events often precede the first major episode of depression. I needed to establish to what extent Anna's brain biochemistry had been disrupted in response to this difficult turn in her life.

But hormonal shifts are also significant in triggering depression. And so I thought we should examine Anna's hormonal history, too. Yet when I asked my colleague about Anna's previous responses to oral contraceptives and whether she had experienced premenstrual symptoms, he told me, "I have no information about those aspects of her history." Then, expressing surprise about these questions, he wondered, "What bearing does this have on my patient's improvement?"

I reassured him that it's not unusual for a clinician to be bewildered about the role that hormones play in a patient's recovery. And then I pushed a bit further. "Do you know if this woman has ever been pregnant?"

"Well, she had a baby a few months ago," he replied.

Now it was my turn to be astonished. I was shocked that such a momentous hormonal and emotional event for a woman—giving birth—had been factored out of the equation. In fact, this piece of information changed the whole evaluation, leading to a much better assessment. Close questioning about how Anna had fared in the first days and weeks of birth would, in and of itself, bring her diagnosis into stark relief. While her father's death three years earlier might have paved the way for her current condition, today she was suffering from postpartum depression.

The Elephant in the Middle of the Room

The female reproductive hormones estrogen and progesterone can dramatically affect the brain's biochemistry, yet unfortunately most clinicians rarely discuss this relationship. Indeed, as with the elephant in the middle of the room that everyone ignores and carefully steps around, clinicians seldom ask about (or they simply ignore) any of the critical points in a woman's reproductive life—her demeanor through a pregnancy, her reaction to birth-control pills, or her premenstrual symptoms—that might hint at some preexisting hormonal vulnerabilities. Yet, without assessing these important elements, it is difficult, if not impossible, to paint a comprehensive picture of a woman's emotional health.

Often we have received urgent calls from mental-health clinicians seeking help with a case that might take a turn for the worse. When we ask a few pointed questions, we find that the patient is currently in labor and the clinician has only now thought about the mental-health complications that might arise after delivery. Until this moment he or she had thought very little about impending problems and risks.

This is far too late to look for assistance. We usually try to bite our tongues, but it is hard not to ask, "And how long is it you say that this woman has been pregnant?" It seems incredible that a mental-health practitioner could sit opposite a woman struggling with depression and/or anxiety for nine months and ignore her expanding abdomen. All too often women who have suffered from mood disturbances before conception are not told that these conditions may worsen during and after the pregnancy, and few preparations are made to deal with more severe problems should they arise. Screening for risk of mood and anxiety disorders is critical during the pregnancy, so that clinicians can formulate strategies for early intervention in case they're needed later.

In a study published in the *British Journal of Psychiatry* in 1987 that correlated and analyzed data from thousands of women, researchers showed that a woman is at greatest risk for the onset of psychiatric illness during the first three months after she delivers a baby.[1] The rate of admission to psychiatric hospitals increases substantially during this period of susceptibility. Yet childbirth educators, obstetricians, midwives, pediatricians, family practitioners, and psychiatrists—in short, anyone who cares for women during the childbearing years—hardly ever considers this information or shares it with women who are experiencing problems.

It's frustrating that although research on these topics does exist, mainstream psychiatry has yet to incorporate these findings into general practice. As a result, women often come to us for help after searching for months and even years for answers to symptoms that other clinicians have treated as inconsequential.

Penelope's case is typical. She came into our office after an eminent psychiatrist had "treated" her for depression for two years. She reported to us that early in her treatment she had explained to her psychiatrist, "For one week before my period, I get irritable, edgy, and have racing thoughts. I have no energy—I feel really depleted—and my husband knows he should stay away from me. These changes in my mood are causing family problems and interfering with my life. I feel this must have something to do with my menstrual cycle. Maybe I have PMS."

Disputing Penelope's intuition about the source of her feelings, her physician told her, "Your symptoms have nothing to do with your menstrual cycle. You have ongoing depression because you are not confronting the problems in your marriage."

"But my symptoms started after the birth of my third child," Penelope explained. "Before that, I was fine."

"This depression has nothing to do with delivering your baby," the psychiatrist persisted. "You are still depressed, and your child is two and half years old now."

After two years of continuing difficulties with her moods, Penelope became frustrated with her treatment. She felt sure that somehow there was a connection between her symptoms and biological events that had occurred in her life. Trusting her instincts, she found the energy to seek a second opinion and called our offices to set up a consultation.

Penelope wasted two years in a therapy that took no notice of how her illness first occurred or how her condition routinely worsened in the middle of her cycle and premenstrually. Certain mood problems occur in very specific patterns after giving birth, and these patterns provide important clues to diagnosis. Although Penelope knew intuitively that there was a correlation between her mood and her menstrual cycle, her doctor did not listen to her. He discounted her sense of herself and her body. In fact, when the depression did not respond to treatment, he blamed *her* for not confronting her issues. He did not evaluate her as a whole person.

When the psychiatric and medical evaluation of a woman does not fully take into account her hormonal cycling, clinicians can misinterpret aspects of her depressive disorder, implementing the wrong therapy. It is a sad commentary that clinicians who treat women in this decade of sophisticated medical and psychiatric knowledge rarely ask about or integrate critical biological elements into their assessment and treatment plans. Our medical system has tragically ignored the effects of female biology in the emotional lives of women.

It is as though these essential components are pervasively invisible. This fact becomes doubly shameful when you consider that psychiatrists are not treating a minority population. Women have twice the rate of depressive and anxiety disorders as men, so there are significantly more women represented in psychiatrists' offices and clinics. To so persistently marginalize and overlook issues that are intrinsic to every woman's well-being is nothing short of an outrage.

Why a Man Can't Be More Like a Woman

Why is a woman's biology still invisible to mental-health professionals? Perhaps it is because today esteemed professional journals and national organizations charged with setting guidelines for psychiatric care continue to do little to improve this state of ignorance. In fact, the biological dimensions of women's mental health are still absent from the latest guidelines on the evaluation and treatment of mental disorders.

For instance, in 1995 the American Psychiatric Association published its *Comprehensive Guidelines for Psychiatric Evaluation*. These purport to provide a clinician with a review of all the basic information he or she needs to gather from a new patient at their first meeting. As you can imagine, this is a crucial conversation. Yet, shockingly, these guidelines do not take into account women's unique physiology. There is not one mention of a woman's menstrual cycle; her use of hormones in birth control, fertility treatments, or hormone-replacement therapy (HRT); her history of abortion, miscarriage, or stillbirth; her pregnancy and postpartum experiences; or her status during menopause.

Similarly, the *Practice Guidelines for the Treatment of Major Depression*, also published by the American Psychiatric Association, ignores gender differences. There is no discussion of women's different rates of absorbing and metabolizing antidepressant and mood-stabilizing medications during their menstrual cycle. Moreover, despite the fact that certain extensively used medications like lithium and Depakote can cause birth defects, rarely is a woman's need for appropriate contraception addressed.

In 1998 *The Journal of Clinical Psychiatry* published the *Guidelines for the Treatment of Bipolar Disorder*. Bipolar disorder is also known as manic-depressive illness (see Chapter 4). But again there is not one reference in these guidelines to how women with this disorder are affected by their menstrual cycle, oral contraceptives, pregnancy, the postpartum period, or menopause, despite the fact that since 1988 a significant number of articles highlighting these concerns have been published.

Sadly, women who have bipolar disorder typically suffer more episodes of depression than do men, experience a more problematic rapid-cycling variant of the disorder (which is difficult to stabilize), and are often exquisitely sensitive to hormonal shifts or interventions such as oral contraceptives or fertility treatments. Severe mood problems frequently occur premenstrually: It is not unusual for women who have bipolar disorder to become destabilized or psychotic before their period, often requiring hospitalization. Yet when these women are admitted, no clinician connects the phase of their menstrual cycle with the deterioration in their condition. As a result, they are rehospitalized month after month, incurring heavy health-care expenses.

Moreover, although women represent two thirds of the population who receive the medications that are now extensively used in psychiatry, they have been largely excluded from drug studies. Results from studies in men have simply been applied to women, but this can be perilous.

Women have a 15-percent-greater blood flow through their brains. Antidepressants and antianxiety agents tend to reach higher blood levels in women, and these medications will affect women's brains faster. They may have an exaggerated impact and can reach toxic levels much more rapidly. More women than men experience troublesome side effects from medications, perhaps because of the cumulative effects of these differences. Yet these issues are rarely addressed when physicians prescribe for women.

Rates of absorption of medications in women even vary according to which phase of the menstrual cycle the women are in. For some, levels of antidepressant and mood-stabilizing drugs in the blood are lower during the last two weeks of the menstrual cycle. This underscores the need to measure levels of medication throughout the menstrual cycle for the best treatment. Unfortunately, such monitoring is rarely undertaken, despite comprehensive reviews published by noted researchers in the field drawing attention to a woman's unique needs.[2]

Moreover, if a woman is taking medication to relieve a mood disturbance prior to conception, her clinician is likely to recommend discontinuing her treatment throughout gestation without considering her risk of becoming ill during the pregnancy and postpartum period.

Dr. Ellen Leibenluft, a scientist at the National Institute of Mental Health in Bethesda, Maryland, reports that most psychiatric researchers do not ascertain menstrual-cycle phases when constructing studies of depressive illness in women. She believes that this information is so important in the interpretation of research results that she discounts conclusions from any studies that do not take into account where a woman is in her cycle.[3]

Most recently Dr. Leibenluft reiterated her concerns about the need for attention to these issues. "The conclusion that gender is irrelevant is untenable for two reasons," she wrote in *The Journal of Clinical Psychiatry*. "Depressive illness follows a different course in women than in men, and female reproductive events not only affect the course of illness, they also influence treatment decisions."[4]

The fact that all of these recently published diagnosis and treatment guidelines do not address women's concerns indicates that attention is not being paid to our unique biology. It seems that where treatment of women is concerned, it takes a long time for the prevailing ignorance to change.

What This Ignorance Can Mean to You

Such ignorance can have grave health consequences in terms of misdiagnosis, mistreatment, and general well-being. For instance, although it is widely recognized that birth-control pills affect a woman's response to medications commonly used in treating diabetes, high blood pressure, seizure disorders, and pain, few clinicians address these concerns when they prescribe the Pill.

Contraceptives can influence the blood levels of antidepressants, mood stabilizers, and thyroid medications, but again physicians seldom take this into account or discuss these issues with their patients. Consequently medications may be misprescribed or problematic side effects may occur without being properly addressed.

Fifty percent of women who use oral contraceptives will experience depression due to the effects of the hormones they contain. Yet women who develop depression while taking the Pill are often uninformed that they may be vulnerable to a recurrence of the illness later in life, particularly after childbirth and at menopause.

We frequently evaluate patients who are referred to us because they appear to have depressive illnesses that don't respond to the usual antidepressants. When we take a history, we discover that a woman had been placed on birth-control pills months and even years before, and became depressed as a result. Not one clinician has asked the patient about this, so the unfortunate woman has been treated with numerous medications with little success.

When we discontinue the birth-control pill, the patient often experiences improvement within a few weeks. We quickly discover that she never needed antidepressants in the first place. The Pill was the culprit!

If a woman becomes depressed in her late forties, a psychiatrist may see her over many months or even years and treat her with every antidepressant available. Yet rarely is she asked if she is on hormone-replacement therapy or experiencing menopausal symptoms. Even if the clinician does note this, it doesn't occur to him or her that some component of the HRT might be one cause or even at the root of the depression. In postmenopausal women HRT can induce PMS-type symptoms that may be mistaken for depression. Estrogen and progesterone use can worsen the mood states of bipolar women to the extent that their condition may become impossible to stabilize.

As we mentioned in Chapter 1, fertility medications that stimulate egg production, such as Clomid and Pergonal, can create significant mood and anxiety problems. When on these drugs, women have estrogen levels ten times higher than during natural menstrual cycles. This is what increases the probability of mood shifts. Even when women undergoing treatment are warned about these dangers, the degree and severity of their emotional reactions frequently upset them.[5] This suggests that their reactions are severe.

Fertility medications work in the areas of the brain responsible for coordinating the menstrual cycle. These same areas are connected to pathways involved in mood regulation, memory, and stability. So why should we be surprised when women complain about these symptoms?

Ignorance can be dangerous. Early in her treatment with Clomid, twenty-nine-year-old Rachel reported to her doctor that her mood had changed from her usual cheerfulness to a feeling of blackness and doom. She was constantly shaky and tearful. Her physician responded, "Those feelings are nothing to worry about. They'll settle." One morning her mood had deteriorated so severely, she decided there was no further reason to continue living, and she attempted suicide.

Fortunately, Rachel did not succeed in ending her life, but her medical team ignored her distress about her worsening depressive symptoms and their link to the medication until a near-tragedy occurred.

The Cost to Society
The ignorance about a female's unique emotional needs exacts a terrible personal toll on millions of women who continue to suffer need-

lessly, but it also weighs heavily on society in general. Depression is an enormous and an expensive public health problem. A study conducted jointly in 1990 by Paul Greenberg and Ernst Berndt at the Massachusetts Institute of Technology and the National Bureau of Economic Research calculated that depression costs the United States $43.7 billion each year in work absenteeism, treatment, hospitalization, chronic disability, and death. Various studies have shown that fifteen to twenty million Americans suffer from depression. At least 10 percent of the population is affected by this condition.

In 1977 Myrna Weissman and Gerald Klerman found that women had twice the rate of depression than men during their adult lives. Women between the ages of eighteen and forty-four are the most vulnerable. More recently, Ronald Kessler reconfirmed these findings, gathering data on more than eighteen thousand people from different communities all over the United States. More than ten million women in America will experience problems with depression at some time in their lives.

Failure to acknowledge the special mental-health concerns of women in the childbearing years is very expensive. In 1995 we undertook a study of women who had been hospitalized in the mother-baby unit we helped to establish at a local psychiatric hospital. Of the first thirty women admitted to the unit, we were astonished to find that fully twenty-five carried specific identifying characteristics that would have predicted a severe emotional illness requiring a stay in the hospital. Had their doctors identified and treated these women earlier, the hospitalizations could have been avoided. Each admission cost the medical-insurance company about $10,000, or a total of $250,000 for the twenty-five avoidable cases. Multiplying that amount each year over numerous patients and hospitals across the United States, you can see how costs needlessly run into the billions.

Women who have difficulties with depression appear to be at risk for other medical problems as well. Studies have shown that women with a history of depression carry a significant risk of bone thinning far earlier in their lives than would otherwise be expected.[6] Osteoporosis can lead to serious fractures in hips, thighs, and the spine. Depression has also been implicated in the occurrence of heart attacks, although it is unclear whether heart disease arises from the secretion of stress hormones in those who are depressed (which could cause erratic heartbeat and affect cholesterol levels) or whether those who are depressed are simply less likely to take good care of themselves. They may fail to watch their diet, adhere to a medication schedule, or manage their high blood pressure, all of which could predispose them to heart attacks.[7]

Yet despite the army of women sufferers and the costs, relatively few receive sufficient treatment. Steven Hyman, the director of the National Institute of Mental Health, noted in 1996 that most people who suffer with depressive illness don't get the treatment they need, and even when they do, it is often inadequate.[8] It is generally known in the medical world that primary-care physicians often do not treat depression adequately or for a long enough time.

The problem is not confined to the United States alone. Recent studies in more than nine countries, including Canada, Puerto Rico, France, West Germany, Italy, Lebanon, Korea, New Zealand, and Taiwan, show that the rate of depression for women in those countries is also double that among men. These transcultural data suggest that the experience of depressive suffering for the family of women is universal and defies culture. The female hormones and the different chemical components of women's brains are implicated in these higher rates of mental illness in both the United States and other countries.

Reproductive hormones act in the brain to stimulate the cyclical process of menstruation. In addition, areas of the brain involved in the expression and regulation of emotions actively respond to different hormonal states. Unfortunately, these connections between female hormones and brain biochemistry remain invisible for most women and their health-care providers if and when they become emotionally ill. Ironically, the very physiology associated with the potential to bear and nurture children brings with it an increased risk for mood and anxiety complications.

When Ignorance Leads to Tragedy

Pregnancy and childbearing are often viewed in our culture as times of great joy and anticipation. Yet it is an unacknowledged reality that when a woman becomes pregnant, she enters a vulnerable period during which she is more likely to experience a mood or anxiety problem. Indeed, some women never seem to recover the same emotional wellness they had prior to having their children. It appears that the process of having borne children may alter important aspects of some women's mood biology.

Rampant ignorance about how ill women can become during pregnancy and after delivery sometimes results in tragic, preventable deaths. Leanne Pitts developed severe depression during the last ten weeks of her first pregnancy. She told a social worker that she was not thinking clearly, couldn't sleep, and was feeling suicidal. The social worker replied, "You need to deal with your issues about becoming a mother," and left it at that.

Within a week of delivery Leanne's depression worsened. She became unable to differentiate reality from her increasingly dangerous paranoia. She began to believe that parts of her body were rotting away. She was unaware of her son's existence as a separate being and therefore believed that he was also decomposing. Her doctors didn't take her symptoms seriously. But feeling that she was evil, Leanne concluded that she had no right to live. It was then that she smothered her baby and tried to shoot herself.

Leanne was failed by the system. When a woman becomes depressed during pregnancy, the likelihood of her condition worsening after delivery is high.[9] Had Leanne's medical team recognized her symptoms, they could have involved the psychiatric team during her pregnancy, averting this tragedy.

The judicial system then failed to listen and appreciate that Leanne, being psychotic, was not responsible for what had happened. She was sentenced to prison. Leanne is now a prisoner instead of a patient. Her biology, the medical system, and the judicial system have triply victimized her. As a society we are paying dearly for the ignorance of her health team and the judicial system. There are hundreds of similar cases throughout the United States.

Women's Brains Are Different!

Why is it that women have so many unique psychiatric and medical needs? Why are they more likely to become depressed or anxious or even, as in Leanne's case, psychotic? Certainly our hormones play an important part. But the truth of the matter is, we are just beginning to learn that women's brains are structured differently from men's as well.

Bestselling relationship expert John Gray states in the title of his book that *Men Are from Mars, Women Are from Venus*. Well, John, although at times it may feel as if we come from different planets, actually we don't! But we have evolved to use areas of our brains differently. These differences have emerged from the needs and survival of the species.

Since new techniques of examining how the brain functions have developed, science is on the brink of identifying structural, functional and metabolic differences in the brains of men and women that may account for our unique ways of thinking and expressing ourselves. There is a reason for everything women are able to do, and the differences between women and men become apparent at young ages.

It is widely acknowledged that girls are more verbal, have better language skills, and focus more on relationships than boys, whereas boys focus on how things work and on the mastery of tasks at the expense of relationships. Recent findings about the structure and functioning of women's brains are beginning to clarify why women like to talk, why they need to feel emotionally connected, and why they view the world differently from men.

Jenny Harasty, a pathologist, and her colleagues at the University of Sydney, Australia, have shown that the parts of the brain responsible for language, called Broca's and Wernicke's areas, are 30 percent larger in women than in men.[10] She suggests that these anatomical differences correlate with women's superior language abilities.

Roger Gorski and Laura Allen, neuroscientists at the University of California, Los Angeles, examined 146 brains and found that in women the thick bridge of tissue (called the *corpus callosum*) that connects the two halves or hemispheres of the brain appears to be 23 percent larger in women than in men. If this connecting bridge and the areas serving language are larger, it suggests why the developmental ability to cater to many different demands at the same time—today we refer to this as "multitasking"—seems to be easier for women than men.

The common lament of women in relationships is "I want to talk and he doesn't." Most men just don't feel the same urge as women to express themselves verbally about issues. Women's brains, with their extensive language skills, are firing away, invoking a complex exchange of information between right and left hemispheres, and women feel compelled to articulate this information. The man's brain will be much more preoccupied with accomplishing the task at hand than with talking about how it will be done. For women the process is important; for men, achieving the cherished goal is.

With the technique of positron-emission tomography, also known as PET scanning, we can take a picture of the brain while it's in action. It becomes a spectacular splash of color on a computer screen, providing the first inklings as to which parts are activated during specific activities.

Utilizing PET scans, Ruben and Raquel Gur, researchers at the University of Pennsylvania, have found that when men and women make their minds a blank, a certain area of the brain demonstrates different levels of activity in men as compared to women. For instance, in women the *paralimbic cortex*—a more recently and highly evolved area of the brain—lights up, registering significantly more activity than in men. One purpose of this brain area is to filter emotional reactions to the environment. There is some research to suggest that maternal behavior emanates from this area. In contrast, when men were asked to empty their minds, more activity registered in older parts of their brains. This suggests that even when women are at rest, their paralimbic cortex remains active as an emotional barometer, vigilant to interpret and respond to what's happening around them. This may also account for women's intuitive sixth sense.

In another set of studies conducted by the Gurs, men and women were asked to pick out happy faces. They all did this successfully. But when asked to identify sadness on women's faces, women were correct 90 percent of the time, whereas men were right 70 percent of the time. (Interestingly, though, men were able to distinguish sadness on other men's faces 90 percent of the time!)

Another fascinating finding emerged from this study. Judging from the activity in the women's brains, they did not appear to be working very hard at identifying sadness on the faces, whereas the men, as seen on the PET scans, seemed to expend more brain energy in the same task. Perhaps identifying emotional states is easier for women than it is for men.

Evoking sad or sorrowful states seems to involve a greater brain area in women. Since sadness and mood are expressed in similar areas of the brain, this may also provide another explanation for why women are more prone to depression than men.

Researcher Mark George at the National Institute of Mental Health has shown that when women are asked to recall sad experiences, the front of the paralimbic area shows significant activity. In fact, women in his study exhibited eight times more activity in this area than men who were asked to perform the same task. Dr. George suggests that sorrowful states induced by loss or grief activate these parts of the brain. But when the grief is unresolved, this mood state can be followed by depression, in which these same areas subsequently show decreased activity. Dr. George states that in men these brain regions are not activated in the same way.

Brain Differences Exist for a Reason

These gender differences in brain functioning exist for significant reasons. Traditionally, men have been the protectors of the community. For their own and the group's survival, it has been important that they retain aggressive and dominant drives. They have had much less need to develop and use their paralimbic-cortex abilities. This may account for their greater propensity to jump into physical altercations rather than use their verbal skills.

In contrast, it is likely that women have developed a more active paralimbic area in response to their infants' cues and emotional needs. As women's role of mother-nurturer evolved, the brain areas serving these abilities became more responsive. Consequently, women have developed an innate capacity for paying attention to emotional details. Evolution required this, and the biology evolved to provide it. Where there is a need, nature finds a way.

The primary relationship of the early years, the mother-infant bond, depends solely on this powerful biological and biochemical tie. A mother's connection with her infant forms the basis of all relationships later in the youngster's life. Children who lack a stable early attachment to their mothers seem never able to fully repair the loss. Without these powerful affiliations humankind would not have survived.

It is likely that a woman's brain functioning has evolved in response to the need for a secure primary attachment with her baby, and thus the propagation of the species. Women's powerful ability to connect emotionally is linked to their different and distinct behavior and thought patterns. Yet, ironically, women have been seen as inferior or weak as a result. Moreover, paradoxically, this innate capacity for empathic connection—a highly evolved human trait—also puts women at greater risk for sadness and depression.

Estrogen and progesterone attachment sites abound in all the brain areas serving emotion, yet the capacity for women's hormonal cycles to influence mood has been grossly underappreciated. It is imperative that clinicians pay greater attention to hormonal changes that occur across a woman's life cycle and to the impact of these hormones on her mental health.

In the chapters that follow, we will look more closely at women's brains and the mental illnesses that commonly occur during their reproductive years. We'll show you how the integration of the bio-chemistry, life stressors, and hormonal functions can help predict the status of a woman's mental-health. We will render visible what has remained invisible for so many years.

Chapter 3

YOUR BRAIN: THE CORNERSTONE OF YOUR
EMOTIONAL HEALTH

Many years ago I met with Sarah, a thirty-five-year-old woman who was severely depressed. This was her first contact with a mental-health clinician. In our initial phone conversation she asked me, "What are you going to do to me? I mean, what happens during the hour?" She was clearly terrified about what it meant to see a psychiatrist.

I told her that we would just talk about her problems and put together a picture of how she came to this point in her life. Then I would make some recommendations about treatment.

Although Sarah was somewhat reassured, she immediately responded, "Well, I don't want to take any medication."

I acknowledged the hesitancy and fear that this call and her impending visit evoked for her, but then I said, "I hope you'll come in, and together we can discuss what you need."

Sarah was indeed clinically depressed. She had not slept well for more than two months and had lost about ten pounds. She felt restless, anxious, and overwhelmed and was beginning to notice that her thinking was less clear than usual. She had recently started to feel that her life was not worth living, and she wasn't sure what she was going to do about that feeling.

Untreated, major depression can be lethal because of the risk of suicide. In fact, suicidal thoughts or plans represent a form of "brain failure." The suicidal individual is no longer able to understand clearly that these are irrational thoughts emerging from an ill brain.

Because of this danger, I knew that I couldn't let Sarah out of my office without starting her on medication. I was also aware that this was going to be a hard sell. However, the symptoms Sarah described hinted at changes in the chemistry of her brain's mood pathways, putting her at risk for more serious suicidal thoughts if the depression worsened. Regardless of the events that had led Sarah to this state, she needed medical intervention.

Once we met, I understood why Sarah had felt anxious about using medication. Her aunt had suffered with depression all her life and had been hospitalized a few times. Sarah had seen her oversedated, listless, and zombielike.

"I don't know exactly what happened to your aunt," I told my new patient, "but it sounds as if she may have been given too much medication. Today antidepressants are much improved, and there are fewer side effects and problems arising from long-term use. I know it is hard for you to hear that you may need medication, but it is important for you to get well, and beginning medication is one of my recommendations."

Sarah sat up straight and shook her head. To her, medication meant that she was starting down "the slippery slope of mental illness," and all she could visualize was a replication of her aunt's predicament.

At that moment I decided to take Sarah on a journey through her brain structure and physiology. I felt I had to show her how her symptoms had occurred in response to the changes in her brain biochemistry and how medication could eliminate some of the symptoms that were getting in the way of her daily life.

I took out a sheet of blank paper and asked Sarah to pull up her chair alongside mine. "I would like to show you what is going on in your brain and what I am aiming to do with medication treatment."

I began by drawing what we know about the mood-pathway anatomy in the brain, pointing out the various parts from which symptoms emerged. I showed Sarah how and where we believe the medications work to treat her depressive symptoms. Her eyes followed every mark I made on the paper.

At one point I heard her inhale deeply. Turning my attention back to her, I noticed that her eyes had filled with tears. As she exhaled through quivering lips, she said, "You mean, I did not make this happen?"

"No, of course not," I replied.

"I've felt so ashamed of myself," she went on tearfully. "I've felt so weak and unable to control my emotions. I thought if I tried hard enough, I could will these feelings away."

We hear such statements all the time from women who experience depression. Overwhelmed by feelings of worthlessness, they often believe they possess a character flaw that has led to this terrible state. Afraid of being judged, they let internal guilt keep them from treatment. At other times they have told us they didn't want to sound as if they were "complaining," so they never told their primary-care physicians how they felt. In addition, the stereotypes of mental illness can keep them away from treatment. Like Sarah, they feel as if seeking help might mean that they, too, would head down a slippery slope from which there is no return.

Sarah sighed and told me that my explanation was helpful; she was beginning to understand. She wanted to get better. "I'll try the medication, but can I call you if I get frightened?"

"Of course you can. I want to see you weekly to support you during this initial phase of treatment."

After this session with Sarah, I realized that all of our patients need information about the areas of the brain involved in mood and anxiety disturbances. They need an understanding of how the different parts of the brain may be miscommunicating and how medications can correct the communication system. In addition, they need to learn about psychotherapy and where and how it works as a part of their treatment plan. You, too, can benefit from this information.

Your Amazing Brain

Your brain is a sensitive, complex organ with more power and ability than you can imagine. It is the master computer that regulates your breathing, heart rate, movement, balance and coordination, digestion, sleep, appetite, metabolism, immune responses, and menstrual cycle—and those are just a few of the processes hinging on its optimal functioning!

We know that the brain orchestrates your physiological life, but it is also intimately involved in how you relate and respond to the world. It is continuously adjusting to internal and external conditions, organizing your behaviors in response to stressors through your moods, actions, thinking, planning, memory, and decision-making and problem-solving abilities. From its lowest, most primitive areas to its highest-functioning, most recently developed parts and throughout its pathways and many structures, your brain is equipped to mobilize whatever you need physiologically and biochemically all day long.

When Your Brain Is in Distress

Usually when a part of your body is in distress, you become aware of it through the symptoms of pain, discomfort, fever, and malaise. If you have bronchitis, you cough, wheeze, and suffer chest pains. If you have a urinary-tract infection, you feel burning when you urinate and must do so frequently. These symptoms force you to take care of the problem because they are uncomfortable. Indeed, they send you straight to your health-care provider, where you will receive medication that targets the biological cause.

But have you ever thought about the signals your brain gives to show it is in distress? Most people are unaware of what their brains tell them regarding the state of its internal functioning. Yet responding to signals that your brain is in trouble is one of the first lines of defense in mood and anxiety disturbances. This, too, should send you to your mental-health care provider, seeking relief and treatment.

How does your brain tell you that it is hurting? Brain tissue itself does not feel pain, so there is no simple way to know. Yet a brain in distress does produce a range of symptoms. Like my patient Sarah, you may experience these as the emotions of fear, anger, sorrow, or depression. Or they may manifest themselves physically, as chest tightness and heart-rate changes, nausea and vomiting, abdominal pain and diarrhea, sleep and appetite disturbances, lethargy, frequent urination, muscle tension, and general aches and pains.

These symptoms are some of the ways that the brain tells you it is overloaded. In fact, a simple way of understanding depressive or anxiety disorders is to think of them as the brain's slowing down in response to being biochemically overburdened.

The Biochemically Challenged Brain

As you can imagine, your brain needs to wind down and rest at some point during a twenty-four-hour day. This is the function of sleep. It allows your brain to recharge itself. In fact, the brain has enormous self-regulating abilities, but unfortunately you may prevent this recharging from occurring. A frenetic lifestyle acts against your brain's self-regulating abilities, as does the use of alcohol, tobacco, and drugs. You may overwork, eat on the run, stay up too late, and just plain overdo. In addition, as you will see, life events and reproductive hormones can affect your brain as well.

Your brain may be the most challenged, taken-for-granted, and—dare we say—abused organ in your body. In essence, we live in a society that fails to recognize the importance of the brain and therefore fails to care for this amazing organ. Sad but true, the current pace of life has made us a population of what we like to call "biochemically challenged brains."

Depressive and anxiety disorders can be accompanied by many physical symptoms. Unfortunately, these complaints can lead you—and often your doctor—to look only to the specific organ generating the discomfort. For instance, irritable-bowel syndrome stems from a stressed brain. The biochemically challenged brain, as the mediator of these symptoms, remains elusive and concealed—and therefore often goes untreated.

In response to this lack of care your brain can become subject to chemical dysregulation. Over time it becomes increasingly difficult for the brain, in its role as grand coordinator, to maintain physiological balance. This results in the sensations you may understand as the early symptoms of an anxiety or a depressive disturbance.

How Your Powerful Brain Evolved

Mental wellness is governed by the normal functioning of billions of brain cells and depends on the orderly operation of millions of high-speed electrical and chemical circuits in the brain that carry information to and from specific destinations. Although science is a long way from understanding all the determinants of emotions and where in the brain we might locate feeling states, we have uncovered some fundamental elements.

In many ways what ails us in the present is rooted in our past. We are old creatures, strongly linked to animals and other primates through the earliest, most primitive parts of our brain. Much human behavior remains quite uncivilized, driven by powerful instincts to survive. In many respects we are still not very different from animals.

Our powerful brain evolved from the inside out. Billions of years ago our brains began in lower animals as a shaft called the *brain stem* that contains nerve cells purely responsible for the automatic functions of breathing, heartbeat, and digestion. The brain stem is located at the base of our brains and connects to the spinal cord.

Around and out of this primitive shaft evolved a ring of brain structures called the *limbic brain* (also known as the reptilian brain). It is responsible for appetite, thirst, the sleep-wake cycle, sex drive, aggressive impulses, memory, body temperature, and control of the menstrual cycle—all functions that sustain and protect life. These functions are vastly more sophisticated than those of the brain stem, but the limbic brain still does not confer the abilities of thought, language, or complex abstract processes so characteristic of humans. Bear in mind, however, that in depression most of these limbic functions are disturbed.

We evolved into sophisticated animals with language and the ability to make judgments and think in abstract ways through the development of the *cerebral cortex* or *cortical brain*—the proverbial "gray matter." The cortex was formed by the growth of billions of brain cells that had spread around and grown over the older limbic-brain structures and the brain stem, each layer densely packed with billions of cells lying on top of one another. You acquire your full complement of cortical brain cells by the eighteenth week of gestation, and you never get any more! These cells continuously communicate with each other and other parts of the brain, and over time they become more complex in their connections. The cortex is responsible for our higher intellectual reasoning.

In essence the old limbic brain with the embedded brain stem and the new cortical brain on top fit together like a brain within a brain within a brain. However, all three parts vigorously exchange information, even from before birth. The two parts of the brain that interest us most when it comes to the relationship between your hormones and moods are the limbic and cortical areas, so let's explore those further.

Your Limbic Brain

The limbic brain serves your primitive drives for survival, as noted above, but it also functions as a major relay station for receiving information from the outside and integrating it with information from the cortex and brain stem. When you encounter an object or event, your limbic brain must decide within milliseconds whether it represents a threat. In fact, your survival is linked to your ability to react immediately to a perceived external danger. This process of awareness and reaction occurs spontaneously and continuously.

If the object or event is perceived as nonthreatening, your limbic brain remains quiet. If it is unsure, then its biochemical response may lead to increased vigilance and a sense of being on guard. If the object or event is potentially harmful, your limbic brain's biological response is quite specific. It stimulates a cascade of biochemical changes that mobilize the secretion of a series of stress hormones that activate your body to respond in one of three ways: you may flee, stand and fight, or become "frozen" with fear. These are primordial responses.

Imagine that you are fourteen years old and that you are walking down the street. Someone jumps from behind a doorway, holds a knife to your back, and demands your wallet. The immediate and universal biological reaction is for your limbic brain to tell you that you are in danger and to mobilize every organ system you need to survive. Your heart races; you breathe heavily; you may feel nauseous, light-headed, or anxious; your mouth goes dry; your pupils dilate; and your blood sugar rises to provide your muscles with immediate energy to protect yourself. You are now in the most hyperalert physiological state possible. You are ready to respond.

Another of our most primitive drives, the necessity to reproduce, is also regulated in the limbic brain. Since sexual activity is vital to the survival of our species, it is often the most difficult drive to control, despite the best of intentions. Men and women are intrinsically sexual beings, which is why celibacy is so difficult to achieve. (See Illustration 1.)

Your Cortex

It may help you to understand the interrelation of your limbic brain with your cerebral cortex by observing children's developing behavior. In fact, you can think of youngsters as little limbic brains running amok. They are impulsive, reactive, aggressive, and spontaneous. They demand immediate attention. Parents often function as their young child's interim "cortex," setting limits and modeling the use of intellectual skills such as problem solving, emotional containment, patience, and negotiation.

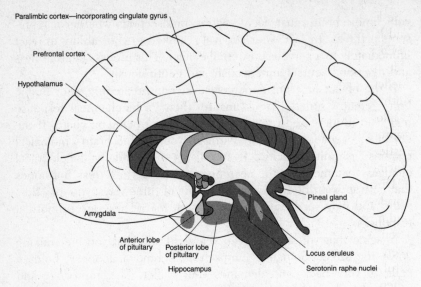

Illustration 1. The cortex and the limbic brain

As the child's brain matures, it develops multiple, intricate nerve networks and pathways between the structures of the limbic brain and the cortex. Eventually the child's own cortex is able to inhibit some of the more primitive drives. The maturation process also allows the cells to relay messages more quickly, so that thoughtful judgment and purposeful behavior become more sophisticated.

As a result we say that the child has been "socialized" to fit into the adult world. When a parent does not model these behaviors, the child never learns how to use sophisticated intellectual skills. One of the tasks of psychotherapy is to help a patient restrain her own impulses, evaluate her behavior, and develop analytical thinking so that old, maladaptive behavior patterns can change. This work involves the engagement of the intellectual abilities that reside in the cortex.

As we explained in Chapter 2, the cortex is divided into halves or hemispheres, and each holds a different function. The right side is more involved in spatial relations (such as the ability to understand and perceive three-dimensional objects), artistic development, music and other nonlanguage sounds, intuitive thought, and the expression of emotions. It also has the capacity to see the big picture, as opposed to focusing on details, which is the domain of the left cortical brain.

The left brain also specializes in analytical skills, mathematics, logic, and language.

Each half of the cortex is also involved in mood states. The right side tends to be responsible for negative, unhappy emotions, while the left side serves positive, even euphoric feelings. Working together, both sides produce a balanced mood. When the right side is damaged, it allows the left side to dominate, so that one's mood becomes inappropriately jocular. An injury to the left side of the brain leads to restless depression because its contribution to the balance is removed, leaving the right side to predominate.

During the evolutionary process the cortex grew larger, and we developed the capacity to control our emotions, inhibit aggression, and modify impulses emanating from the more primitive limbic brain. Even though we have evolved enormous cortical-brain abilities, however, there are times when the cortex inadequately inhibits our powerful emotional drives and we manage these impulses less well, as when rage erupts into violence.

When symptoms of depression and anxiety occur, they originate from our limbic brain, but they involve the cortex as well, since severe depression is associated with diminished insight, poor judgment, lack of motivation, and attention deficits—all functions of the higher levels of brain.

The Limbic Brain and Depression

Although the limbic brain is quite complex, we would like to explain a few of its specific structures that relate to mood or anxiety disorders: the *amygdala, hippocampus,* and *hypothalamus.* Together with the cortex, these structures recall, correlate, store, and impart emotion to all of your experiences, whether consciously or unconsciously.

THE AMYGDALA

By relaying nerve signals related to emotions and stress, this almond-shaped structure regulates emotion and fear responses and participates in the establishment of memory. The amygdala notes threats in the environment and decides whether you should freeze, flee, or fight.

The amygdala is thought to modulate the production of the neurotransmitters serotonin and norepinephrine. Indeed, researchers have found also that the amygdala can be overactive in people who are depressed. The greater the activity, the deeper the depression.[1]

THE HIPPOCAMPUS

This seahorse-shaped structure is implicated in how memories are made, stored, and retrieved and in the modulation of stress responses and emotions. It may also play a role in immunity.

THE HYPOTHALAMUS

Connected by a stalk to the pituitary gland beneath it, the hypothalamus is a kind of concertmaster, orchestrating the menstrual cycle, thyroid function, physiological stress responses, body temperature, sleep-wake cycle, appetite, growth, and production of milk. It does so by secreting special hormones, called releasing factors, which in turn stimulate the release of hormones from the pituitary gland. It manages stress hormones and other bodily functions required during fearful encounters.

Fear—real or perceived—is a fundamental emotion that colors experience. Pervasive, difficult to control, and incapacitating, anxiety is a frequent symptom of depression.

The Paralimbic Cortex

When the cortex developed by wrapping around the limbic brain, the first layers to appear comprise what we now call the *paralimbic cortex*. Not surprisingly, these were the first areas to inhibit primitive limbic drives. The development of the paralimbic cortex bestowed upon us the ability to impart emotional coloring to experiences. It works collaboratively with the structures in the limbic brain.

An important area in the paralimbic cortex is the *cingulate gyrus*. This connects to our fight-or-flight reaction when we face danger. And it may be responsible for the dread and anxiety that surface when a person with OCD is unable fulfill her obsessions.

Maternal bonding, another step forward in the evolutionary process, is also dependent on the cingulate gyrus. Without this primal emotional bond between mother and offspring, we would not have survived. To mother is to feel, not only for ourselves but also for others, in the form of empathy. This is what gives us humanity.

Paul MacLean, an eminent neuroscientist,[2] explains that the evolution of the cingulate gyrus allowed for the development of bonding behaviors between early mammals that were related to one another—thus the family was born. These first attachments were driven by the development of a cry the infant made when it became separated from its mother. The mother could then respond to this "separation cry," which may represent the earliest and most basic vocalization in mammals. In time the offspring's separation cry must have sealed the attachment process. The mother would stay close to her infant, communicate with it, nourish it with her milk, and nurture it toward independence.

In 1981 MacLean and his colleagues found that if they destroyed a specific area of the cingulate gyrus in newborn hamsters, the animals grew and developed normally, but the females showed no evidence of maternal behavior when they delivered pups.[3]

He proposed that because the cingulate gyrus localizes the separation cry and also is richly innervated by cells involved in the perception of pain, separation from its mother might actually evoke a feeling of physical pain in the offspring.

Just think for a minute about an infant's cry. It summons a response in the mother or caregiver—the urge to pick up and comfort the baby. But if the baby is left to cry, what happens at the cellular level in his or her brain? Does the baby learn and record at a preverbal level that emotional distress feels like physical pain?

This calls into question the strategy of letting babies cry for long periods of time in the hope that they will ultimately learn to soothe themselves. More likely the infants become emotionally distressed and feel abandoned—separated from the only security they know. Indeed, they may even feel physical pain in the process. Perhaps the cingulate gyrus establishes a connection between emotional distress and pain early in life, leading to the experience of pain with separation issues as we grow older.

The cingulate gyrus may be implicated in the occurrence of postpartum OCD because it is involved anatomically with the fight-or-flight response, mood regulation, and the maternal bonding process.

The Emotional Brain and Memory

The most significant experiences in life are emotional. Emotions are feeling states usually not under your control. Although you may choose to hide the extent of your feelings from others, the emotional experience is nevertheless there, fully experienced in your body.

You experience many different emotional states, including joy, sorrow, frustration, satisfaction, rage, contentment, bliss, and pain. Everything that you remember as meaningful in your life is imbued with a particular emotion, and each such experience is recorded and embedded in your brain, becoming intrinsically part of you.

Very recent investigations of how the brain functions in severe depression involve the limbic and paralimbic areas as well as two other sites—the *prefrontal cortex,* located directly above the eyes, and the *frontal cortex,* located behind the forehead.

When the prefrontal cortex is damaged, judgment is impaired, emotions become shallow and blunted, and motivation and drive disappear. People become irritable and easily enraged, and their moods can be depressed or lacking in interest. They may disregard socially acceptable behavior, and their thinking can lose depth. Generally, a state of apathy or confusion may set in. Many of these characteristics are present in the illness of depression.

Brain scans have shown decreased activity in the prefrontal cortex of individuals with depression. And this area seems to be smaller than average in individuals who suffer from depression and bipolar illness, although we don't yet know if this deviation is at the root of or the result of these illnesses.[4]

The limbic area and its connections to the paralimbic brain and the prefrontal cortex are fundamental parts of the emotional brain. At our office we call this system the *prefrontal-limbic complex,* and it plays a large role in the processing of emotion, the regulation of moods, and the storage of memories. It is here that are fixed the powerful emotional recollections from childhood, which can shape your development and adult life. (See Illustration 2.)

Although you may be unaware of the ongoing process or its role in shaping your vision of and relationship to the world, from earliest childhood onward this area is laying down memories and the emotions attached to them. You can have good memories, of course. For instance, if as a child you spent wonderful times baking chocolate-chip cookies with a parent, the aroma will become emotionally connected to your warm and loving experience with that parent. As an adult, when you smell chocolate-chip cookies, your prefrontal-limbic complex will immediately retrieve those warm and loving emotional connections.

The aroma itself, other than being pleasant, has little meaning. But the affection and good feelings associated with it many years ago will give it an emotional meaning. Of course it is also true that if an aroma is associated with a memory of a bad experience, it will in the same way generate a negative response.

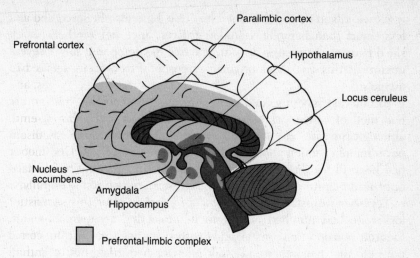

Illustration 2. Areas of the brain responsible for mood

Smells and sounds can trigger memories as well as emotions. If the experience was painful, both are often stored in a fragmented fashion. This may happen because the amygdala and the hippocampus, which mediate response to stress, record painful experiences in a piecemeal rather than a cohesive fashion. As a result the prefrontal-limbic complex recognizes only portions of the experience, not the entire episode, and will most often recognize the emotion before any associated memory is retrieved.

This explains why you may become distressed when confronted with a certain smell or color but may be unable to recall the meaning of the association. It may also explain why traumatic memories are often only incoherently or partially accessible to conscious memory.

Depression and the Lost Memory of Sorrow

As a second-year medical student, Kate had contacted us because she had become depressed. She complained of a sense of emptiness in her life. She had gained a good deal of weight in three months, and along with her appetite increase, her state of sadness and withdrawal indicated that she was suffering from major depression. When these symptoms occur, it means that biochemically there has been a disruption in some of the brain pathways responsible for mood stability.

As we talked, it also became clear that Kate also believed she was less smart than her fellow students. Ever since her mother's death she'd had an unwavering drive to practice medicine, but now she was unsure of this goal. Her original, intensely driven focus seemed to dwindle.

In our first meeting Kate sobbed as she revealed that her mother had died of cancer when Kate was ten. It was still a raw wound, although the loss had occurred nearly twenty years earlier. Kate did not remember much about her life before the age of ten. Her mother had been ill for three years prior to her death, and Kate had blotted out these painful memories and the associated distressing emotions.

Together we established that for a long time after this significant loss Kate had numbed herself to it, projecting a supercompetent, focused persona that was at odds with her grief state within. It did not help that her father and other relatives had urged her to "put all the bad stuff behind her and keep a stiff upper lip." She had never been allowed to grieve.

Carrying this internal load, Kate cried herself to sleep for years following her mother's death. During the day she often felt as if she wore a mask, and that the real Kate had also died.

At a young age Kate's brain already revealed that it had difficulty managing such a great loss. Lack of attention to her grief meant that her brain was shouldering this heavy chemical load without help. This can take a later toll, since it may establish permanent alterations in the mood pathways. It is well documented that significant loss early in life can precipitate depression in adulthood. A child carrying a load of chronic grief inevitably experiences some form of depression later. When you are not permitted to focus on the death of a parent and deal openly with your sorrow, the internal strain on the brain's biochemistry grows larger by the year.

Kate's "masklike" mood states during childhood may well have indicated the early flickerings of depression that emerged full-blown some twenty years later. A great student and model daughter who selflessly nurtured her young siblings, Kate began to feel as if she were an actress. In time, with psychotherapy, she would have to confront her fear of removing the mask. As I explained to her, "One of the hardest things to do in life is to be yourself, especially when those who mean the world to you are telling you to do otherwise."

My task was to treat Kate's current depression and help her understand that the emptiness she was feeling was related to the premature shortening of the vital relationship to her mother. We needed to coax back into consciousness the emotions of her early life, however painful. Therapy prods the brain's apparatus for feelings, learning, and memory to retrieve and reunite the fractured recollections of early childhood. Kate needed to recover the memories of the thwarted emotional connection to her mother that were stored in her prefrontal-limbic complex. Along with appropriate medication, her treatment involved discussion of her early life experiences and how the feelings they aroused were still present.

The Prefrontal-Limbic Complex in Action

The unconscious embedding of childhood events within the prefrontal-limbic complex is the most powerful determinant of your emotions and behaviors later in life. Your choice of a partner in a serious love relationship is a good example of the prefrontal-limbic complex in action.

At the beginning of the relationship, although you may feel a strong attraction, it may be unclear to you that your new love repeats some of your parents' personality characteristics. As the relationship develops, however, features emerge in your lover—both good and bad— that remind you of your parents. You have unconsciously gravitated to this person because something feels familiar. These are the elements that were imprinted in your prefrontal-limbic complex during your childhood experiences.

This may be why women from abusive homes tend to choose abusive partners. Indeed, they may stay in damaging relationships until they become aware of how they are repeating their painful childhoods by being drawn back to an emotional ambience they know so well.

Another sign of your prefrontal-limbic complex at work occurs when you are driving down the highway and someone cuts you off. Your limbic response is to drive the offender off the road. Ideally, your paralimbic cortex will buffer your road rage long enough for your cortical or intellectual skills to kick in and tell you that this would be foolish. Using the cortex to control an impulse is a learned, maturational skill, one that unfortunately many adults have not fully mastered.

In depression and premenstrual syndrome you may experience rage, anger, irritability, and hostility. In these mood states the chemical functioning within the limbic-brain area that extends into the cortex

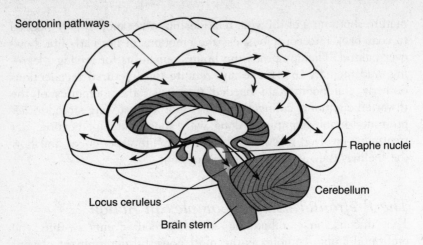

Illustration 3. The serotonin pathways

has been altered. It is as if the cortex, challenged by premenstrual hormonal fluctuations, is no longer able to inhibit angry and aggressive impulses. The chemical dysregulation within the mood pathways overcomes the buffering effects of the cortex, and the difficult behavior breaks through. Or as some patients have said to us, "I just don't understand why I snap at my children at this time!"

Mental health can be destabilized if the chemical equilibrium between the cortex and paralimbic areas is disrupted. When the condition is treated and the chemistry in the pathway is stabilized, the impulses, despondency, and anger melt away. Once the disruption in limbic pathways is soothed, the cortex can again do its job.

The Chemical Messengers

How do the billions of nerve cells within the brain communicate with each other? One way is through the amazing molecules called chemical messengers or *neurotransmitters*. These substances are made within each nerve cell and are secreted into the *synapse,* the space between one cell and the next. The "mood pathways" in the brain that we have been referring to consist of the chemical messenger systems that travel through and innervate the prefrontal-limbic complex. (See Illustration 3.)

Of the three main classes of chemical messengers,[5] we will focus on those that are called the *monoamines*. Serotonin is the best known of this class. It is heavily implicated in depression, anxiety disorders, and obsessional states. Others in this class are dopamine, norepinephrine, and acetylcholine. All four of these neurotransmitters are involved in the expression of mood, anxiety, memory, movement, and stress and in the *regulation of the menstrual cycle*.

Scientists have found that normal serotonin levels are associated with emotional balance and normal moods and behaviors. Insufficient serotonin can lead to the sleep disturbances, agitation, worry, lethargy, and hopelessness involved in depression.[6] Not surprisingly, mild premenstrual symptoms also have been linked to disruptions in the serotonin pathways. Women's brains have been shown to have higher levels of serotonin than men's.

Insufficient serotonin levels may be linked to suicidal behavior. Autopsies of suicide victims have shown that they have less serotonin in the fluid surrounding the brain and spinal cord than normal. What's more, their frontal-cortex brain cells have more receptors for serotonin, as if to make up for the inadequate supply.

These chemical messengers originate in the lower, most primitive brain-stem areas, extend into the limbic area, and move from there into the paralimbic and then on to the rest of the cortex. Because the extensive serotonin circuit is implicated in depression, anxiety, and other disorders, we will focus on it. But remember that this neurotransmitter pathway constitutes only one part of the depression process.

Serotonin is made from *tryptophan*, a basic protein building block, and is stored in granules in nerve cells. An electrical firing of the nerve[7] activates its release from the storage granules and into the synapse, or space between the nerve cells, where it attaches to a specific site or *receptor* on the neighboring nerve cell, much as a key fits into a lock. This attachment induces firing of the next cell, and then the next and the next, millions of times over. (See Illustration 4.)

Serotonin levels are regulated in various ways, including absorption back into the nerve cell, breakdown within the nerve space, the availability of storage, timing of release, and the number of receptors. Levels even correlate with the amount of tryptophan in your daily diet. A few studies have shown that when people are given a drink that experimentally depletes tryptophan, a depressive state quickly ensues. Estrogen promotes tryptophan availability in the brain.

Changes occurring at each of these points can alter the dynamics of serotonin, which can lead to depression and anxiety. For women the serotonin pathway is also highly influenced by hormonal shifts

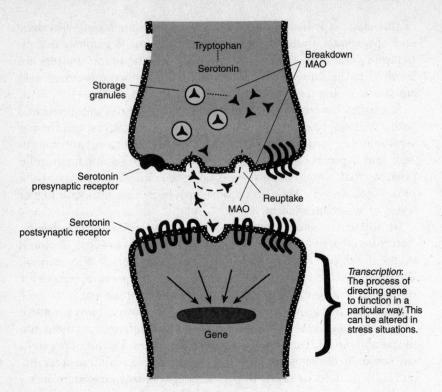

Illustration 4. Cascading events in the synaptic space

that occur normally during the menstrual cycle. Thus, the integrity of this pathway is jeopardized while estrogen pursues its role in reproduction every month.

The Impact of Estrogen

Brain biochemistry in women is designed and organized to be highly receptive to hormones. A woman's brain carries countless receptor sites for the female sex hormones estrogen and progesterone, where they can fasten and exert their effects far from the cells that made and secreted them. There are estrogen and progesterone receptors all over the brain, but they can be found most densely in the limbic area.

Through their multitude of impacts in the brain, estrogen and progesterone can induce changes in all the neurochemical pathways involved in mood disturbances. *This is the critical, vital component of women's mental health that remains invisible and unacknowledged.*

Estrogen maintains the orderly firing rates of the serotonin, dopamine, acetylcholine, and norepinephrine nerve cells. This promotes positive moods, thinking, memory, perception, motivation, appetite, sex drive, anxiety, and stress responses. It can slow the breakdown of the neurotransmitters, alter the number of receptors on the nerve cells, and enhance their sensitivity. Estrogen also strongly enhances glutamate activity. Glutamate is a neurotransmitter that accelerates nerve communication in the brain. This also encourages mood stability.

There is evidence that estrogen can promote the growth of nerve cells containing acetylcholine, particularly in the hippocampus. Since intact memory function is dependent on adequate acetylcholine levels, this heightens mental acuity, sustains memory functions, and enhances connections with other nerve cells. When estrogen levels decline at menopause, acetylcholine levels decrease also. This helps to explain why estrogen-replacement therapy in menopausal women helps to prevent difficulties with memory and word-retrieval skills (see Chapter 18).

When estrogen levels rise, their overall effect is to increase the amount of serotonin available in the spaces between the nerve cells, thereby contributing to mood stability. Within the brain estrogen may in fact act as a natural antidepressant and mood stabilizer. When estrogen levels drop, a reversal of this antidepressant effect presumably occurs. *In this way the fluctuations of estrogen across the menstrual cycle and at other points in a woman's reproductive life may disrupt the balance of the neurotransmitters and affect a woman's mood stability.* Estrogen can be regarded as having a protective effect against depression in women.

Of course, not all women experience mood changes during their menstrual cycle. It is likely that the receptors and cells in these women's brains have the resiliency to withstand the impact of hormonal changes. This may in part be caused by differences in genetic makeup. Perhaps these women's brains come equipped with chemical "circuit breakers" that allow them to reregulate serotonin when estrogen and progesterone levels fluctuate.

Many women do not experience the onset of premenstrual symptoms until their thirties and forties. The delay in the onset of symptoms may be due to the normal aging process or to changes in hormonal levels in response to life events and stressors.

Progesterone, the other female sex hormone, decreases the number of available estrogen receptors, which may be one of the mechanisms by which it can induce depression. There is evidence that at the end of the menstrual cycle progesterone can actually dismantle the nerve connections that estrogen established at the beginning of the cycle. Perhaps this is why the progesterone component of birth-control pills and hormone-replacement therapy can produce feelings of distress and depression in some women.

Testosterone, the male hormone, is produced in small amounts in the synthesis of estrogen and affects the limbic brain, stimulating libido and aggressive behavior.

Stress, Brain Chemistry, and Depression

Think back to the hypothetical situation we posed earlier. You've been held up at knifepoint and your heart raced, your mouth became dry, and your stomach churned. You may wonder how all that happened so quickly. Your response to stress is a lightning-fast yet highly complex cascade of chemical and biological events in your brain and body.

A nucleus in your old brain called the *locus ceruleus* is the brain's main depot for the neurotransmitter *norepinephrine*. Norepinephrine activates serotonin and cortisol-releasing hormone from structures in the limbic brain,[8] and prompts the pituitary gland to release *adrenocorticotropic hormone* (ACTH) into the bloodstream. ACTH tells the adrenal glands, which sit atop the kidneys, to secrete cortisol and adrenaline, the body's stress hormones, which in turn send your heart pumping, your stomach churning, and so on. As complicated as this may sound, amazingly the entire circuit is activated within milliseconds.

Every part of this stress circuit (what's called the *hypothalamus-pituitary-adrenal* circuit or HPA) is pumping to biochemically enable you to respond. You are now primed to meet the crisis.

When the robbery is over, you may be left without your wallet, but your body will remain on alert for a while. Eventually your heart rate will slow, your breathing will return to normal, and you will feel relieved. Your brain, however, will continue to stay "armed" for a few days in response to the event. You may find that you startle easily or feel a bit anxious for a time, but ultimately your body will reregulate and resume normal functioning.

The brain has intrinsic mechanisms for switching off the stress response and allowing recovery to take place. Once the original threat is gone, adrenaline and cortisol tell the pituitary and the limbic brain (in particular the hippocampus) to stop secreting ACTH and other stress hormones. When this occurs, the locus ceruleus replenishes the depleted norepinephrine, serotonin normalizes, cortisol drops, and the HPA circuit quiets. *The hyperalert state settles because the brain has biochemical mechanisms to bring it back into balance.* This chemical ability to "switch off" is vital. Yet in women's brains estrogen and progesterone appear to delay the ability to switch off the stress response.

Although traumatic, fortunately, the robbery doesn't limit your life, and you go on without further repercussions. You cope because you had some power over your destiny. The act of willingly surrendering your wallet was a key factor in your surviving the attack, and that provides you with a sense of control.

But the repetition of difficult life stressors such as these can chemically "load" the brain. For instance, suppose now that you're seventeen and your best friend is killed in a car accident. The same stress reaction that occurred during the robbery cascades through your body, but this time your anxiety persists.

It's not as easy for your cortex to process this event as it did the robbery; your brain is unable to switch off your stress-hormone response. Serotonin levels become depleted, and your HPA circuit, taking on a life of its own, goes into overdrive and stimulates the overproduction of stress hormones from the adrenal gland. As a result, no matter what you do, your cortex cannot calm the primitive limbic responses as easily as it did before. You begin to have symptoms of chemical dysregulation: difficulty sleeping, loss of appetite, problems concentrating.

Four months later you are still not feeling yourself. You eat poorly and have lost fifteen pounds. Your sleep is disturbed, you are easily irritated, and you find that it is harder to get going in the morning. It looks and sounds as though you are in a major depression. Because the onset of these feelings coincides with the death of your friend, you tell yourself that in time you will feel better and your symptoms will settle on their own.

But when they do subside and your brain has finally been able to switch off the stress response, it is not without cost to you. Your brain's biology has probably changed. The nerve cells activated by the stress of your friend's death may now be sensitized by complex factors affecting their genetic coding, so that they learn to function as if stress were present all the time.[9]

The Effects of Repetitive Stress

Therefore, when another traumatic event occurs, even if it is not as severe as your friend's death, your HPA circuit may become more easily disturbed because it has already "learned" how to do so. A changed biology is now part of who you are.

So, for instance, at eighteen you go away to college. During the first semester you begin to experience the same symptoms you had when your friend died, but this time there is no tragedy. Even though you had looked forward to going away to school, the normal developmental stress of leaving home triggers a biological response. It starts to feel like a crisis, and you have another depressive episode. You seek therapy with a college counselor. Over several months you adjust to college life. For the first time, however, you notice premenstrual feelings of moodiness, irritability, and insomnia. But within a few days after you get your period you're back to your old self again.

Even though you have recovered from the stress of going away to college, the circuits in a number of your chemical pathways may have been altered. Although now reregulated, they have the capacity to dysregulate premenstrually. And as estrogen levels fluctuate within the normal menstrual cycle (see Chapter 5), they have an impact on the now-sensitized serotonin pathways. Your biology easily tips into the dysregulated state that it learned in response to previous life stressors, and your premenstrual phase now includes symptoms of a mild depression.

Now suppose that at twenty-five, after ending a serious love relationship, you suffer another bout of depression. Despite counseling, this episode lasts for a year, and your premenstrual symptoms worsen noticeably. Eventually the depression lifts, and you feel better. At twenty-eight you have yet another depressive episode. This time, however, there is no obvious trigger.

The series of stressful events we have proposed has loaded, strained, and eventually changed your brain's mood pathways. Ultimately this sensitization becomes so profound that a normal female event such as the premenstrual period can easily trigger the biochemical disruption that leads to depression. The result: You bring a chemically altered brain into your adult years and are at risk for mood and anxiety problems throughout your reproductive life.

It seems not to matter whether the stress emanates from an external life event, an internal psychological concern, or the hormonal fluctuations that can come with PMS, childbirth, or menopause. Stress is stress, and the brain responds to protect you. Life has a biological impact on your brain.

Helping Kate to Heal

As our client Kate came closer to greater independence and accomplishment in medical school, the unresolved grief surrounding her mother's premature death reemerged. Kate's brain chemistry might have been altered when her mother died, then further loaded over time, as she was never allowed to fully mourn. Now, as Kate began to reexperience the sorrow, biochemistry was finally breaking through her mask to produce symptoms of depression. She was enduring an emotional earthquake.

She could not move on successfully until she dealt with this large piece of unfinished business. Life felt meaningless to her, because its meaning had drained away a long time ago. Kate's work was just beginning. She would find her true competence only when she stripped away the mask of false competence she had been wearing for so many years.

Our treatment plan was aimed at different levels of brain functioning. First we wanted to correct Kate's brain biochemistry. When biology is erupting, it's hard to achieve effective or meaningful psychotherapy. Consider the aftermath of an earthquake. If injured people are trapped in buildings, that is not the time to analyze the geological forces causing the upheaval! We must attend to basic injuries first. Only then can we examine the larger surrounding events.

To stabilize Kate's biology we started her on the antidepressant Prozac, which enhances mood-stabilizing serotonin levels in the brain. At the same time, in psychotherapy sessions, she recollected memories of her mother before she had died. This was the means by which we addressed the "mask," allowing Kate to feel more authentic in her interactions with the world. Once she could acknowledge her feelings of grief, rage, fear, loss, and helplessness, she no longer needed the mask. She could then direct the energy she had used in creating and maintaining it toward effective progress in her life.

Finally we taught Kate how this experience carried implications for her mood states in the future, especially with the advent of hormonally based reproductive events. Now she could be on the alert for any recurrence of depressive feelings and take steps to stop them before they became entrenched.

Women's brains can become biochemically and psychologically overloaded in childhood and adolescence. As a result of traumatic experiences and physiological brain responses, millions of women arrive at adulthood biochemically at risk, despite the fact that they have coped and survived. These biochemical changes can set them up for the emergence of serious depression in response to various reproductive events later in life.

Childhood trauma carries a hidden toll, slowly encoded within your biochemistry, which can reemerge later. For Kate it was a mother's death, ungrieved and unresolved. For you it may be some form of emotional, physical, or sexual abuse. As you read the chapters that follow, remember that the brain you bring into your adult years may be different from the brain with which you were born.

Chapter 4

"WHAT I'M FEELING HAS A NAME?"
MENTAL ILLNESSES AFFECTED BY HORMONES

How can you tell if you are susceptible to hormonally induced mental-health problems? In truth, all of the symptoms of a full syndrome need not be present for a vulnerability to exist.

For instance, you may have come to your childbearing years with mild or occasional symptoms of mood and anxiety disorders that could indicate a predisposition to these problems, but these may have gone unrecognized. Common "hidden" precursors that occur during adolescence include alterations in sleep or eating patterns, fatigue, and, if times are hard, some passing fantasies about death. Because of the tiredness, you might have found it harder to mobilize yourself, so your grades might have fallen off, or perhaps you maintained your grades but gradually dropped out of other activities. Or maybe you've struggled through bouts of depression each month as your period approached or while you were taking birth-control pills.

When we listen to women's accounts of their lives, we want to know whether they've experienced these symptoms because that helps us to pinpoint the onset of the disturbance. To ascertain if our patients have a special vulnerability to hormonal change, we look for:

- evidence of puberty-related depression
- evidence of premenstrual depressive symptoms
- an adverse response to oral contraceptives

- depression or anxiety while taking fertility-enhancing drugs
- signs of illness during pregnancy, including mood changes in the first few weeks
- changes in demeanor in the last few weeks of pregnancy
- problems in the delivery or the baby's health that could contribute to mood changes later
- obsessional thoughts of harming the baby
- changes in disposition before and after taking hormone-replacement therapy

When a woman develops symptoms of mood or anxiety disorders in relation to a reproductive event, be it menstrual periods, taking birth-control pills, having a baby, or entering menopause, it means that something within her brain's capacity to regulate itself has become disturbed. Our first step is to evaluate any previous symptoms that would tell us what set the stage for the hormonal upset to occur. We treat our patient, observe her progress, and then make educated predictions about the future.

Depending on your biochemical vulnerability, preexisting emotional problems can recur or worsen with future reproductive hormonal events. And once your brain biochemistry has responded to these hormonal events, it is likely that it will continue to respond in similar fashion for the rest of your life. If, for instance, you suffered from major depression after your baby was born, you may also experience premenstrual dysphoric disorder (also known as PMS) before each period and mood changes as you approach menopause.

Forewarned is forearmed. In Chapter 7 you will learn about the NURSE Program. It has all the elements you need to help you take care of your brain and its delicate functions. Control the elements that you can and learn to let go of what you can't. This is not a moral issue but rather just what is. If you have a diagnosable illness that has become chronic, you must learn to live within the givens of your biochemical makeup, recognizing that the condition is unlikely to disappear. Your brain will, however, respond to preventive measures and care.

The Framework We Commonly Use
The framework we use for defining the different syndromes and disorders that women exhibit is *The Diagnostic and Statistical Manual*

of Mental Disorders (4th Edition) or the DSM-IV, published by the American Psychiatric Association.[1] The DSM-IV acts as a sort of diagnostic "bible" for mental-health providers. It was first conceptualized, developed, and published in the early 1950s by a group of psychiatrists as a way to define and describe psychiatric disorders.

Unfortunately, the DSM-IV is by no means comprehensive. Acting only as a road map to help us understand the range of symptoms that may occur, it tells us nothing about a woman's life or her soul.

Also bear in mind that you do not have to have every symptom listed to have a problem requiring treatment. That is why we should regard a manual of emotional illnesses only as a guide. Still, it is helpful to understand how mental illnesses can manifest themselves so that you may seek appropriate treatment.

Mood Disorders

You may already have a sense from some of the women's stories we have presented that there are several types of mood disorders. It is important for us to specify these mood states, because women who have them can be quite vulnerable to hormonal changes through the childbearing years. If we can understand what type of mood problem they have, then treatment is much more accurate, aimed at resolving the problem and not just chasing symptoms.

It is the responsibility of the clinician treating you to distinguish what kind of disorder you may be experiencing. This process involves the clinician's diagnostic skills coupled with your honest sharing of symptoms, as well as a discussion of the intensity and duration of your distress. Your clinician can make the correct diagnosis and initiate the appropriate treatment only with a complete and thorough assessment of your history, complaints, and concerns.

MAJOR DEPRESSION

The most commonly known mood disorder is major (also called "clinical") depression. It is important to distinguish major depression from being in a sad mood or "having the blues." The blues encompass a sense of feeling unhappy in response to a transient stressor, disappointment, or loss. For example, you may feel sad after your youngest child has gone off to college or in response to a work conflict or a poor showing on an exam. Although you are down in the dumps, you can identify the cause and know that you will feel better after a short time. You call on your coping skills, and soon the sad mood lifts.

Major depression is quite different. It involves a continuing downward spiral associated with changes in other bodily functions such as appetite, concentration, sleep-wake cycles, and energy level. This type of depression appears to be the result of a chemical dysregulation in the brain. Unfortunately, people suffering from a major depressive disorder often do not seek help when they first feel despondent because of the shame involved. It is a myth that you can shake these feelings by being busy and carrying on as usual with a big smile on your face. Unlike having the blues, if you are depressed, more often than not you can't just "snap out of it!"

The symptoms of major depression include persistent sadness and melancholy coupled with the loss of interest in all or most of your usual activities. This mood state must be present continually for at least two weeks or more and be associated with at least *five* of the following additional symptoms:

- increased or decreased appetite
- weight gain or loss
- agitation and restlessness or lethargy
- the onset of panic attacks or pervasive anxiety
- difficulty with sleep, sleeping either too much or not enough
- feelings of hopelessness, worthlessness, or inappropriate guilt and shame
- difficulty thinking, concentrating, or making decisions
- recurrent thoughts of death or suicide

Some people with major depression are severely ill and unable to function, while others meet the criteria for this disorder and still function from day to day. However, the latter will say that they are performing in a diminished way.

Some women can experience depression in relation to the seasons or even to fluctuations in daylight and darkness. These women may feel better and better as the day goes on, but their moods will worsen at night or when the weather turns gloomy. They are also more depressed in the winter than in the summer, especially if they live in northern latitudes. This suggests that their sleep-wake clocks are sensitive to light and dark. Perhaps the secretion of the sleep hormone melatonin is linked to their mood disorder. This is called seasonal affective disorder (SAD) and is a variant of major depression.

Nanette was a tall, slim, twenty-eight-year-old woman who came to our offices. She shared her many concerns with Jeanne. "I feel like I am losing my mind. I am losing weight, and I'm terrified all the time. My doctor can't find anything wrong with me. I was referred to you because I feel so lousy. Am I crazy?"

Externally Nanette looked good. She was neatly dressed, she smiled, and Jeanne noted her beautiful blue eyes. But we have learned that looks can be deceiving. As Jeanne listened sympathetically, the full story emerged. "I can't sleep. The world feels so dark— it's like black clouds follow me wherever I go," Nanette confessed, tears rolling down her cheeks. "I cry all the time, and I feel like I want to jump out of my skin. I can't sit still; I have to keep moving. I'm like the Energizer Bunny, but I have no interest in going anywhere! I am really scared and don't know why this is happening. My life felt quite fine before, but now I feel as though it has come to an end."

Nanette was experiencing a serious depression. Her symptoms included the loss of her sex drive, poor appetite, insomnia, irritability, fear, constant anxiety, and restlessness. In addition, there were times when she felt sad, alone, and unfocused. She had lost any sense of caring about her work, family, and life in general. These are the hallmarks of major depression.

DYSTHYMIA (MINOR DEPRESSION)

Women with dysthymia describe themselves as feeling "low," "down in the dumps," or just plain unhappy. They may also experience excessive fatigue and find that life does not hold the enjoyment it previously had. Often these symptoms have become so ingrained in everyday living that our patients say, "I've always been this way." They cannot remember when life felt good to them.

With this type of depression you may suffer from a continuing, chronically depressed mood that occurs some days of the week, often for a number of months or years. According to the DSM-IV, during these periods of depressed mood at least *two* of the following additional symptoms must be present:

- poor or increased appetite
- low self-esteem

- low energy
- poor concentration
- difficulty making decisions
- disruptions in sleep patterns: being unable to fall asleep or an increased need for sleep
- self-criticism
- feelings of hopelessness

Occasionally, symptom-free periods can occur for a few months at a time, but then the old pattern resumes.

Many women with dysthymia experience premenstrual worsening of their depressive symptoms. However, they often identify the premenstrual period as the problem, not their chronic mood state. They are so used to living with a continuing state of low-level depression that they fail to see the mood as the primary problem. In fact, people with dysthymia often describe having dull, heavy feelings since childhood or adolescence. Unfortunately, the disorder was never recognized.

Consequently, women with dysthymia can be in psychotherapy for long periods before their continuing depressed mood state is identified as needing some antidepressant medications to correct the errant biochemistry. Women with dysthymic disorders are at particular risk for premenstrual, postpartum, and menopausal mood disturbances.

Shirley, a thirty-two-year-old woman, came for help after the birth of her first baby. Although she told us that this was the first time she had ever experienced such feelings of tearfulness, insomnia, loss of confidence, and difficulty concentrating, after several psychotherapy sessions she realized that in the past she had had difficulty mobilizing herself. Her cycles of oversleeping, overeating, feelings of low self-esteem, and fatigue were indeed symptomatic of dysthymia. Despite these hindrances, however, Shirley had maintained herself through college and work situations.

PREMENSTRUAL DYSPHORIC DISORDER (PMDD)

Susan came to our office complaining, "For a few days before my period I feel jittery and keyed up. My husband says I'm impatient with him, and I can't just 'let things go.' I'm more likely to snap at him for small things, although my mood doesn't feel particularly sad or down." Susan finds it harder to get to sleep premenstrually, and she craves sweets, particularly chocolate. She gets a little "bloated," and her breasts become tender premenstrually, but she tolerates these discomforts. "The funny thing is," she continued, "within an hour or so of starting my period, I feel much better, and after a few hours I'm back to myself." Susan presents us with an example of mild premenstrual dysphoric disorder (also known as PMDD or PMS for premenstrual syndrome).

Women with premenstrual dysphoric disorder complain that they have difficulty with their moods before their periods. At times they can become quite short-tempered or irritable, or they describe a day or days of feeling excessive fatigue, when they are unable to accomplish anything. Ordinary events seem intensely sad; they weep at television commercials and overreact to their husband's glance or to the way he butters his toast or loads the dishwasher. But when their periods start, these symptoms evaporate, and they regain their normal energy level.

BIPOLAR 1 DISORDER (MANIC DEPRESSION)
Grace was an attractive twenty-eight-year-old woman who had been married for three years. Her husband, a law-school student, spent most of his time with his studies. Grace had worked full-time until she delivered their first child, two years earlier—a planned pregnancy that had been quite normal. She'd had a good deal of nausea in the first twelve weeks—distressing in itself—but she tolerated it, as most women do. After the nausea dissipated, she felt, in her words, "wonderful."

"What do you mean by 'wonderful'?" I asked when I interviewed her in her hospital room.

"Oh, I had lots of energy," Grace told me. "I never got tired! I worked two jobs until the day I went into labor."

This made me immediately suspicious. Although many women feel a mild euphoria—they're energized and joyful—in the second trimester of pregnancy, this is likely due to the antidepressant effect of high levels of estrogen circulating in the blood. But having huge stores of energy is out of character for the last trimester of pregnancy, when most women feel tired and uncomfortable.

"How did you manage two jobs?" I probed further. "What were your hours?"

"Oh," Grace replied, "I worked my day job from seven A.M. till four P.M., then went to my second job from seven P.M. until midnight."

"Really? How were you able to cope with such long hours in your pregnant condition?"

"I felt quite well and wasn't tired at all," she said.

"How much sleep did you get?"

"Well, not much. Probably about five hours."

"Weren't you ever curious about your boundless energy?" I continued. "That's when most other pregnant women complain about aches and pains.

"No, I just did what I needed to do," Grace replied blithely.

But Grace's situation was nothing to be blithe about. It was too extreme. In fact, I had been called in to treat her after she had attempted suicide upon weaning her toddler. Her mood had swung from the euphoria of her pregnancy to a deep depression when she stopped breast-feeding him. She was suffering from bipolar illness (also called manic depression), a disorder that affects between 0.5 percent to 1.6 percent of the total population.

Bipolar illness often begins during adolescence or early adulthood. In its most severe form, people experience marked changes in mood, from normal or depressed to excessive elevations that we term mania. The symptoms that characterize such manic behavior include:

- enormous energy
- elated mood
- feeling able to conquer the world
- grandiosity
- nonstop activity, frequently around the clock
- very little need for sleep
- nonstop, rapid talking
- racing thoughts and ideas
- inability to conduct a conversation that reaches a goal
- delusions: false beliefs about who one is
- hallucinations
- paranoia and fearful thoughts
- poor judgment, shopping binges, promiscuity, and/or illegal behavior

There can be varying degrees of mood elevation or good feelings, and people in the early stages of mania are often quite charming.

Usually they don't want to consider these mood states problematic because they feel great. Those in the throes of mania have a strong sense of accomplishment and describe how they get a lot done. Unless a clinician asks about the types of symptoms listed above, bipolar illness may be missed, leading to inaccurate diagnosis and perhaps inappropriate treatment. Indeed, some women who have attempted suicide during the postpartum period may be misdiagnosed as having been depressed because the mental-health professional has missed the manic phase of the illness.

If the manic mood devolves into a delusional state, a sufferer can become frightening. A woman experiencing delusions may believe that she is the president or even the Virgin Mary. Hallucinations can take the form of seeing images or hearing voices that order her to perform acts harmful to herself or others, including her baby.

At the other pole of this disorder is a severely depressed mood. Patients become withdrawn and isolated. They feel unable to get out of bed. Devoid of hope and self-worth, they believe that the world is black. Every day is a significant struggle. This state looks like major depression and carries a high risk of suicide if untreated. Sometimes the first evidence of bipolar disorder appears in adolescents as major depression, and the manic episode occurs later. But once one manic episode takes place, most sufferers will experience recurrent problems and require ongoing medication.

Morgan was fifteen years old when she came to our attention. Her case clearly illustrates how ignorance of reproductive-hormonal events and misdiagnosis can combine to exacerbate the symptoms of bipolar 1 illness in women.

After her first menstrual period Morgan became increasingly animated, needing less and less sleep. Soon she acquired four boyfriends and was sexually active with three of them. She took on more and more projects at school, feeling that nothing was too much for her. She also started to use alcohol and often became intoxicated. This behavior continued for about six months.

Then Morgan's mood suddenly shifted: She was unable to get out of bed to go to school, she sobbed uncontrollably, and she stopped taking care of herself. Her parents took her to a psychiatrist, who diagnosed depression and prescribed an antidepressant. He did not ask about her menstrual history or about the preceding six months. He also did not inquire about her sexual activity or the fact that she was on the Pill. Within two weeks of starting the antidepressant Morgan began to feel wonderful again. She had lots of energy (in fact, too much of it), little use for sleep, and once again believed she was going to save the earth.

In this completely manic state, her judgment was impaired and her activities spun dangerously out of control. She was admitted to a psychiatric hospital. That's where a new diagnosis of bipolar disorder was made. But for Morgan a complete evaluation should have taken into account the possibility that the birth-control pills she was taking were contributing to her instability and that the medications used to stabilize her mood were improperly correlated with her menstrual cycle. Nor was attention paid to the fact that her reckless sexual behavior was putting her at great risk for sexually transmitted diseases. In short, Morgan was not receiving the most effective treatment, one cognizant of her female biology, her general health, and its relationship to her care and healing processes.

Over the next several months Morgan was admitted every month to the inpatient unit because she continued to become irritable and manic before her period. Although this occurred four times in four months, nobody recognized that each time she was admitted, she was premenstrual. This is commonly a time when women who have problems with bipolar illness fly out of control. Additionally, blood levels of her medication should have been measured across her menstrual cycle to ascertain their fluctuations. Until all of these issues were addressed, Morgan could not hope for proper stability of her bipolar episodes.

A woman with bipolar 1 disorder is at extreme risk for mental illness during pregnancy. She should be considered a high-risk patient, just as a woman with diabetes would be. This does not mean that bipolar disorder cannot be managed at this time. Rather it means that a woman with this disorder must receive serious attention. If the illness is not controlled, it can constitute a risk to the mother and her unborn baby.

Risks for these women after they deliver are also quite high because they can become seriously ill with mania and delusions or, like Grace, with severe depression. This, too, presents a danger to mother and baby. It is when they are in the grip of severe depressive or manic illness that some women have killed their infants and/or attempted suicide. Unfortunately, many women who face their first episode of illness after they deliver find this diagnosis hard to accept and may test it out in their own, discontinuing their medications, only to find that they become ill again.

A woman with bipolar 1 disorder requires close medical care.

BIPOLAR 2 DISORDER

When most people encounter the term "manic depression," they think of the severe symptoms we have just described. But there is another, less extreme form of this illness, called bipolar 2 disorder, with which most of us are less familiar. Still, this condition affects substantial numbers of women and causes significant disruption and unhappiness in their lives and the lives of their loved ones.

The hallmark of bipolar 2 disorder is the recurrence of depressive episodes severe enough to meet the criteria for major depression, coupled with short *hypomanic* swings. Less severe than mania, a hypomanic phase is characterized by an abnormally and persistently elevated, expansive, or irritable mood. Although the DSM-IV states that hypomanic episodes should last for four days, we have found that they can range from a few hours to more than four days in someone with this disorder. The mood stops spontaneously and reverts to normal or to depression.

Hypomania is also accompanied by some of the following symptoms:

- inflated self-esteem
- decreased need for sleep
- irritability
- talkativeness and rapid speech
- flight of ideas or racing thoughts
- distractibility, with attention easily diverted
- going on buying sprees or making foolish investments

People do not get hallucinations or delusions in hypomania.

Women with bipolar 2 illness were frequently irritable or impulsive as kids. They can also be hyperactive, extremely emotionally reactive, moody, tremendously creative, highly productive, and accomplished in their lives. They are often involved in many activities and seen as having an excitable, demanding temperament from early on.

Although mild symptoms may have existed for years, some women who have this type of mood disturbance first become seriously ill after they've had a baby. They experience an initial hypomanic phase immediately after the birth, which then swings into a severe depression. But most often when a woman has bipolar 2 disorder, it has been present since adolescence, affecting her relationships and her life.

In some women the mood swings of bipolar 2 disorder occur in relation to the menstrual cycle. Some become irascible and irritable. They seem agitated and experience increased activity and decreased sleep before menstruation. Others become more depressed premenstrually, and may be more energetic in the first two weeks of their cycle. Because bipolar 2 disorder manifests itself as severe irritability and mood swings premenstrually, it is often mistaken for a premenstrual mood disorder.

At twenty-six, Kelly complained of symptoms of premenstrual mood problems. She explained that seven days before her period she became a "wild" woman. "I feel irritable, out of control, undirected, and I lose my sense of purpose," she told Jeanne. "I get angry easily, become unrealistic, and can't solve problems with any kind of rationality. I also have temper tantrums, which are ridiculous! When my period starts, I feel even worse. I'm quite down and sluggish for a few days, but then I feel better. I have a few cramps, but no other real physical problems. This has been happening to me for as long as I can remember."

Kelly went on to say that she had always been told she was a behavior problem in school and at home. "I guess I'm just hyper and impulsive," she continued. "There are times when I have so much energy; I can get so much done. I hardly need any sleep, and I feel great. I get really talkative, and I have a great sense of humor. I could party all night!" Kelly explained that she had lots of creative ideas at those times.

These periods would last a few days and then settle down. Often, following this great burst of energy, Kelly would became lethargic and would need more sleep. She would have a hard time getting out of bed and would feel much less motivated. "I could cry if you looked at me in a way that feels funny to me," she told Jeanne. Then these mood changes would just lift. Kelly attributed these periods of instability variously to her personal life and her work situation.

Kelly provided Jeanne with evidence that she had experienced hyperactive, impulsive mood states as a child. Many women who have bipolar 2 disorder describe this type of childhood behavior, often indicating mood-swing problems early in life. After Kelly started menstruating, her mood swings became more apparent. Her anger and irritability worsened premenstrually, sometimes to the point where she couldn't get out of bed for a few days at a time. As a result, her relationships deteriorated significantly.

As she entered her twenties, the mood swings took on clear periods of hypomania. (Very often, impulsive behaviors accompany this mood state, and unfortunately some women believe these are due to attention-deficit problems rather than bipolar disorder.) Because her mood swings had existed for much of Kelly's life, she thought they were normal and believed that she needed help only with her premenstrual symptoms.

When it comes to bipolar 2 disorder, it is easy to be confused. This is the most unrecognized and undertreated mood problem we encounter in our practice. In fact, some researchers estimate that 4 to 5 percent of the population suffer from it.[2] We are always on the lookout for it, since misdiagnosis can lead to worsening of the condition. The brain pathways in a woman with bipolar 2 disorder are exquisitely sensitive to the fluctuation of hormones. It often becomes evident at puberty and can worsen with the use of oral contraceptives. In fact, when Kelly took birth-control pills, she became depressed immediately. She was tearful and unable to mobilize herself at all. Once she stopped the Pill, she felt better within a few days.

The condition may improve during pregnancy, but then deteriorate into serious depression in the postpartum period. These women usually report significant PMS symptoms and then a worsening of symptoms around menopause.

Unless this disorder is diagnosed, women who suffer from it have a difficult time with their moods throughout their childbearing years. They often complain of intense irritability, anger, and restlessness as their hormones fluctuate. Their relationships can be stormy.

Anxiety Disorders

When in the grip of an anxiety disorder, you may feel excessive, incapacitating fear that inhibits your daily activities. There are several types of anxiety disorders, each with differing degrees of physical, emotional, and fearful symptoms. These symptoms can even start in childhood. Indeed, some studies have noted that toddlers under two years of age whose mothers have been diagnosed with panic disorder show high degrees of inhibited behavior. This suggests that the propensity for an anxiety disorder is part of our genetic inheritance and may be reflected in the children's general temperament and behavior.

Let's look at some of these anxiety disorders more closely.

PANIC DISORDER

People with panic disorder experience the acute onset (within a period of ten minutes) of a panic attack as a sensation of intense fear, anxiety, or discomfort that is often accompanied by a sense of impending doom and the urge to escape. According to the DSM-IV, during these periods of panic at least *four* of the following additional symptoms must be present:

- palpitations, pounding heart, or rapid heart rate
- sweating
- trembling or shaking
- sensations of shortness of breath or smothering
- feeling of choking
- chest pain or discomfort
- nausea or abdominal distress
- feeling dizzy, unsteady, light-headed, or faint
- feelings of unreality or feeling detached from oneself
- fear of losing control or going crazy
- fear of dying
- numbness or tingling sensations
- chills or hot flashes

When a person has panic disorder, she experiences at least one attack a week for four weeks associated with symptoms of continuing or ongoing fear and anxiety during this period. She will also persistently worry that the attack will recur and will often institute behavioral changes to cope with the fear. For instance, she may refuse to go out because she dreads having a panic attack at the supermarket, or she may refrain from driving since the last attack she had was in the car. Many patients with panic attacks have periods of generalized anxiety and are often fearful of going to places they believe may trigger an attack.

The panic attacks might occur with little regularity. For instance, many people can experience a few panic attacks during the first weeks of the condition and then the symptoms will settle; weeks or months can pass with no symptoms. Some will experience limited attacks in which fewer than four of the symptoms are present, but at other times they will experience a more full-blown attack.

Physicians often miss the syndrome of panic attacks. As you can see from the symptom list, physical symptoms predominate, so often many medical tests are ordered and nothing is found to be abnormal. We have had patients who complain only of the dizziness, detached feelings—which they frequently call "spaciness"—numbness, light-headedness, and nausea. These are more difficult to diagnose, but we are alert to these women because they suffer greatly. Unfortunately, other doctors usually label them hypochondriacs, because their symptoms are so elusive and their blood work and brain scans always come back normal.

Many women enter their childbearing years not knowing that there is a name for their symptoms and that they are experiencing anxiety. Anxiety symptoms are likely to worsen at specific times during these years such as premenstrually, during pregnancy, and postpartum.

PHOBIAS

The hallmark of this disorder is a sudden or persistent *unreasonable* fear brought on by the presence or the anticipation of a specific object or situation. You might have a phobia about heights, deep water, snakes, or germs. One of our clients developed a phobia regarding catching HIV from water fountains after she attended an educational workshop on the virus for her professional work. Some women develop tremendous phobias that their babies will contract some horrible disease if they leave the house.

When the person experiences the phobic situation or place, she has an immediate anxiety response that may lead to a panic attack. Usually she knows that this fear is excessive and unreasonable, but her intellectual knowledge does not stop the intense feelings. As you can imagine, having a phobia can interfere with your normal daily living.

OBSESSIVE COMPULSIVE DISORDER (OCD)

Many people suffer with obsessive-compulsive disorder, often termed OCD, although relatively few seek or receive treatment for it. In the general population, obsessive-compulsive disorder is usually diagnosed in young adults. It is typified by repetitive thoughts and behaviors that have no particular meaning and over which sufferers have little or no control.

People with OCD have recurrent *obsessions* (persistent, intrusive, and inappropriate ideas, impulses, or images that cause much distress and/or anxiety) and *compulsions* (repetitive behaviors or mental acts aimed at preventing or reducing the anxiety or distress). These symptoms can cause significant impairment in a person's life. A person experiencing this disorder knows that the thoughts and behaviors are excessive and make no sense, but she can't stop them. She also knows that the feelings are coming from inside, but she can't figure out why.

Obsessions might include fears about leaving the gas stove or electrical appliances turned on, leaving the door unlocked, contracting illnesses, having personal effects out of order, and so on. Consequently, the most common compulsions include checking appliances or locks, washing hands, cleaning, counting, requesting or demanding assurances, repeating actions, or placing objects into some kind of preordained order.

In postpartum women we have seen the onset of intrusive, strange thoughts that something might hurt their baby. The woman knows that her thoughts and worries are extreme and improbable, but they don't go away. Prior to their deliveries, these women had led normal, loving, and functioning lives with no history of mental illness. They were not psychotic, since they were well aware that their thoughts made no sense, even while being unable to stop them. They did everything they could to protect their babies from harm, often by avoiding them. Some locked their bedroom doors for fear that they might act out their thoughts during the night. Others made sure they were never left alone with their infants. One woman even sent her newborn to live with her parents. They stopped reading newspapers and watching television, lest violent news act as a trigger for their thoughts. They lived in constant fear of exposure, which might lead to their husbands, parents, or social agencies removing their children from them.

One of our patients described her disorder as "funny hormonal pictures that would come into my mind that I could harm my baby . . . drop her or something." Another woman described that she was cutting up a chicken, "and then all of a sudden I thought that I was cutting up my baby. . . . I almost died. I dropped the knife and ran to the baby. She was sound asleep in her room, but it was a horrible thought!"

POST-TRAUMATIC STRESS DISORDER

The media has been doing a fine job of informing the public about post-traumatic stress disorder (PTSD), and you may have heard a lot about it in relation to war veterans and the response to rape and sexual trauma.

Anyone can develop symptoms of PTSD. They usually follow an extremely traumatic event involving an experience that might have threatened a person with death or caused serious injury or some other risk to the person's integrity. PTSD may also occur in response to witnessing an event that involves threat, injury, or death to another person. Traumatic events include being a victim of or observing rape, incest, physical abuse, sexual abuse, car accidents, bombings, war, or even a difficult childbirth. Someone experiencing or witnessing this event may feel intense fear, helplessness, or horror.

One of the hallmarks of PTSD is that the sufferer reexperiences the trauma continuously. She may have:

- recurrent and intrusive recollections of the event, including images, thoughts, and perceptions
- recurrent dreams and nightmares
- a feeling that the event is happening at this moment (flashbacks)
- intense psychological and physiological distress and reactivity to some object or event that symbolizes or resembles the traumatic event

People with PTSD often try to avoid situations, places, or people that remind them of the initial trauma. They may withdraw from activities, feel dull or numb, and may be unable to foresee a positive future. They often describe a hypervigilant sense of anxiety or worry. They may have difficulty falling asleep, feel irritable, experience explosive outbursts of anger and an exaggerated startle response, and have trouble concentrating.

As you will come to learn, women with a history of PTSD are at high risk for worsening their anxiety disorder or depressions during the childbearing years. There is also a group of women who enter pregnancy with no history of trauma, but who may experience PTSD in response to an extremely difficult birth experience.

GENERALIZED ANXIETY DISORDER

Generalized anxiety disorder is characterized by an excessive worry—which nothing seems to quell—that occurs for the majority of days over a period of six months or more. A person with generalized anxiety disorder cannot control her fears and usually complains of:

- restlessness or always feeling "on edge"
- exhaustion
- difficulty concentrating or her mind "going blank"
- irritability
- muscle tension
- sleep problems

The continual anxiety and physical distress get in the way of day-to-day living. Often such problems emerge in childhood or adolescence. With hormonal cycling, the anxiety disorder can worsen premenstrually. Interestingly, these women are at risk for the emergence of depression at significant hormonal points later in their lives.

Diana was thirty-four years old and pregnant with her first baby when she came to see us. She needed help because she had become "increasingly anxious and exhausted and was having difficulty falling asleep." She and her husband had recently moved to the area, a few months before she became pregnant. Diana had resigned from her job in New York as an editor to move to New England so that her husband could advance professionally.

I learned that their families were on the West Coast and that Diana's husband worked long hours at his new job. She had made a few new friends in their new neighborhood, but nevertheless felt quite lost and thought that maybe the stress of moving had contributed to her loneliness and sense of disconnection.

Diana had begun to express anger at her husband for moving. "I feel so out of control. I threw a cup of tea at him one morning, which is so out of character for me. I don't know what is going on." She described that her husband was the quiet type, who did not talk very much or express his feelings. She had begun to feel that he didn't care about her and the baby.

As the pregnancy progressed, she had become tearful and described feeling "constantly worried, like something bad is going to happen." Tense, irritable, and discouraged, she stated that her appetite had fallen off, though she was pushing herself to eat. Diana was suffering from generalized anxiety disorder, and without proper intervention she was also at risk for major depression.

POSTPARTUM PSYCHOSIS

Postpartum psychosis affects from one to three per thousand of child-bearing women and is an emergency situation. This illness can occur in women already diagnosed with bipolar disorder, but it often occurs "without warning" in a woman who has been otherwise well. The prevailing information among researchers and clinicians who treat many numbers of women is that it occurs out of the blue.

A woman suffering from postpartum psychosis experiences extreme agitation, confusion, hallucinations, delusions, and the inability to sleep, eat, or maintain a coherent conversation. Her moods may swing wildly from euphoria to profound depression and back again. It is within the depths of these depressions that new mothers make sui-cide attempts. Sadly, many succeed.

When a woman is in the delusional state of a postpartum psychosis, she may believe that she or her infant must die. Perhaps God has cho-sen her to be Mary or some other figure who will remove Satan from the world. If the mother embroils her baby in the delusion and identifies him or her as the "devil," the infant is at great risk. Unfortunately, ba-bies can be harmed or killed as a result of this delusional thinking. Both the severity of the depression and the psychosis contribute to the ur-gency to hospitalize the mother at this time and treat her aggressively with mood-stabilizing and antipsychotic medications.

Here is how one woman characterized her descent into psychosis:

I was lying on my bed with my three-week-old baby. My husband was out of town on a business trip and would be away for another week. My last phone conversation with him had not felt right. Some-how what I wanted to say did not come out of my mouth. I felt as if I was disconnected from my brain, and I began to feel as if I was floating into a sea of ephemeral haze. A fog was descending, sweeping me up. I became weightless, looking down at my baby. He seemed so sweet and innocent lying there. Like a little sacrificial lamb.

There seemed to be voices coming from every direction, each giving me instructions. To which voice should I listen? It is hard just hearing a voice and no body. My thoughts are becoming more disconnected and distracted. I'm struggling to keep my mind on the task at hand, which in my mind is to carry out the sacrifice. Must put a body to a voice, you must join the parts. Need to discuss things first. Negotiate, that's it—negotiate, don't take the crap—amazing, wherever you are, there is the same crap. Everybody has an opinion. I want to follow my own mind.

Most people don't understand that postpartum psychosis is a brain-chemical illness related to mood-swing disorders. We believe it is initiated by a number of varying hormone alterations that can occur after a woman gives birth. Although the rapid drop of estrogen levels after delivery seems to be strongly implicated as a trigger to the brain events, some psychiatrists feel that altered thyroid and stress-hormone levels also contribute to the psychotic reaction. It is our belief that postpartum psychosis is a bipolar disorder that should be treated with mood stabilizers as well as antipsychotic medications (see Chapter 16).

In women with this disorder, there is usually indication of mood problems prior to pregnancy. With careful assessment, treatment can be instituted either during a pregnancy or postpartum so that severe postpartum-psychotic reactions do not have to happen. There is no need for women to suffer. This and many other disorders are treatable.

As you move through this book, you will read more about these diagnoses, the interventions we have prescribed in response, and the results of the healing process for many women. In each situation we stress the importance of having a proper diagnosis—it's crucial for your clinician to understand what type of mood or anxiety disorder you are struggling with. We also bring into consideration the impact of hormonal contributions and reproductive phases. In making an evaluation and prescribing treatment, we look at the whole woman, and you should expect no less from your care provider.

Chapter 5

DEMYSTIFYING THE MENSTRUAL CYCLE

Beth, a married thirty-two-year-old third-grade teacher, complained to Jeanne about her premenstrual situation. "For five to seven days before my period," she explained, "I feel totally revved up. I start to get bloated and tired, and I just don't seem to think as clearly. I have to repeat things to myself or reread them before my brain gets it. I find that I eat more junk carbohydrates, and I really crave chocolate and desserts.

"Sometimes when I arrive at school, I find it difficult to organize myself and get focused. The noise the children make really bothers me before my period. I get impatient with them, and I think I'm less tolerant in general. Occasionally I've been known to 'lose it' with a student, and I feel terrible remorse afterward, because I know I over-reacted."

Noting that she sometimes drops a cup of coffee or bumps into furniture at home, Beth acknowledged that her coordination skills change at this time, too. "My body just doesn't feel the same in space. I head for the kitchen and stub my toe as I negotiate the sofa, even though I see it and try to avoid it!

"I snap at my husband for silly things—about how the color scheme of his clothes bothers me, for example. Even my skin feels more sensitive to touch, so I don't want Jim to be affectionate or embrace me. I tell him he should just 'stay away,' but my choice of words is usually not so polite. My sexual desire disappears anyway at that time of the month. Jim understands that this is the way I am, and fortunately he doesn't make demands on me.

"But then, within hours of my period beginning, it feels as if a veil has been lifted. I start to feel better, and my troubles are gone by the second day."

Beth's symptoms of premenstrual dysphoric disorder (PMDD, popularly known as PMS) are mild to moderate. And although her symptoms are not disabling—after all, she gets herself up and to work during this time of the month—they clearly interfere with her usual functioning and relationships. She does not consider herself to be sick, but having to be so vigilant about her moods and behavior creates additional stress in her life. These bothersome mood changes are what brought her to see Jeanne. Unfortunately, many women suffer PMDD in silence and at the expense of their important relationships.

In order to be absolutely sure that Beth was experiencing PMDD, Jeanne took a careful personal and family history and a series of blood tests and was able to rule out other disorders. She also asked Beth to record her symptoms for two months on a daily rating chart (see Chapter 8), so her experience could be tracked more precisely. When Beth returned with her charts, they showed graphically that she was indeed quite well for the three weeks and that her symptoms emerged, just as she had described, one week prior to her menstrual period. This was a picture of pure PMDD—a condition that is triggered by the hormonal fluctuations of the menstrual cycle.

Mood, Mind, and the Menstrual Cycle

One of the primary treatment goals in our practice is to educate our patients about their brains and biochemistry. In collaboration with our patients, we routinely develop a visual representation of the critical threads in their lives that combines their genetic predisposition, life events or stresses, and their menstrual cycle (see Chapter 6). This graph demonstrates how hormonal fluctuations of the normal menstrual process interact with a woman's life events to affect her brain biochemistry. It demystifies the process by which mood problems arise and shifts the stigma of mental illness or emotional disorders from silence and shame to insight and empowerment.

Knowledge is empowering. In this chapter we will help you to understand one of these crucial threads—the menstrual cycle—in the context of PMDD. You will discover how your premenstrual symptoms and emotions may be linked to hormonal mechanisms and biochemical changes that can translate into emotional responses.

No longer will premenstrual symptoms feel as threatening or "crazy," as if they were emanating from some amorphous place. There is a reason for the way you feel. Understanding and embracing your unique physiology is important in mobilizing you to seek help if you need it.

The Menstrual Conversation

The menstrual cycle presents the picture of a constantly changing hormonal environment. It would be nice if you didn't have to experience the ups and downs that your cycle brings, but that's not the reality of your biology. In fact, your cycle is the result of an intricate, precise dialogue between your brain and your ovaries. It must occur in order for hormonal events to be accurately timed, so that if and when a sperm fertilizes one of your eggs, the proper milieu exists to support the pregnancy and facilitate the growth of the fetus.

This communication between the brain and the ovaries culminates at puberty with your first menstrual period. That is why we ask our patients about their first periods and how they felt around that time. Interestingly, during the early teenage years, the awakening of the ovary can be associated with the first emergence of anxiety or depressive symptoms. Research has shown that the first time depression becomes a problem for adolescent girls is when they are between the ages of thirteen and fifteen, and that teenage boys have lower depression rates than girls.

Even though in our society girls feel great pressure about their appearance and their body and may experience stress as a result, we often neglect to recognize the menstrual cycle's contribution to the emergence of depression and anxiety symptoms at this age. The impact of a teenage girl's hormones may worsen whatever effect outside events may exert her on brain.

Although the biochemical conversation between your brain and your ovaries begins at puberty, the framework for it was set into place long before. In fact, it began prior to your birth, shortly after you were conceived. At that time your fetal brain began secreting hormones known as releasing hormones or *gonadotropins* (GnRH). These hormones eventually precipitated and now control your menstrual cycling. The cluster of nerve cells that produce these gonadotropins is located in the limbic area of the brain within the hypothalamus gland (see Chapter 3).[1]

After your birth, the GnRH levels in your body dropped and remained low until your brain emitted a signal (what triggers this process is not yet quite understood) that told your ovaries to "wake up." That awakening constituted puberty—the development of breasts, a womanly body, and menarche—your first period. And from that point until menopause, the dialogue between your ovaries and brain has occurred on a cyclical basis. The dialogue is always precise and polite, with each participant having a specific role. When things go wrong, it means that one of the parties has spoken out of turn, and the conversation is either cut short or lengthened, and so your menstrual cycle runs long or short.

As you mature, adult levels of estrogen are eventually reached, and for most women this cycling establishes a stable monthly pattern. You could say that by then the conversation between ovary and brain has evolved into a courteous and respectful interchange that continues until you approach menopause (see Chapter 17).

Your Ovaries

At birth your ovaries carried about three hundred thousand eggs. During each menstrual cycle, follicle-stimulating hormone (FSH) activates many little sacs (*follicles*), each containing an egg, to grow toward the surface of the ovary. Only one follicle per month matures enough to release its egg. This release is called *ovulation*. After the egg is released, the other follicles disintegrate. For every follicle that releases an egg, about a thousand do not make it. Nature can be extravagant! By the end of your reproductive life, your ovaries are depleted of eggs, and menopause occurs.

The Three Phases of the Menstrual Cycle

The average length of the menstrual cycle is twenty-eight days. The first day correlates with the first day of bleeding or menses, and you count from there. In most women's lives, menstruation is a monthly event. If there is no pregnancy, the lining of the uterus is sloughed off and secreted via the vagina. Once this occurs, the process begins again.

The menstrual cycle is divided into three phases: the follicular phase, the ovulation phase, and the luteal phase.

THE FOLLICULAR PHASE

The follicular phase occurs when messages are being sent back and forth between the ovary, the hypothalamus in the limbic brain, and the pituitary gland (located below the hypothalamus) to induce the development of the follicle and the release of an egg. This phase usually lasts from day one to day fourteen, although the actual length of the phase can vary, depending on the time it takes for messages to be sent and received.

The dialogue between brain and ovary goes something like this: On day one of the menstrual cycle, the hypothalamus gland[2] secretes gonadotropin-releasing hormone (GnRH). This "tells" the pituitary gland to release follicle-stimulating hormone (FSH). The FSH is carried in the bloodstream to the ovaries, where it prompts certain follicles to enlarge and mature. As they do so, they secrete the female hormone, estrogen.

THE OVULATION PHASE

The rising estrogen levels tell the hypothalamus to slowly turn down the secretion of GnRH and FSH. It is a gradual process, much like the action of a dimmer switch on a light. As the FSH decreases, estrogen levels from the maturing follicles rise abruptly. This sharp rise tells the pituitary gland to release luteinizing hormone (LH), which causes one mature follicle to release its egg.

Ovulation will not occur if there is insufficient estrogen in your system to trigger LH or if the proper level of estrogen is not maintained for the correct time.[3] The timing of ovulation is quite exact. It occurs within thirty-six hours after the surge of LH. There is much to be said for the exquisite nature of this communication system!

At the same time, just before ovulation, the follicles generate a rapid rise in progesterone, the other female hormone. Progesterone prepares the lining of the uterus (the *endometrium*) for the implantation of a fertilized egg. The endometrium will support the fertilized egg until the placenta grows and takes over. If there is no fertilization, this lining will slough off as menstrual flow.

The rise in progesterone also appears to keep FSH secretion going long enough to allow the full maturation of the follicle. The rise in progesterone must be exact, too, since abnormally high levels will prevent ovulation.[4] In fact, given the need for such precision, it is amazing that pregnancy ever takes place at all.

While estrogen rises in the first two weeks, the release in the brain of substances called *endorphins*[5] also occurs. These are the body's own natural analgesics or painkillers. But in addition to their pain-killing function, they have the ability to elevate your mood.

Endorphins increase from low levels during the first half of the menstrual cycle to their highest levels at ovulation. They then decrease during the third, or luteal, phase of the cycle. Endorphins affect your appetite, thirst, breathing rate, regulation of pain, memory, learning, and sexual behavior. They work together with estrogen to switch off the hypothalamus's production of the follicle-stimulating hormone (FSH) and GnRH. They also help the brain's capacity to withstand the potentially dysregulating effects of stress hormones.

That's why exercise, which releases endorphins, is a wonderful way to take care of your brain at any time of the month and why we include it in the NURSE Program! Endorphins are also released during acupuncture treatment, which is why the symptoms of what we call "brain strain"—anxiety, fatigue, and insomnia—can be improved with this technique.

At the same time that the hypothalamus is shutting down the release of FSH, substances called *prostaglandins* increase in the follicle just before rupture. It is thought that the prostaglandins may help expel the egg by breaking down the follicle wall and causing contraction of smooth muscle tissue cells in the ovary. Prostaglandins are also believed to be the cause of menstrual cramps later in the cycle.

Many women can actually feel when they ovulate. Their abdomens become a bit distended, and they experience a pain on the right or left side. This is known as *mittelschmerz*, German for "middle pain." Also, your body temperature rises from 0.5 to 1 degree Fahrenheit at the point of ovulation. These symptoms allow women who are trying to become pregnant to document the moment when they are the most fertile.

Testosterone levels increase progressively and are highest at mid-cycle, after which they decrease. That is why many women report increased sex drive at this time.

THE LUTEAL PHASE

After ovulation, estrogen levels plunge, and the luteal phase begins. Now the empty follicle in the ovary forms the *corpus luteum,* or "yellow body," which secretes progesterone and estrogen. Consequently, estrogen levels start to rise again, but fall a second time during the last or premenstrual week of the cycle. If there is no pregnancy, this luteal phase lasts exactly two weeks after ovulation.

So there are actually *two* estrogen drops or *withdrawal states* in one menstrual cycle. This is a key point. We believe that the first drop in estrogen sets the stage for the impact in the brain of the second drop. Each decrease in estrogen creates an estrogen withdrawal state as this hormone unbinds from the estrogen receptors in the brain.

The truth of the matter is, estrogen and serotonin are two of our natural feel-good "drugs." Estrogen withdrawal can feel like coming down off a drug. During this withdrawal process, cascades of biochemical reactions occur, and signals in the nerve pathways are altered. These reactions can lead to alterations in mood health because serotonin, as well as the other neurotransmitters, may be depleted by the process of estrogen withdrawal. Serotonin depletion is most often implicated in depression.

Peter Schmidt and David Rubinow, researchers at the National Institute of Mental Health, have shown that when they deliberately shorten the luteal phase of the menstrual cycle by using RU486 (better known as the French abortion pill), women still developed symptoms of PMDD despite the fact that they had skipped the phase during which these symptoms usually appear. The researchers concluded that whatever sets the process of PMDD in motion occurs earlier than the last two weeks of the cycle. Because all of the women in this study ovulated, we believe that the estrogen fluctuations that occur at ovulation begin the serotonin problem. Although the precise mechanism is still unclear, ovulation seems to be associated with PMDD. (You have to ovulate in order to get it!)

Drs. Schmidt and Rubinow's findings support our clinical belief that the first drop in estrogen right after ovulation seems to prime or sensitize the serotonin receptors in the brain. The second drop exacerbates the reaction, and so the symptoms of PMDD emerge. *Whenever there are hormonal changes in the blood, no matter how small, they can affect the brain.*

Interestingly, if you measure estrogen levels of someone with PMDD during the luteal phase, they are normal. It appears that it is not the *amount* of estrogen—the high or low levels, per se—but rather the *rapid change* in the levels—how steep or gradual the drop in the blood—that induces the dysregulation in the brain, causing mood and anxiety symptoms. That means you can have the same hormone levels as another woman but still have PMDD while she doesn't. This is why blood tests alone can't tell the full story of PMDD. Many women are informed, "Your hormone levels are normal," yet they still have PMDD. (See Illustration 5.)

It All Makes Sense

Think about the many biochemical changes that occur during your menstrual cycle. During the first two weeks your estrogen and endorphin levels are rising. This probably contributes to the stability of your moods by affecting positively the pathways of several mood-regulating neurotransmitters such as serotonin, dopamine, and norepinephrine. In response to the high estrogen and endorphin levels, these mood-elevating neurotransmitter levels are probably high, too.

At midcycle, approximately two weeks before your period begins, you experience a rapid rise but then a sudden drop in estrogen. This constitutes a quickly induced "withdrawal state." If your mood pathways are more sensitized, either because outside events have induced stress-related changes or because these pathways are vulnerable due to your genetic constitution, your brain-cell receptors have the potential to be more reactive to this withdrawal state.

After ovulation your moods stabilize for a while because estrogen is rising again. However, now progesterone levels rise quickly to a peak at eight days after ovulation and then begin to decline in days nine through eleven. Progesterone can induce mood stability by binding to certain receptors (called the GABA receptors) that slow the nerve firing in the brain. Interactions between progesterone, GABA, and serotonin may contribute further to stable mood states.

Then, during the last week of the menstrual cycle, estrogen starts to drop, as do progesterone and the endorphins. A remarkable situation ensues. These three vital substances begin to unbind from their dense attachments in the limbic brain. When sensitive receptors and firing mechanisms in the brain experience this withdrawal, they protest temporarily by short-circuiting the pathway.

Myriad mood changes can follow. Often irritability, anger, sensitivity, or sadness emerges. You may also experience clumsiness, memory and perceptual difficulties, carbohydrate cravings, isolating behavior, and decreased libido. These symptoms may indicate that there is less serotonin available to the limbic and prefrontal brain, inducing short-circuiting and causing the range of symptoms that you recognize as

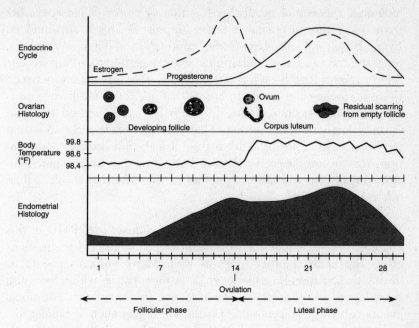

Illustration 5. Menstrual-cycle events

PMDD and even depression. When menstruation begins and estrogen levels begin to rise as part of your next cycle, the short-circuiting situation reverses itself, and your mood stabilizes once more.

The Limbic Brain Runs Amok

"It gets very complicated, doesn't it?" Beth commented to Jeanne. "Even though I am aware of my irritability and how I abruptly snap at my husband and students, some part of me just does not function when I'm premenstrual. I'm unable to be myself. The area of my brain that allows me to curb my irritability just seems to switch off. I always recognize the behavior and feel sorry afterward, but it's so difficult to control myself in the heat of the moment. It's so impulsive! I feel as if I've lost my mind!"

No, Beth hasn't lost her mind, but at this time in her cycle she is having more difficulty connecting with her cerebral cortex—those intellectual skills that might help her curb her behavior. Indeed, her description reveals how, during the premenstrual phase, she feels as if she has only a primitive limbic brain, severed from the greater judgment capacity of her higher-functioning cortex. What keeps her from being able to tame her limbic impulses? This is still unclear. Even though we now have some information about how estrogen, progesterone, and the endorphins work together to influence the brain's chemical pathways, there are many other interactions between these hormones and brain structures that are yet to be discovered.

If you have been suffering from PMDD, rest assured that you haven't "lost your mind" either. These symptoms are real and have a chemical basis. They arise from the intricate but normal "conversation" that occurs in every woman's body. Some of us are more sensitive to the rise and fall in "volume" of these hormonal voices than others.

We have focused on the menstrual cycle's impact on PPMD in this chapter, but it's important to remember that hormonal fluctuations affect the brain at other times as well. Many women come to us during the postpartum experience or at menopause, which have also been identified as times of increased risk for depression. Hormonal events can trigger diagnosable psychiatric illness such as bipolar disorder. Indeed, if previous life experiences have shifted or affected brain biochemistry, a significant hormonal event such as pregnancy or menopause may be the final factor that triggers an emotional earthquake. We will explore these issues further in succeeding chapters.

Chapter 6

PUTTING IT ALL TOGETHER

When I consider my own life, I realize that my vulnerability to mood disorder began when I was nine years old. My beloved father died suddenly of a heart attack. In no way was I able to cope with the impact of his death.

I remember how that day unfolded with its stark gravity and how my life veered violently off course after that. The chaotic events indelibly imprinted themselves in my memory like a terrifying movie— my mother trying to resuscitate him, while between breaths she screamed at me to get a doctor. Me running frantically up the road to find a local internist. God knows why we didn't phone him. It was, however, too late. My protector, inspiration, hero, and source of joy was no more. I couldn't believe it.

My dad had always called me his "tawny lion" because of my gold-streaked auburn hair. How could he leave his tawny lion? I remember my thoughts as I looked at his lifeless body. Was there life after this? If he was gone, was I gone, too? The first act was over, the curtain came down, and from then on I had to make up the script as I went along.

I probably had an unusually close relationship with my father. In fact, much of what I remember of my existence before nine years of age was my life with him. As an anesthesiologist, he would often take me on his evening rounds to check on patients before surgery. I remember padding along beside him, holding his big, gentle hand when we walked into the patients' wards together, and listening to his kind reassurances to them. At other times he took me with him when he ran a blood-transfusion service. I helped the nurses test the blood. I felt so special.

He was also a wonderful jazz pianist. He would often lift me onto his lap and play boogie-woogie and Scott Joplin rags, both of us counting out the beat. Sometimes we would study the evening sky. By the age of five I knew most of the Southern constellations. Not realizing that he was providing a means for me to cope with his death, he enrolled me in the local swim club.

After he died, I put myself on autopilot. His absence reverberated in my life on a daily basis. Somehow I kept myself going, but it was often a struggle. I don't even remember when the numbness went away. My grief continued well into adulthood.

We were left almost penniless by his death, so life's difficulties were compounded. My mother, having lost her own father as a girl, found it almost impossible to cope. She took out her rage on my younger brother and me. There was little solace at home, so I spent more and more time in the swimming pool. Fortunately, I was good, and I had one of the best trainers in the country—the coach of the South African Swim Team. His coaching was free; otherwise I would never have had that option. He just did it for the love of the sport. He provided a beacon for me, as I felt so adrift in a churning sea.

Home continued to provide anguish; I spent as little time there as possible. I was mostly my own caretaker. The continuing stress was affecting my brain, as we now know. But I hid my internal pain, as so many children and adolescents do. To everybody else I was an extraordinary kid—coping with a difficult life but succeeding at school, at piano, and at swimming. I was mobilizing everything I had, but it came at a hidden cost. At some point I was going to crash. How could I not?

Eventually I represented my country at international swim meets. I went alone to most of the contests—rarely was a family member there to cheer me on. I asked other parents for rides, and sometimes my coach would pick me up.

Looking back, I can see that despite overwhelming odds, I somehow found ways of achieving my goals. I got through medical school. I thank God for a group of wonderful fellow students who have never appreciated what a comfort and support they were to me during those years. They became the first loving family I had since my father died. Somehow I always managed to find caring mentors who also provided solace and inspiration for me, opening doors at times when all seemed hopeless.

After I completed my medical training, my husband and I immigrated to the United States. The culture shock was immense; my brain started to shut down. It just could not handle any more. The grief I still felt became more insistent. Now my depression was evident. I stopped functioning. In desperate need of many years of soul healing, my brain just gave up.

I did not sleep; I did not eat; I did not care. I hated myself. There just seemed no reason for living. Finding a good psychiatrist was another sad story. The first few understood the "issues" but had no clue about medication. One man suggested that I have an affair with him to heal the wounds. I left his office and never returned. At least my ego was strong enough to understand that his "plan" was outside the realm of accepted practice!

Sometimes I experienced severe premenstrual worsening of my mood, but nobody ever asked me about it. If I volunteered the information, all I got was a "hmmm." In fact, not one mental-health clinician I encountered ever posed a question about my menstrual cycle. To them, it had no bearing on mood! How wrongly informed they have been.

At one point, I used a birth-control pill and began to feel suicidal within a week. I stopped, but still my gynecologist never pursued this as an issue. I wondered what it was about the hormones that so quickly led me into despair. Was it the estrogen? The progesterone? What did these substances do in the brain? Nobody knew. Nor did they seem to care.

When I was pregnant and becoming more depressed, I tried to ignore the problem. Again, no one asked about my emotional state. I learned quickly that I was a case of "Physician, heal thyself." Not one doctor whom I have seen—and I have now encountered the "best"— has known anything about hormonal events. And to tell the truth, they probably would not have known what to do with the information even if they had it.

My depression worsened after the emergency cesarean birth of my second child, but no one linked this traumatic experience to my emotional state. I was even told that I did not need any antidepressant medication, that if I worked hard enough in therapy, everything would resolve. I struggled on, under the watchful care of an uninformed psychiatrist. I now call the treatment I received "masterful mismanagement."

Ironically, through all of this, if you had asked me whether I had a history of depression, I never would have considered that I had. "Bad stuff" had happened, but I was living, functioning, and coping. Ostensibly there was nothing amiss. Yes, I was desperately unhappy, but wasn't I handling it? I was overriding my depression with a powerful ego.

But from the time I was very young, my brain had been continually loaded with death, grief, and emotional devastation, which had translated into persistent brain-chemical alterations. It was impossible for me to have come out of such a childhood without an altered brain-mood chemistry. It had changed a long time ago and now was vulnerable to the effects of hormonal shifts, premenstrually, postpartum, and around menopause. Like many of my patients, I had brought a loaded brain into my adult years.

Through Jeanne's and my own work, and with the help of a wonderful, compassionate therapist—the first person who finally "got it"— I now know how to take better care of myself and how experiences earlier in life can have a profound effect on brain chemistry. But I needed to do the grief work and revisit the chaos of my early life in order to move on. After I did so, I became whole.

Difficult Early-Life Events and Depression

My early life experience, painful as it was, is not so different from that of the many women whom we treat in our practice. Many difficult situations occur in the lives of our patients before they find us. Ostensibly they, too, have experienced "no mood or anxiety difficulties" before the illness erupts, but when we question them closely, we find that the antecedents to their current condition have accumulated over time. These earlier events have actually sensitized the brain, loading and straining the biochemistry of its mood pathways.[1]

We often find evidence of minor or more significant mood disturbances or anxiety in our patients' histories. Since these mood and anxiety changes appeared subsequent to a stressful event in their lives, our patients usually take their reactions to be a "normal" response to an overwhelming situation. When they feel unhappy, find it difficult to cope, and have sleep difficulties and exhaustion, they do not attribute these experiences to a mood disturbance. They never think of these previous reactions as a "psychiatric history." In fact, however, these symptoms are precursors to the current episode that has brought them to consult us.

For example, when Jeanne helped Nanette (the twenty-eight-year-old woman with depression whom we met in Chapter 4) go back into her childhood to recall feelings of sadness or apathy, Nanette revealed the following:

> When I was twelve years old, my four-year-old younger sister died of cancer. My parents and I could barely cope with it. My mom and dad went for counseling for a while; then my dad was promoted, and we had to relocate from Arizona to the East Coast. They thought this would be a good move, since it would take them out of the area where Emma had grown up. I did, too, but when we got there, I hated it. It was a horrible experience.
>
> I had become an only child, and I really hated leaving all my friends in Arizona. I remember feeling sad for what seemed like a long time. I would cry myself to sleep. My parents told me I should be happy; they were trying so hard, but things in the house never really returned to the way they had been before. Although she tried to pretend that she was fine, I heard Mom crying from time to time. My dad buried himself in his work, so we never saw him.
>
> Dad was making lots of money, and we could now afford new things, but I didn't really care. All I knew was how unhappy I was, and I couldn't tell my parents. I was trying to show them that at least I was still alive and okay. I felt that if I really showed them how bad I was feeling, I would become an extra burden to them, and things would be worse.

Yet when Jeanne asked Nanette whether she had a psychiatric history, she said no. She also denied any family history of emotional or mental illness. This is why careful, sensitive questioning is needed in order to trace a problem to its true beginnings.

Stressful life events like those that occurred early in my and Nanette's lives helped shape our chemical brains and laid the groundwork for our subsequent depressions. We have known for a long time that these situations can precipitate depression. Although each person has her own threshold for coping with distress, some situations are universally injurious. These—like the death of a parent, a sibling, or a child; severe medical illness; divorce; the loss of a job; rape, incest, or other serious psychological challenges to one's sense of integrity—are known to carry a significant "emotional weight." Often an initial episode of depression follows such a severe, identifiable crisis.

Unfortunately for many women, their first encounter with depression occurred during adolescence and even before, but neither they nor their parents recognized it, and so they did not seek help. Or if it was recognized, their clinicians elected talk therapy instead of therapy coupled with medication. Few want to undertake this more aggressive treatment with a young person to actually stop a depressive episode dead in its tracks, because there is a lack of understanding about how depression threatens to permanently alter brain chemistry.

Yet allowing depressive symptoms to continue for a long time may well be doing the worst harm possible. During that time the brain pathways are being trained to function in the dysregulated state.

Women and Trauma

Stress and depression are highly interrelated. In Chapter 3 we saw how traumatic life events can permanently alter the brain's delicate mood pathways. In fact, research from laboratories all over the world have found that at least half the people who suffer from depressive disturbances also have disruptions in their stress-hormone levels. This has led to the theory that depression is one way in which the brain responds to stress.

Traumatic events evoke the stress response—that complex cascade of cortisol and other hormones—in your brain and body. In fact, when the emotions are powerful and prolonged, the stress response can overwhelm your brain's self-regulatory capacity, which is usually able to counter it. Cortisol levels remain high, and for reasons that we don't yet understand, they don't shut off.

Cortisol is necessary for our survival. It mobilizes us when we are in danger. But when the stress response continues unabated, certain nerve cells are tricked into believing that they still need to keep this response going, so they maintain a high level of activity, even though the precipitating event may have ended. The brain's own neurochemical brakes fail. Paradoxically, the protective stress response begins to undermine and exhaust us, as we remain perpetually hypervigilant chemically.

Many women come from backgrounds of persistent verbal, physical, or sexual abuse. They may emerge from violent or alcoholic families with negative feelings about themselves and their abilities. Living in constant fear of being hurt or traumatized and hiding chronically low self-esteem are the worst possible assaults on a young girl's brain.

In fact, Dr. Bessel van der Kolk, a leading researcher on post-traumatic stress disorder (PTSD) at Harvard Medical School, suggests that chronic ongoing abuse constitutes the most severe stress to which a human being can be subjected. Children are most likely to be victims of long-term emotional and physical abuse, and they are the least likely to be able handle these situations. They are our most vulnerable, least armored human beings. Maltreated children later find themselves coping with serious depression, anxiety, and eating disorders as teenagers and adults. It is likely that the painful aspects of their lives have permanently affected their brain chemistry.

Depression as a Chronic Illness

You may experience just one depressive event in your lifetime and recover without any more episodes. In most first-time situations the mood pathways revert to normal. But a serious bout of depression can generate long-term changes within the cells of the mood pathways, leaving an "imprint" that may predispose you to subsequent relapses. And most people do encounter more than one stressful event in their lives.

When the next stressor occurs, the brain cells readily revert to an altered way of functioning because they have already learned how to do so. The second stressor need not be as severe as the original one, and usually it isn't. But a new "normal" has been established within the brain—one that can leave you vulnerable to mood and anxiety changes. In fact, eventually the cells don't even require a stressful event to dysregulate. They will do so seemingly out of the blue. You may complain, "But nothing bad has happened in my life lately!" and you are right. Nothing untoward has occurred, but now the cells function spontaneously only in the dysregulated state—they have learned to respond to stress in that way.

This is why depression often becomes a recurring illness. Indeed, more than 70 percent of those who have experienced one episode will go on to have another. Millions of people struggle with persistent depressive problems for the rest of their lives. For them, the illness has become a long-term medical disorder, just like other biological conditions such as high blood pressure or diabetes.

Regardless of their origin, when depression symptoms are present, we now know that *changes in brain biochemistry drive them*. And those who experience recurrent episodes of depression or manic depression are almost always able to identify a particularly stressful event that preceded their first episode.

It's important to realize that depression is not a transient mood change. It is a brain illness that compromises the brain's ability to regulate its own chemical functioning. We could understand depression as a form of partial brain failure.

What Happened? Allostasis and Brain Strain

Bruce McEwen, a neuroscientist at Rockefeller University in New York, explains how the brain that slowly becomes overloaded with stress eventually loses its ability to cope. He calls this process *allostatic loading*. Allostasis refers to the body's ability to adapt when it is subjected to an increased workload. It does so by mobilizing itself to support a new reality in the face of increased demands.

Each of your organs is equipped to deal with additional demands that may be placed on them from time to time; we would not have survived without these adaptive mechanisms. For example, when you don't have enough to drink, your kidneys cope with the extra demand by altering their excretion mechanisms to reabsorb water. As a result, your urine becomes more concentrated, but the fluid in your body is conserved. However, if the fluid deprivation persists, there is a point at which your kidneys can no longer overcome this adversity, and kidney failure occurs. Similarly, a large portion of your liver must be damaged before you experience liver failure. There is a good deal of powerful reserve built in to each organ's functional capacity.

The brain has the same adaptive abilities, but it has its limits, too. Over a long time it mobilizes all the hormone systems to help you cope with financial problems, a poor marriage, social isolation, chronic low self-esteem, caring for sick family members, and so on. The sorrow, grief, hurt, anger, shame, guilt, or jealousy that these stressful situations generate carries a high emotional valence and has a significant effect on stress pathways in the brain.

Over time the persistence of such feelings constitutes a continuing load on the brain's self-regulatory systems. Eventually they deplete or dysregulate the brain's coping mechanisms. When this occurs, the strain overcomes the brain's capacity to compensate. In effect, the brain goes on strike.

Bruce McEwen uses the analogy of a seesaw to explain the concept of allostasis. Imagine that each side of the seesaw is loaded equally so that it remains balanced. If the load on both sides increases proportionately, equilibrium will be maintained, but the seesaw may bend with the increased weight. Eventually, if the load gets too heavy, the seesaw will break. In the end, either a small or large load may finally cause it to give way.

The seesaw's breaking point is determined by the weight of the load but also by its own intrinsic qualities—the strength of the wood, for instance, or its resilience to extremes of weather. This tells you that the seesaw's innate properties must be factored into how it handles stress. As you will see, this baseline becomes important when we talk about your genetic susceptibility to mental illness. What you inherited from your parents is also part of your brain's basic makeup.

As we noted, Bruce McEwen terms this ongoing burdening, allostatic loading. We call it *brain strain*. Brain strain manifests itself in physical ailments like headaches, anxiety, fatigue, as well as difficulty concentrating and feeling overwhelmed. It is the brain's way of warning you that it's headed for trouble.

Brain Strain and Daily Life

Consider the degree of brain strain that our supercharged, hyperlinked, productivity-consumed world constantly confers on all of us. Cell phones, pagers, faxes, e-mail—our brains are being asked to mobilize and maintain a state of high alertness for long hours every day. For women in particular, the hidden costs of juggling work, children, and household needs can cause brain strain. Moreover, premenstrual, postpartum, fertility drug–related, or menopausal hormonal events can tip the balance, causing you to develop overt symptoms of depressive and anxiety disorders.

Indeed, your daily life coupled with your hormonal life may constitute a biochemical challenge to your brain—a perfect example of allostatic loading. This powerful concept helps us understand why, although most of the women we see in our practices say they have "no psychiatric history," they in fact have usually contended with significant life stressors and traumas that have loaded and strained their brains. We know this because they describe symptoms of mood and anxiety disorders long before they have finally come for help.

To endure this hyperalert state, the brain copes by mobilizing all the chemical factors necessary to survive. Doing so, however, takes a toll on the brain's chemistry, leading eventually to a state of chronic dysregulation. We believe that this is why so many people need anti-depressants merely to go on with their lives today. Our brains are not equipped to guard against the battering impact of modern culture, and these medications act as brain-stress stabilizers.

Brain strain has profound ramifications for our society. Because of soaring stress levels and stress-related illnesses in our high-tech world, it is entirely likely that more and more people will experience bio-chemical changes that can lead to depression. Even Aldous Huxley did not anticipate such a hectic pace in his *Brave New World*! Our brains are just not equipped to cope with the intrusively strident demands of modern living, and we are paying for it with dysregulated and altered brains.

Peek inside the waiting rooms of primary-care doctors and you'll find them filled with exhausted, harried people suffering from stress-related disorders. Yet the physicians treat only the symptoms. Rarely do they look for the one problem that is causing all the others. A patient will be given antacids for reflux, painkillers for headaches, sleeping pills for insomnia, tranquilizers for anxiety, and so on. All this will be prescribed after masses of blood work, scans, bowel and stomach investigations, and X rays.

Rarely, too, are patients counseled about how to reduce stress. In fact, if the physician talks for any length of time to the patient, it falls into the realm of "alternative medicine"! Medical students are now sent to alternative-medicine courses to learn how to talk to pa-tients and find, to their great amazement, that when they do this, they might just uncover what is going on in the patient's life to ac-count for the headaches and insomnia. They also learn that there is healing value in the doctor-patient relationship!

I recall two maxims I learned in medical school: "Common illnesses occur commonly" and "Always look for the one pathology that ac-counts for all the symptoms." Stress and depression occur simulta-neously, often explaining many of the physical ailments that bring people to physicians' offices. Yet physicians still do not readily link the two.

In light of these far-reaching discoveries about how the brain

"learns" depression, mood and anxiety problems clearly require aggressive treatment so that brain chemistry is quickly stabilized. The
longer the chemistry remains dysregulated, the more likely it is that
long-term changes will occur in the brain.

The Hormonal Connection

As we have seen in Chapter 5, a woman's unique reproductive cycle
has the capacity to destabilize the delicate balance of brain chemistry
much as stressful situations do. Many women experience their first
problems with depression or anxiety in their adult years during pregnancy, the postpartum period, or menopause. Some have problematic
premenstrual mood symptoms. If previous life traumas and stressors
have shifted the biochemistry, these profound hormonal events can
be the final blow that pushes the system into disruption. *In fact,
hormonal events are powerful enough on their own to thrust the brain
biochemistry into dysregulation.* The reproductive events in and of
themselves do not constitute an abnormality. Rather it's the impact
of these "normal" hormonal fluctuations on loaded neurochemistry
that can create the problem. (See Illustration 6.)

The Genetic Link

Your genetic heritage may contribute to the vulnerability of your biochemical system, which may be primed and waiting for a hormonal
event or life stressor to set off a depressive episode.

Your life story began when you were conceived. Your inherited
biochemistry—the biology with which you were born—provides the
genetic foundation or hardwiring for your brain. Hardwiring is an
electrical-engineering term that mental-health practitioners have bor-
rowed to explain how parts of the brain are connected to each other,
much like the wiring in electrical circuits. Sometimes, if the circuits
are overloaded, a fuse blows and the power is lost.

In families that do not have histories of mood or anxiety problems,
it is possible that under stressful conditions the brain circuits experience loading, but do not short-circuit or result in symptoms. Or if
symptoms do occur, they may be mild and the biology may correct
itself spontaneously. It is as if the brain has come equipped with its
own automatic-reset button.

Perhaps the brains of people who are not genetically at risk are
able to shut off the oversecretion of stress hormones when these are

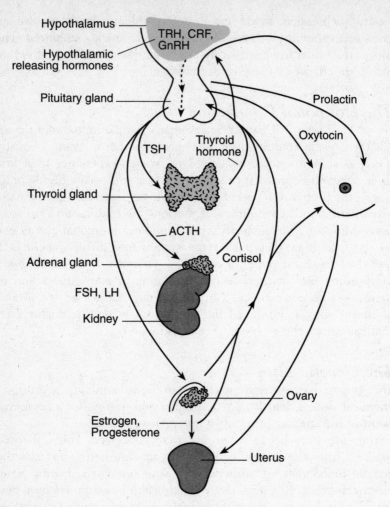

Illustration 6. Hormonal relationships in the woman

no longer required, thus rendering their chemistry intrinsically more resilient. Or perhaps these brains have an ability to withstand the chemical flooding without overloading. We do not know. But it is important to understand that life events, if serious enough, can alter the brain chemistry of people who do not have a genetic history of depression. If the situation is desperate enough, they, too, may become depressed.

Genetic links make themselves known in various ways. If a woman has a family history of mood disturbances, for instance, she may experience her first inkling of depression in the premenstrual period. In our practice we have also observed that women with PMDD symptoms are more prone to serious mood disturbance later in their lives. PMDD hints at the degree of brain-chemical reactivity likely to be dormant.

Bipolar disorders often run in families, so if a woman suffers from bipolar illness, usually other family members have these symptoms, too. Often at least one parent has had diagnosed mood difficulties. If a member of the family has committed suicide, this also indicates the presence of a severe depressive disorder, which other family members may carry genetically.

The Earthquake

When women experience the onset of a mood or anxiety problem, they often say it feels as if they are in the midst of a sudden major disruption in their lives. "Everything is falling apart," they tell us.

An earthquake is a perfect analogy to describe what is happening in our patients' lives. Earthquakes occur when the internal pressures on a weakened subterranean fault line become overwhelmed. To relieve the intense pressure, the fault line gives way with great force and the earthquake erupts, breaking through the earth's surface and creating chaos and destruction above. When all has settled, the fault line shifts into a new position, vulnerable to the pressures of the rock adjacent to it and in a state of altered quiescence, while the cycle of pressure builds again.

Smaller tremors prior to an earthquake indicate that there are indeed pressures building on the unstable rock formations underground. These induce modest but detectable shudders above ground, reminding residents of the instability below.

Our basic brain biochemistry can be equated with the fault line beneath the earth's crust. As the surface of the earth above the fault line appears intact, so, too, do women, as they often portray themselves as feeling "fine" even if their brains are suffering from overloading and strain. Eventually the burdens of stressful life and/or hormonal events can disrupt this delicate balance of brain biochemistry (just as the pressures created by geophysical forces affect the geologic fault line) and an emotional earthquake occurs.

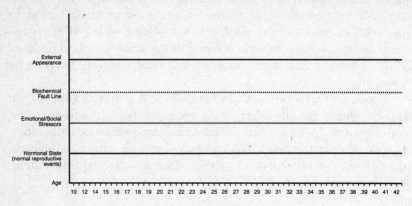

Illustration 7. The Earthquake-Assessment Chart

Some women experience periods of short-lived, minor mood and anxiety symptoms. We could characterize these as tremors. They indicate a slight biochemical dysregulation beneath the surface. But eventually an earthquake occurs, often in response to a compounding of these smaller events.

When women come to see us, it is usually in response to an earthquake. They are in the throes of distressing symptoms that interfere significantly with their ability to function. Although they have survived many previous tremors and coped sometimes on their own and at other times with counseling, stress management, and yoga or meditation, we now know that this has come at a cost to their brain biochemistry.

Mapping the Fault Lines

We help patients visualize the many factors contributing to their current condition by mapping with them their underlying fault lines. Three themes are critical for charting the wellness/illness continuum: genetic brain biochemistry, reproductive hormonal biology, and life events or stressors—predictable, unpredictable, or traumatic. (See Illustration 7.)

But above all of these, we must put a "public appearance" line. It is like the earth's surface, covering all the other factors. A woman's external appearance can reveal little about what is taking place in her brain biochemistry, unless she complains of symptoms that have pushed through to the surface. Beneath the external-appearance lines, we place the brain biochemistry, the life events, and the hormonal lines.

The only way we know that there is brain trouble is by symptoms we can see, that is, changes in the external-appearance line. This line is brain strain made visible.

Understanding Nanette's Fault Lines

Let's return to our example of Nanette. In order for Jeanne to understand Nanette's current depressive symptoms, the two of them mapped what had happened to her over time. This information helped them ascertain the nature and severity of Nanette's brain strain and also gave them the answer to why the earthquake had occurred now. It would assist them in planning Nanette's treatment.

Nanette's collection of symptoms (loss of sex drive, poor appetite, insomnia, irritability, fear, constant anxiety, and restlessness) suggested that her brain biochemistry had been pushed to levels where symptoms appear above the surface—an earthquake. Yet her demeanor revealed little of what was bubbling beneath.

As so often happens, Nanette denied any personal psychiatric or family history of emotional or mental illness. But Jeanne knew that when there is an earthquake, a patient usually has survived earlier tremors. And so, with a few questions, the sad story of Nanette's disrupted childhood and her sister's death emerged. Nanette was living with continual family stress at a young age. Her early adolescence was fraught with uncertainty and loss, and denial was the family's major coping mechanism. This is a significant degree of stress for a preteen girl, but she got up every day, and life went on. Nanette's despondent feelings lasted for several months—until she became involved in her school's theater group. This process of withdrawal from family closeness and focus on school activities is common in many teenagers when there are unspoken family conflicts.

Within this framework Nanette became self-sufficient. While the family presented an external picture of a cohesive, happy, affluent group, they were all emotionally devastated. This was a period of depression—a large tremor—but Nanette got no professional help. She coped and survived.

Jeanne asked Nanette if she could recall other times when she felt changes in her mood over the ensuing years. "In college I met Fred, and we dated for three years," she replied. "I really thought I would marry him, but then I found out that he was cheating on me, and we broke up. I was devastated; I felt so betrayed."

Nanette's expression was sad and drawn. This loss was alive for her; she still was pained by that experience.

Was this another tremor or a full-blown earthquake? Nanette acknowledged that she shut down for the rest of the semester. "I couldn't focus or study, so I took Incompletes in all my courses," she continued. "I couldn't sleep. I felt restless all the time, and I lost twenty pounds without even trying. I found that if I had a few glasses of wine before I went to bed, that helped me fall asleep.

"I saw a college counselor for twelve weeks to deal with the grief and loss of the relationship, but I don't remember that I ever really felt great during that time. Eventually I found that I could focus better, and after a few months off from school, I was able to go back. I carried additional credits in my senior year so I could graduate with my class. It was a tough time."

Nanette had had an earthquake. Her disrupted brain chemistry had finally pushed through the surface, giving rise to symptoms that interfered with her everyday living.

Jeanne needed to assess the final thread—Nanette's hormonal status. "I started my period at about thirteen," Nanette revealed. "It was no big deal." Gently, Jeanne continued to probe as to whether her patient had had any difficulties with irritability or mood changes around her menstrual period.

"Well, initially I just had cramps, but as I got older, especially after I stopped birth-control pills in college, I noticed that I was really irritable for about ten days before my period. My roommates could always tell when I was going to get my period. In our house everyone said, 'Watch out for Nanette. The broom is out, and she is flying!' I tried everything—evening-primrose oil, Vitamin B$_6$, aerobic exercise. I even stopped eating chocolate, but nothing helped.

"It was tough then, and it's still tough. My husband travels a lot, and he's glad when a trip coincides with my period so he doesn't have to live with me through that time."

"Nanette, have you ever been pregnant?" Jeanne asked.

With tears gently rolling down her cheeks, she replied, "I was pregnant with Freddy's baby." Electing to terminate the pregnancy, Nanette described that afterward she could hardly get out of bed each day. "That also added to my sadness," she said. "I told you that was a bad time."

Pregnancy and abortion can significantly add to depression. The pieces of the puzzle were coming together. "Nanette, I feel that you are experiencing the symptoms of a major depression," Jeanne explained. "Let me share with you how I believe this has happened. In our practice we use the analogy of an earthquake to describe how events can lead to a major depression. When you were twelve, you described a tremor. Your sister died, and your family's intact structure disintegrated. The members of your family retreated to their corners, nursing their own wounds, imposing on you a persistent loneliness and isolation. We understand this as chronic internal loading. You coped, but there was a hidden cost.

"Eventually your symptoms went away, and life went on. Then you had another major disruption in college with the pregnancy, abortion, and breakup with your boyfriend. In fact, I would say that you experienced an earthquake at that time—a major depression.

"You've had mood changes both on and off birth-control pills, and your moods shift premenstrually. This suggests your brain chemistry's underlying vulnerability to fluctuations in your reproductive hormonal levels. We know that this sensitivity occurred as a result of the loading process following your first episode of depression when your sister died. And that left you more vulnerable as a twenty-year-old, when you had your second episode of depression."

On a sheet of paper Jeanne began to chart the critical lines of Nanette's life to show her how she had come to this "earthquake" episode of major depression. (See Illustration 8.)

"Nanette, can you see how the biology of the brain, your hormones, and the stressors in your life have combined to trigger this episode of depression?" Jeanne asked. "We are not able to pinpoint a specific triggering event at this time, but enough loading occurred in your past to account for how this episode occurred spontaneously."

Nanette nodded. "Am I going to feel better? Am I going crazy?"

Jeanne sat forward in her chair and said firmly, "You are not crazy. This is a biological problem, and we will work together to help you feel better." She went on to describe a suggested treatment plan: medication and psychotherapy.

As you can see, brain chemistry is a dynamically changing frontier; there is nothing static about it! The earthquake model is an ideal way for you to understand what has occurred in your life to bring you to where you are now. It is also a way for you to visualize clearly that

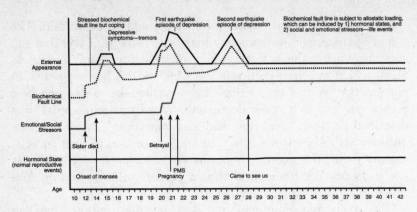

Illustration 8. Nanette's Earthquake-Assessment Chart

the brain you were born with is not the same brain you have today.

When we implement the earthquake analogy with our patients, they feel less ashamed about their emotions. They discover why they feel the way they do, and what they can do to move toward emotional balance and well-being. Those are the first important steps toward healing.

Chapter 7

HAVE YOU TAKEN CARE OF YOUR
BRAIN TODAY?

Imagine you are running your own business that is dependent on the proper functioning of an enormous computer. Would you not care for and repair this vital piece of equipment? After all, your livelihood and that of your family and employees depend on it. You are probably quite assiduous about noting when it tells you that something is wrong. Before anything else malfunctions, you correct the problem and do what you must to maintain it. So why not pay the same attention to the master computer in your body?

Since your brain's health is central to your emotional and physical wellness, and since its well-being is compromised in mood and anxiety disorders, a program of brain care is fundamental to a healthy life. Indeed, no "women's health program"—be it a menopause clinic or a gynecologic, obstetric, or fertility service—is complete without the inclusion of your mental health. If you ignore your brain, you discount a good portion of your physical health. When your brain is in pain, so is your body!

When you learn how to take care of your brain, you will go a long way toward helping it to reregulate itself. This, in turn, improves your responses, not only to everyday living but also to self-care therapies such as yoga, meditation, or other stress-reduction techniques. By learning ways of taking care of your brain, you may even protect yourself against depressive or anxiety illness. You need to take care of your brain daily, whether you're coping with premenstrual mood problems, postpartum mood and anxiety disturbances, menopausal distress, or any other stress- or hormonally based emotional disorder.

In the preceding chapters you learned about the anatomical structures important in emotions and how the nerve cells communicate. You also learned how reproductive hormones act in those very same brain areas. Another part of the treatment process is to know what you can do to help your brain maintain its own self-regulating potential. If you have already experienced a mood or anxiety problem, this chapter will teach you what you can do to maximize your response to other treatments. Many people are afraid of seeing psychiatric clinicians; we also hope to demystify the process of evaluation and treatment here.

How Does Your Brain Reregulate Itself?

Although your brain interacts with many mechanisms when you encounter a stressful event, it also does everything it can to avoid overfiring so that you can maintain a normal mood. Many different chemical "brakes," in the form of receptors and hormones, are built into each pathway to slow the volume and intensity of the stress response. The brain self-regulates by using this system of accelerators and brakes. In fact, a different chemical brake exists for each neurotransmitter, and some structures in the limbic brain also serve as deterrents.

One very important element involved in slowing the stress response is the hippocampus, the seahorse-shaped limbic structure implicated in the way memories are made, stored, retrieved and in the modulation of stress responses and emotions. Sometimes when we are feeling stressed at the office, we joke that we need to give our seahorses a break! But actually stress reduction is a serious business. It is imperative to find ways to reduce the chemical loading on the brain, and specifically on the hippocampus, in order to protect your brain from its own chemical responses to stress.

Indeed, the hippocampus is a key determinant in the brain's ability to fine-tune the stress response. It seems that if the hippocampus cannot switch off the oversecretion of cortisol, damage to its nerve cells can occur, eventually leading to depression and memory problems. According to Dr. Bruce McEwen, the very process of wear and tear on the hippocampus can eventually lead to its dysregulation and damage.

Use the NURSE *Program to Reduce the Stress Load on Your Brain*

By understanding how your brain biochemistry is interconnected with your reproductive hormones and stress responses, you and your mental-health clinician can begin to develop a care plan that is unique to your life situation. You can employ many care strategies to maintain your brain's optimal functioning in spite of its inherent vulnerability.

In our practice we base our treatment on the critical lines of the earthquake model: external appearance (symptoms), biochemical fault line, hormonal status, and stressful life events. Our goal is to provide our patients with the tools they need to nurse their brains back to emotional balance and to maintain that balance at an optimal level. We call our care plan the NURSE Program.

If you look up the word "nurse" in the dictionary, you will learn that it means "to attend, to minister, to sustain, to cultivate, and to nourish." These action words are important in every woman's self-care. You need to attend, minister, sustain, cultivate, and nourish your brain, your body, and your soul in order to enjoy life to its fullest.

If you are living with ongoing mood and anxiety problems, consider this program an adjunct to any other treatment you might be receiving. We have found that it often allows for the reduction in medication dosages, while improving our patients' sense of well-being and self-esteem.

Each letter in the word NURSE stands for the critical concepts of brain care:

- Nourishment and Needs
- Understanding
- Rest and Relaxation
- Spirituality
- Exercise

Using this program, you can develop an individualized care plan in collaboration with your mental-health clinician.

Nourishment and Needs

In order to protect your mood health, it's essential to maintain basic nutrition using the research-based food guidelines developed by the United States Department of Agriculture and supported by the Department of Health and Human Services. These guidelines suggest that you:

- eat a variety of foods to get the energy, protein, minerals, and fiber necessary for optimal health. That includes:
  - fats and oils used only sparingly
  - two to three servings daily of dairy products
  - two to three servings per day of meat, poultry, fish, eggs, and nuts
  - two to four servings per day of fruit
  - three to five servings per day of vegetables
  - six to eleven servings per day of bread, grains, cereal, rice, or pasta (One slice of bread or one ounce of cereal equals one serving.)
- moderate your intake of sugars and salt, and include plenty of grain products, vegetables and fruits.
- keep your consumption of cholesterol-rich foods low.

These recommendations are based on the Food Guide Pyramid (see Illustration 9). (This information is contained in a booklet that can be obtained from the Consumer Information Center, United States Department of Agriculture: Center of Nutrition Policy and Promotion, 1120 20th St., N.W., Suite 200, North Lobby, Washington, D.C. 20036-3475.)

It's also important to eliminate alcohol, which acts as a depressant in the brain and compromises the treatment plans. Additionally, reassess your caffeine intake and cigarette smoking. Caffeine and nicotine can exacerbate anxiety and complicate diagnosis. It becomes difficult to sort out how much anxiety comes from the disorder and how much is being induced by the substance.

Because diets often don't provide adequate vitamins, it makes sense to supplement with a daily multivitamin. A recent editorial in the *Journal of the American Medical Association* (December 1993) indicated that even with healthy diets, vitamin intake is often insufficient. In addition, women are often deficient in iron. Have your care pro-

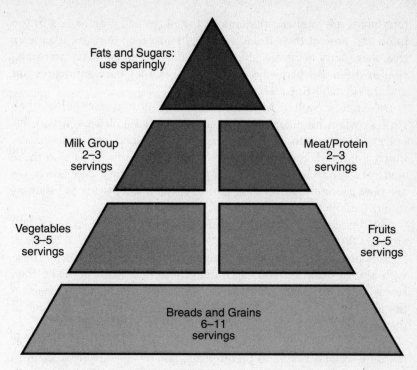

Illustration 9. The Food Guide Pyramid

vider check for anemia. You may benefit from iron supplementation, if needed. Folic-acid deficiency during pregnancy has been found to be associated with the birth defect spina bifida. Folate supplementation decreases the risk of spina bifida and other neural tube defects by 70 percent. Low folic acid has also been associated with other neurological disorders in women who are not pregnant. Since some medications deplete folate, we ask our patients to include a dietary supplement of 1 milligram of folate daily to enhance their stores.

Calcium is a critical nutrient for healthy bones, so it is wise for all women from the age of thirty-five onward to increase their calcium intake. This will help your bones maintain optimal density levels as you reach your forties, heading into the perimenopausal years. You need 1,000 to 1,500 milligrams of calcium per day before and after menopause.

New research suggests that the alpha-omega-3 polyunsaturated fatty acids are vital components of the nerve-cell membranes in the brain and protect the cardiac vessels. In adequate dosages, it appears that these fatty acids are able to modulate chemical nerve transmission in the mood pathways in the brain, so they have antidepressant and mood-stabilizing effects.

Dr. Andrew Stoll at McLean Hospital in Boston reported startling success when he augmented the diets of men and women with bipolar disorder with alpha-omega-3 acids. Mood stabilization was much improved. As a result of this and other indications that these acids play a role in the protection of the brain against depression, we are now routinely prescribing alpha-omega-3 fatty acids as adjuncts to our patients' treatment regimes.

The dosages Dr. Stoll used in his study were high—between 6,000 and 10,000 milligrams per day. We recommend 3,000 to 6,000 milligrams per day for women with depression and higher doses for those with bipolar disorder. You can obtain these fatty acids in health-food stores as components of flaxseed and fish oils. Check the dose on the label, as there is a wide range of dosages available, depending on the brand.

Finally, if we feel that our patients would benefit, for whatever reason—weight loss, food preferences, and so on—we refer them to nutritionists for individual counseling. You, too, might seek the advice of a registered dietician.

Medications for the brain such as antidepressants, mood-balancing agents, antianxiety pills, and hormone supplements act as nourishment at the biochemical level. You may need them to support, replenish, regulate, and enhance your brain's disrupted biochemistry.

In fact, we believe that first and second episodes of depression should be aggressively identified and treated with medication. Drug treatment ought to be instituted early and maintained for much longer periods than most mental-health practitioners have been doing, in the hope that the biochemistry can be retrained to function normally. Indeed, as you will see, psychotherapy is important in healing, but the use of medication may be the key ingredient to support and quickly restore the brain's balance. Once the brain's biochemistry is stable, effective psychotherapy can occur.

That's why we believe strongly that adolescent girls should receive rigorous medical treatment if they are depressed. This might allow their brains to reregulate without becoming adapted to a dysregulated state. Sadly, this does not often happen.

Your emotional needs are also part of Nourishment and Needs. What are you not getting that you should have? What do you need to counterbalance what you put out for everybody else during your day? It is often shocking to consider how little comes in and how often women are even unaware of their depleted state.

We help our patients to better structure their days so they integrate into their busy lives some distinct "down periods" or time for themselves. This may mean simply taking a bath without interruption or sitting in the car for ten minutes at a lake, forest, or even in a parking lot, but just not jumping out and rushing around. As women, we are conditioned to do for others; learning how to do for yourself can be a new (and wonderful) experience. We want you to love and honor yourself rather than feel that if you do something good for yourself, you are being selfish and self-centered.

Understanding

We hope that in the preceding chapters we have provided you with a wealth of information about how your brain and body interact. Your feelings have an anatomy—they are rooted in the brain structures. Once you understand this, you will be better able to seek out the care and nurturing you need to resolve your unique situation without guilt. You can remove blame and shame from your life. You can honor yourself and your personal journey.

But because you are a human being, and not just an illness, treatment with medication alone is limited. You may also need psychotherapy—an important component of your understanding. We strongly believe that you need a safe place to tell your stories, to be heard, and to be validated. You must have the time to sit with what you are feeling and understand how your brain biochemistry has become strained, perhaps from the time you were young.

In psychotherapy you will use your intellectual or cortical-brain skills. For instance, if you have suffered a trauma, your therapist will engage your intellect in the healing process. Although your limbic-brain structures have captured the emotions, smells, and colors of the event, talk therapy will help you make sense of it. Talking about it allows your cortex to comprehend it, and that helps you integrate the experience into your life and go on. Another useful intellectual skill includes writing down what happened and how you felt about it. This, too, helps you put the event into perspective.

Using your cortex in these ways encourages your brain to quiet limbic overactivity, enhancing the effectiveness of physiological braking mechanisms that return your brain chemistry to normal. Psychotherapy, therefore, can be considered a biological therapy, engaging your intellectual skills to work with your physiology.

(It is still unknown, however, whether short-term intensive talk therapy in an acute stress situation can prevent long-term brain changes, or whether long-term psychotherapy is effective enough to protect the brain from future insults.)

Psychotherapy can also help you identify old ways of thinking and behaving that may perpetuate feelings of low self-esteem. It equips you with new strategies for coping. As a result, you acquire a sense of empowerment.

Rest and Relaxation

Relaxation is essential for your brain's health. Sleep is a priority. It is during sleep that the brain biochemically resets itself, allowing hormones, neurotransmitters, and peptides to replenish themselves. Although we know little about all the factors that come into play during this important process, we do know how restorative sleep can feel.

Melatonin plays an important role in the resetting process and is stimulated by the coming of twilight. Released by the pineal gland deep in the center of the brain, and linked to hypothalamic control of the sleep-wake cycle, melatonin helps to maintain your regular sleep cycle. It also protects your body from the harmful effects of chemical byproducts known as *free radicals* by mopping them up. Melatonin enhances the body's ability to fight infection and suppresses potential tumor growth by stimulating the production of T-cells, which are vital immune system defenses.

It stands to reason that if you are chronically sleep-deprived and suffer from diminished levels of melatonin, these protective mechanisms will be reduced.

We also know that oxytocin, the peptide hormone that triggers milk ejection during breast-feeding and causes the uterus to contract during menstruation and labor, has brain-resetting functions. Cort Pederson, a biochemist at the University of North Carolina Medical School, has reported that when oxytocin levels rise toward the afternoon and evening, the daily secretion of cortisol drops. It will be exciting to learn more about how this hormone helps the brain contain stress reactions every day.

In addition to sleep, various stress-reduction techniques such as meditation, visualization, biofeedback, and mindfulness diminish limbic overdrive and enable the cortex to contain the debilitating effects of stress. Incorporating these techniques into your day, even if you do not have a mood or anxiety disorder, can protect you against the deleterious effects of modern life.

Spirituality

For us, spirituality relates less to organized religion than to the meaning of life. We define it as any experiences that help you to feel uplifted and joyful. Relationships, solitude, appreciation of nature, creative endeavors, music, keeping a journal or other reflective practices, and belief in God/Goddess or a higher power all can nourish the soul.

Getting in touch with and reconnecting to your spirituality—the essence of your nature—can require time and effort, but the process is wonderfully rewarding. It may be as simple as buying fresh flowers for your office, listening to classical music, or sitting in your car by the side of the road gazing at an extraordinary view.

Donating your time to a charity that means something to you is another way of getting in touch with your spirituality. Meditation or prayer can help you achieve joy and meaningfulness, too. Enjoy the process of exploration, and find whatever works for you.

Exercise

Exercise heightens levels of endorphins, the body's mood-enhancing substances. Regular exercise such as walking, swimming, running, or any form of aerobics can energize you and reduce jitteriness. Preliminary evidence also suggests that exercise increases levels of serotonin and dopamine in the brain. In essence, exercise helps your brain's innate ability to regulate itself competently. It enhances your ability to withstand daily hassles and stressors.

In addition, exercise elevates levels of T-cells, which are part of the brain's immune function, strengthening your body's defenses against stress-induced immune compromise as well as the ability to withstand viral and/or bacterial infections. This may also account for why exercise has been linked to lower rates of bowel cancers and even breast cancers.

Research suggests that exercise also alleviates premenstrual symptoms and depression in some women. Vigorous exercise at a set time of day is a powerful cue to set the biological clock. It promotes bone formation and is important for the maintenance of strong bones and optimal bone density as you enter menopause. In postmenopausal women, exercise greatly enhances the ability to lower blood cholesterol to safe levels, when diet alone has little effect.

The NURSE *Program in Action*

Louise is a forty-year-old woman who found herself coping with her young son's acute attack of hepatitis. Between taking him to numerous medical appointments, tending to his needs, and trying manage her own job, she found herself becoming overwhelmed, jittery, and irritable. She started sleeping poorly and became unable to concentrate.

Based on a prior episode of depression ten years earlier, when she was successfully treated with psychotherapy and medications, Louise's current symptoms indicated that she was experiencing brain strain. She knew that without attention to this aspect of her biology, she was headed for another episode of depression.

We believed that the quick initiation of the NURSE Program to decrease Louise's stress response and enhance her brain's own self-regulating mechanisms would avert a rapid deterioration.

Louise had been eating far too much junk food from vending machines at the hospital and had been so focused on her son that she often forgot to eat at all. Besides, she reported that her appetite seemed dulled. We reviewed the basic food groups to help her get her diet under control. We also recommended that she start her day with Spiru-tein® (a soy-based protein drink) so that at least she was getting adequate protein and water.

We agreed with Louise that this was indeed a highly stressful time and helped her to structure her days. She needed to get to bed at a regular time, and we encouraged her to use relaxation tapes to help her fall asleep. We also suggested that she ask her employer for a short vacation so she would feel less stressed from being pulled between her work and family. We encouraged her to stop at the market and buy herself some flowers as well as take the dog for a walk every day—if not for his needs, at least for her own. It was good to be out in the fresh air.

After two weeks Louise reported that she was definitely feeling better. She was able to concentrate, she was sleeping more soundly, and she felt more grounded and centered. Fortunately, her son's medical crisis was resolving. Louise is a living example of how the prompt initiation of the NURSE Program can help reregulate your brain biochemistry and reduce the symptoms of brain strain.

Designing your own NURSE Program will help you pay attention on a daily basis to these critical aspects of brain care. As you have learned, your mental-health is made up of the interrelationship of your genes, neurochemistry, reproductive hormones, and life experiences. The NURSE Program is designed to meet you where you are, helping you to achieve the full and balanced life you want and deserve.

Managing Your Condition

How many medical illnesses are actually cured? In truth, most are just managed. Unfortunately, mental-health clinicians and patients continue to believe that a state of "being off medication" is a success. In fact, often it works exactly the other way around. Where ongoing emotional illnesses are concerned, you should not anticipate a "cure" but rather a state of stability maintained with careful medication monitoring and a lifestyle that does not perpetually put you into overwhelming life-stress situations. Once those parts of treatment are achieved, you then need to heal your soul.

Indeed, we have learned that there is no cure for some disorders. With conditions such as bipolar illness and chronic depressive and anxiety illnesses, for instance, we must accept the genetic and physiological givens—that's just the way it is. We cannot put the system back to its pre-illness state. Unfortunately, even with all of our high-tech advances, we do not yet know how to rewire the brain. Your symptoms are your brain's way of telling you, "I'm in pain. I need attention." But with informed life management (taking care of your brain and soul) coupled with good medical management, you can look forward to enhanced brain stability so that you feel better and lead a productive life.

No More Self-Blame!

Our patients often have been led to believe that if they learn to be strong enough or smart enough or if they cope more maturely, their symptoms will disappear. Unfortunately, this is not the way the brain responds. As you now know, your brain chemistry is constantly adapting and mobilizing to meet your needs from moment to moment. Depression, anxiety, and post-traumatic stress responses carry a biochemical price. Once these symptoms have emerged, there is always the risk of their occurring again, especially under certain hormonal conditions.

Often women also believe that they can think or talk themselves into feeling better, but they find that the symptoms do not respond to talking interventions or even worsen over time. When such women require medications, they may feel disappointed or self-critical that they were unable to heal themselves. Yet the symptoms merely mean that the brain is in distress and may need more potent interventions to heal.

At other times talking or other therapies may work well. All situations are different. You must understand your own in the context of what has transpired, both in the present and in the past. Both Jeanne and I had to come to terms with our unique situations, and the process is not always easy.

When Jeanne became symptomatic after her deliveries, she tried to tell people how she felt but was left feeling "bad" for having such shocking thoughts. Had she known about brain biochemistry when her girls were young, her condition would have taken less of an emotional toll. She struggled in silence.

I, too, struggled to understand the true nature of the depressive illness I had experienced. Although many years ago I accepted that this was a biological condition that needed medical management, my full understanding of how this illness evolved fell into place only once I put together the elements of brain strain and loading, altered chemistry, and hormonal impacts.

If you understand your symptoms with this new knowledge, you will feel less ashamed or blamed for something that may be entirely beyond your control. This is a vital step toward breaking the silence and empowering you. When we all appreciate how reproductive events can contribute to mood and anxiety disorders, we will all take a giant step forward in the realm of women's health.

Where Do We Go from Here?

In the next several chapters we will examine mood and anxiety problems that can occur at specific periods in your reproductive life. Focusing on premenstrual syndrome first, we will then move to pregnancy, postpartum, and finally menopause.

As you read about the women we have treated, remember that you are unique. You bring your own distinctive features to any of these junctures. So while the symptoms of certain mood problems may be similar to what you have experienced, you also must factor in an entire inner world and life experience that is yours alone. This is why you cannot assume that others' emotional responses will match your own. Everything must be considered within the context of the relevant concerns of *your* life.

As we have seen, biochemical loading can arise from many sources. Your genetic history helps to determine your brain's resilience to the stresses of life. Your responses to these stresses, in turn, also affect your biochemical brain. What you perceive as traumatic is an individual reality—others may not react in the same way you do. Whether or not you had access to support and care during or after a traumatic event can also influence how your brain responds.

Reproductive events in and of themselves do not constitute an abnormality. Rather it is the impact of these "normal" hormonal fluctuations on your loaded neurochemistry that can trigger emotional symptoms. Predictable female reproductive hormonal cycling includes the onset of the menstrual cycle, its cyclical recurrence, and its cessation at menopause. Depending on your biochemical vulnerability, a new onset or an exacerbation of preexisting emotional problems can occur when you bring your biology and neurochemistry into these events.

Forewarned and forearmed about whether you could be at risk, the NURSE Program is designed to help you take care of your brain with its delicate functions. Control the elements you can and let go of what you cannot. You will learn to live within the givens of your biochemical makeup. If you have a diagnosable illness that has become chronic, you must develop ways to live with it, recognizing that it is unlikely to disappear, but your brain will respond to preventive measures and care. When you recognize symptoms of brain strain, you can forestall relapses by taking good care of yourself—and your brain!

Part II

PREMENSTRUAL PROBLEMS

Chapter 8

PMDD IS A BIOCHEMICAL PROBLEM, NOT AN EMOTIONAL ONE

If you are sitting with a roomful of friends, chatting about the joys and sorrows of the menstrual cycle, chances are that about 80 percent of your cohorts will describe some experience with premenstrual dysphoric disorder (PMDD, known to the world as premenstrual syndrome, or PMS). If you continue this conversation with your friends' partners, husbands, or lovers, you'll find that about 50 to 80 percent will acknowledge that they know what PMDD feels like—but from the other side of the room, or perhaps from the vantage point of the sofa to which they have been relegated for the night!

Premenstrual mood changes are so prevalent that they've become the subject of greeting cards! Women spend millions of dollars each year on products that claim to alleviate PMS distress. In fact, by the time patients come to us with their premenstrual complaints, they have usually investigated vitamins and herbal therapies, creams, oils, and foods. There is, however, little scientific evidence that any one product can consistently alleviate all the symptoms of PMS.

While there are and have been thousands of natural remedies for PMS, the causes of these symptoms still remain a mystery. We still do not know exactly what accounts for the myriad moods, behaviors, and physical symptoms that women exhibit during their menstrual cycles. When women experience the full range of symptoms of PMS, this means that several physiological processes are occurring at once.

And although great numbers of women and men knowingly nod their heads at the mention of PMS, the intensity of the experience varies considerably from one woman to the next.

We do know that the mood and behavioral PMS symptoms emanate from the limbic-brain areas through the limbic brain and up to the cortex. Serotonin, dopamine, acetylcholine, and norepinephrine pathways connect these areas. Any short-circuiting in these pathways can have far-reaching effects on your mood and daily functioning. Aggression, sleep, rage, irritability, appetite, memory—all of these functions come from the limbic brain. Your cortex affects your judgment, attention, concentration, the way you view and interpret the world, and your moods.

Science is on the threshold of validating what women have known for decades: PMS is a real, biochemically driven experience, not an emotional or hysterical reaction. Its biological underpinnings are located in the brain.

Once you appreciate that PMS is a hormonal/brain-biochemistry problem that results in mood and behavioral distress, this allows you to listen to what your brain is telling you through symptoms and behaviors. You can now use your intellectual skills to interpret the messages and institute effective remedies. In this chapter you will learn to care for your brain using various strategies available to all women. You will know why you are using them and what they do for your brain.

Is My Menstrual Cycle Abnormal?

Since your brain and hormones are involved in the symptoms of PMS, it is important to know how they affect each other. (In Chapter 5 we explain the menstrual-cycle/brain-chemistry link in detail.) When you experience symptoms during the week before your period, these represent a temporary chemical dysregulation in the limbic and prefrontal mood pathways induced by the *normal* fluctuation of hormones and peptides across your menstrual cycle. Normal is key here, since there is nothing unusual about the cyclic changes in female reproductive hormones. But it is the impact of these changing hormones on brain biochemistry that generates the symptoms.

What Exactly Is PMS?

There is a wide range of how and what women feel during this time of the month, so one woman's PMS symptoms may not be the same as another's, even though both use the same term. Indeed, "PMS" has become a catchall phrase that can mean anything from "I have menstrual cramps and bloating" to "I am so irritable and out of control, I'm in danger of killing somebody!" The husband of one of our patients has his own definition of PMS. He calls it "time to Pack My Suitcase."

In the psychiatric and medical world the currently accepted term for PMS is "premenstrual dysphoric disorder," or PMDD. PMS was previously called "late-luteal-phase dysphoric disorder," just a fancy way of saying that you experience an uncomfortable mood in the week before menstruation. Indeed, for PMDD to be diagnosed, symptoms must first arise after ovulation has taken place (when an egg is released from the ovary) and must settle completely within a day or two after menstrual bleeding begins.

Also you must experience a 30-percent worsening in the severity of your symptoms during the premenstrual week as compared to the preceding week in order to call your condition PMDD. These symptoms must interfere with your normal functioning, whether at work, socially, or within relationships, and the symptoms must include mood, behavioral, and physical changes.

As you can see, these are stringent criteria for a disorder that so many women describe having! In fact, only 5 percent of those who complain about premenstrual symptoms actually meet the full standards for PMDD.

PMS Symptoms

Most women consider PMS to be a time in their monthly cycle when they experience a variety of symptoms that feel irritating and bothersome. Numerous studies have shown that 30 to 70 percent of women experience some degree of premenstrual symptoms even if they don't have the full-blown syndrome. Though these percentages are large, for the vast majority symptoms are moderate and only mildly debilitating. Most women have learned to "live with" their symptoms, but they also believe that they would be better off without them. Of course, the way a woman copes with the experience can vary, too.

Behavioral symptoms may include food cravings, withdrawal from normal activities, confused or muddled thinking, clumsiness, diminished sex drive, or increased alcohol use. Physical changes can encompass headaches, migraines, abdominal cramps, bloating, weight gain, breast tenderness, hot flashes, fatigue, malaise, nausea, and acne.

Technically, if you suffer "only" from headaches, bloating, weight gain, and cravings for sweets premenstrually, this is not PMDD, although the symptoms may be quite uncomfortable. Certainly, cramps and breast tenderness can be painful and may disrupt your life. But strictly speaking, they don't constitute PMDD because they exclude mood disturbances such as sadness, despair, loss of interest and motivation, irritability, anger, or anxiety. Being overly reactive to situations that at other times would not elicit such a response is also considered a mood-related symptom.

Women experiencing anxiety disorders often find that their symptoms worsen premenstrually. In fact, anxiety problems might declare themselves in the context of the menstrual cycle long before they become fully expressed.

The following is a list of common symptoms that can occur premenstrually. As you see, it is long and varied. In fact, women report about one hundred symptoms associated with the last two weeks of the menstrual cycle, but we have not listed them all!

COMMONLY REPORTED PREMENSTRUAL SYMPTOMS

Physical	Emotional	Behavioral
headaches, migraines	irritability	food cravings
breast tenderness	depression	decreased interest in activities, work, relationships
abdominal cramps	tearfulness	social isolation
bloating, weight gain	anxiety, nervousness	avoidance of activities
skin changes, acne	mood changeability	poor concentration
hot flashes	sadness	clumsiness

Physical	Emotional	Behavioral
diarrhea, constipation	anger, rage, hostility	decreased libido
general malaise, nausea, lack of appetite	oversensitivity, feeling easily overwhelmed	slower, muddled thinking
palpitations	"raw" feelings	increase in alcohol consumption
weight gain	tremulousness	increased food bingeing
fatigue	jumpiness	perception problems

When Do PMDD Symptoms Emerge?

Often premenstrual symptoms first emerge when a woman is in her early thirties. Perhaps at this time brain receptors are not as resilient to hormonal fluctuations as they were in earlier years, or perhaps the process of allostatic loading eventually renders the receptors less able to compensate.

In our clinical practice, however, we do find that women who first experience PMDD in their late thirties and early forties generally have a history of depression, often occurring during the postpartum period. They usually tell us that they were never treated for the mood and anxiety symptoms but rather that "they just went away."

Perhaps the symptoms did ultimately disappear, but as we now know, the brain does not forget. It has incorporated the depression experience into its mood and anxiety pathways and becomes a vulnerable biology just waiting to be pushed again under the influence of the next female hormonal event.

When Brenda, for instance, gave birth to her second child, she experienced a depression that lasted for six to nine months. "I did not go for help," she explained. "I stayed in the house most of the time. It felt as if a screen had come down on my life. I don't know how I made it through. I just knew I had these two little faces to look at every day and that I was the only one who would be there for them."

Further questioning revealed that during this depression Brenda experienced difficulty sleeping, poor appetite and concentration, sadness, and decreased interest in all her activities.

Now, at the age of thirty-eight, Brenda is coping with severe PMDD. Although she is happily married, for the past three years she has had increasing difficulty with premenstrual symptoms, substantially reducing her ability to function. In fact, she cannot plan to do anything socially or at work during the last week of her cycle. She has become so irritable that she is unable to tolerate the slightest disagreement or problem.

Brenda clearly had an earthquake episode of postpartum depression after the birth of her second child, but it went undiagnosed and untreated. Although this was a difficult time, she battled it alone. Perhaps this is why her premenstrual symptoms have erupted now with such severity.

The hormonal fluctuations that take place when estrogen production slows before menopause can cause symptoms that mimic PMDD in middle-aged women, inducing the mood pathways to short-circuit. What looks like late-onset premenstrual symptoms may really be perimenopause (see Chapter 17).

What Your PMDD Symptoms Are Trying to Tell You

When you study the list of PMDD symptoms, one thing becomes immediately apparent. Many are exactly the same as those of mood or anxiety disturbances. When you have PMDD, your brain is telling you that for some reason it is unable to maintain its usual chemical balance during the last week of your cycle. However, when your brain recovers its intrinsic regulating abilities within a day or two of menstruation—lo and behold—you feel well again! Whatever biochemical process induced the temporary short-circuiting has resolved.

The imbalance and its accompanying symptoms have nothing to do with your being good or strong enough. They are simply your brain alerting you to a chemical condition. This is not a moral issue; it is biology. During the last week of your menstrual cycle, under the influence of "normal" hormonal effects, the brain is unable to regulate itself properly. Understanding and embracing your unique physiology is important in mobilizing you to seek help.

Stress and PMDD

Not surprisingly, premenstrual symptoms can worsen when you are under stress. Receptors for estrogen and progesterone are dense in the hypothalamus and limbic area, and this can intensely influence the serotonin, norepinephrine, and dopamine pathways. Together, stress and reproductive hormones can disrupt nerve transmissions there during the menstrual cycle.

In a way, you might consider PMDD a "tremor" in your life—a self-limited mood disturbance that arises as a result of normal hormonal shifts. As such, it opens a window of opportunity for you to observe how your brain chemistry reacts under a specific hormonal challenge. The presence of a PMDD "tremor" suggests that you may be vulnerable to future hormonal challenges like those occurring at pregnancy, postpartum, and menopause.

Because stress tends to worsen PMDD symptoms, we believe that the stress-reduction techniques we advocate in the NURSE Program—such as adequate rest, spiritual renewal, and exercise—are all helpful in modulating your symptoms.

Cramping and Bloating

The physical symptom of cramping is most likely unrelated to fluctuations in estrogen. Rather, it is probably due to the secretion of prostaglandins. These chemicals are produced to help your ovary release the egg during the follicular stage. They cause the smooth muscles in the ovaries and the uterus to contract and therefore are also believed to be responsible for menstrual cramps. That is why anti-prostaglandin medicines like ibuprofen (Advil, Motrin) and fenamates (Ponstel and Meclomen) are highly effective in relieving cramps.

Bloating and fluid retention are not well understood. It is thought that during the last two weeks of the cycle small blood vessels throughout the body are less able to prevent fluid from seeping through to the tissues. Other fluid retention mechanisms probably promote fluid accumulation in the breasts and abdomen. Progesterone causes the smooth muscle of the intestine to relax, which might account for the uncomfortable, distended feelings.

Diuretics, medications that promote fluid loss, are often prescribed for bloating. The most commonly used is spironolactone, which also prevents the loss of potassium. Sometimes bromocriptine is used, but it may not be as effective. Diuretics, however, do not help mood and behavior symptoms.

How Do You Know If You Have PMDD?

Because the symptoms for PMDD can be so variable and because they can be mistaken for other disorders, we have found that a Premenstrual Daily Symptoms Rating Chart is helpful in tracking our patients' symptoms. (See Appendix B.) You can make copies of it and use it to record your daily experience over several months.

This chart allows us to ascertain if other symptoms appear during our patients' cycles, such as elevated, euphoric, or racy mood coupled with a more depressed state. These can point to other types of mood or anxiety disturbances that may be present as well as alert us to any worsening of symptoms. We ask our patients to rate their symptoms daily from 0 to 3, with 0 representing no symptoms and 3 representing the worst they have ever experienced.

Tracking your symptoms over several months will provide you with a graphic representation of your experience. This can also validate that your symptoms are real. It enables you to compare previous cycles and can help you plan treatment interventions with your mental-health practitioner.

For instance, after our patient Susan (in Chapter 4) recorded her symptoms daily for two months, we confirmed that she had a mild case of PMDD. Her chart showed that she became snappish with her husband, had trouble sleeping, and craved chocolate premenstrually.

Using the NURSE Program to Alleviate PMDD

We used the NURSE Program to help Susan deal with her mild symptoms. Over the next few sessions she learned basic brain anatomy, physiology, and how the reproductive events of her menstrual cycle affected her brain biochemistry. This was the Understanding element of Susan's NURSE Program.

Nourishment was a problem for Susan. She admitted that she skipped breakfast, would sometimes grab a cup of soup and a piece of bread for lunch, and then usually ate some pasta at night. She snacked on cookies between meals. Susan was not eating enough vegetables, fruit, or protein. Her brain was starving! We talked about the need for her to adopt a low-fat, high-complex-carbohydrate diet that included adequate protein intake. We also recommended a daily dose of from 4,000 to 8,000 milligrams of alpha-omega-3[1] oil to enable her nerve cells to better withstand the impact of her biology. Susan also embarked on a program of exercise and relaxation, incorporating meditation at least once a day.

With these modest lifestyle adjustments, Susan noticed a difference in her mood and behaviors in just a few weeks. She felt in charge of her life. "This has been an amazing learning experience for me," she told us. "I had no idea that I could do so much with so little. I am becoming aware of what my brain tells me now. It's as if I have explored a whole new dimension in my life." Yet all she had really done was give her brain the tools with which to regulate itself.

By caring for her brain, Susan was able to help it accommodate to normal hormonal changes. Self-care became a priority for Susan, and with it came a sense of improved mental-health.

Treating More Serious PMDD

Beth, the thirty-two-year-old teacher whom we met in Chapter 5, was suffering from more serious PMDD. Although her symptoms were not disabling, they did interfere with her ability to teach and with her relationship with her husband.

Beth described symptoms that occurred cyclically over her menstrual cycle, but Jeanne needed to identify more pieces of this puzzle. Beth's PMDD symptoms were simply a biochemical snapshot at this moment within her menstrual cycle. She had little information about the events in Beth's life that might explain the brain loading underlying the eruption of PMDD.

When Jeanne asked about her family, Beth admitted that her mother had had problems with depression on and off throughout her life but had received no treatment. "For years, my mom saw psychiatric treatment as a failure of character," Beth explained. "She thought it meant she was unable to cope. My sister and I had urged her to get some help, but she never would. She is of the old school."

Sadly, many consumers and health-care professionals do not understand that most psychiatric problems are alterations in brain chemistry, not defects in character. Shame and denial not only prevent sufferers from getting accurate diagnosis and quality care, but also can interfere with their full participation in life.

Beth went on, "When my mom started going through menopause,

her depression became so severe that she didn't really have much of a choice. She now takes a medication called Zoloft, and she's a different person. Today she swears by the slogan 'Better living through chemistry'!"

It is likely that Beth's neurobiological makeup was similar to her mother's, predisposing her to depression at some point in her life. She was born with genetic loading that led her to experience some degree of depressive disturbance, although it was confined to the menstrual cycle.

"What do you think about medication?" Jeanne continued.

"Why do you think I am here? I've tried all that homeopathic and natural stuff. It hasn't worked for me. I've done some reading about Prozac being used to treat PMDD. So I want to ask you about my treatment options."

Before she could make that determination, Jeanne needed more information. Although Beth had not mentioned having any previous episodes of depression, she might have experienced it but not labeled it as such. Since Beth's premenstrual mood changes indicated a vulnerability to small hormonal shifts, Jeanne was looking for signs to help her predict future earthquakes.

"Tell me what it was like living with your mom," Jeanne probed gently. "Given what you've said about her depressive phases, I wonder how it felt growing up with her."

Reluctantly Beth acknowledged that relating to her mother was difficult. As a child, she often felt shut out, confused, and adrift. Her relationship with her father partly compensated for this, but the family never discussed the issues. Each member coped individually, with little mutual support or validation.

When Beth allowed herself to think deeply about her relationship with her mother, it weighed on her, inducing a sense of loss and sadness. She acknowledged periods of unhappiness, during which she was uninterested in getting together with her friends. "Life felt heavy," she said. But just as she had coped as a child, Beth pushed these thoughts away and did not think about them. To distract herself, she used a learned coping skill—she buried herself in activity and her work.

Beth had indeed had periods of what could be termed mild depression. She just called these times of "unhappiness," "emptiness," or "aloneness." But as you now know, there is an emotional cost to "pushing away the thoughts and not thinking about them." The cost is brain strain, which may render the brain more vulnerable to dys-regulation. Behavior, thought patterns, feelings—good and bad—that you have learned as a child, always emerge at some point in your life. The limbic brain eventually yields its secrets.

Although Beth had compensated relatively well, her brain was be-ginning to reveal signs of its vulnerability as it reacted to the normal hormonal events of her menstrual cycle. Not surprisingly, the symp-toms were becoming apparent as she entered her thirties. For Beth, as for many young women, these symptoms may be the first indication of mood problems yet to come.

Finally Jeanne asked Beth to chart her mood and behavioral symp-toms daily for the next two months. Jeanne also ordered some blood tests to rule out any medical or endocrine problems.[2]

Two months later Beth returned with her charts. They showed graphically that her symptoms emerged one week prior to her period, just as she had described. In addition, her blood work was within normal range. Now that it was clear she had PMDD, it was time to talk with Beth about treatment options. (See Illustration 10.)

Jeanne taught Beth about the NURSE Program to help her maximize her brain's intrinsic regulating abilities and enable her brain pathways to withstand the flux of hormones.

Second, Beth thought about how she could reduce stress and adapt to the physiological changes in her brain during her premenstrual days. She decided to increase story time and plan other low-key pro-jects with the children at school. She would also allow her students more time outside, so they could release energy on the playground. Perhaps this would decrease their exuberance in the classroom and their behavior would be less irritating. If Beth felt less stressed, her coping abilities would be enhanced.

Beth promised to come back for a follow-up appointment after implementing this NURSE Program for a few months. If these mea-sures did not work fully, she and Jeanne would then consider medi-cations to stabilize her serotonin brain receptors. Medications can be helpful for individuals with moderate to severe PMDD.

Coping with Severe PMDD

Brenda often found herself screaming at her teenage children during her premenstrual phase. She overreacted to everything. She felt de-pressed, angry, and hostile toward her family. She isolated herself and

Name																														
Day of cycle	1	2	3	4	5	6	7	8	9	10	11	12	13	14	15	16	17	18	19	20	21	22	23	24	25	26	27	28	29	30
Date																														
Menses	M	M	M	M																								M	M	M
Symptoms																														
crying, tearful																														
anxiety, restlessness																					1	1	1	1	2	2				
sadness																														
overwhelmed by things																					1	1	1	1	2	2	1	1		
mood changeability																														
anger, rage attacks																										1	1			
irritability																					1	1	1	1	2	2	1			
overly sensitive																				1	1	2	2	2	2	2	2			
loss of interest																														
loss of enjoyment																							1	1	2	2	2			
feeling tired																				2	2	2	2	2	2	3	3			
feeling guilty																														
blaming self																														
disliking self																														
loss of libido																							1	1	2	2	2			
poor concentration																					1	1	2	2	2	1				
confusion																					1	1	1	1	1	1				
forgetfulness																					1	1	1	2	2	1	1			
social withdrawal																					1	1	2	2	2	1				
appetite: incr/decr																					1	1	1	1	2	2	1			
suicidal thoughts/plan																														
panic attacks																														
obsessional thoughts																														
compulsive behaviors																														
avoidant behavior																														
food cravings																				1	1	2	2	2	2	3	2			
sleep: incr/decr																					1	1	1	2	2	2	2			
nausea																														
abdominal bloating																							1	1	1	2	2			
hot flashes																														
clumsiness																						1	1	1	2	1	1			
breast swelling																				1	1	1	2	2	2	2	1			
abdominal cramps																														
headaches													1								1	1	1	1	1	1				
increased energy																														
hyperactivity																														
talkative																														
start many projects																														
racing thoughts																														
buying sprees																														
elevated mood																														
euphoria																														
alcohol intake											✓		✓																	
medications																														
doses																														
other pertinent events																														

Scale: 1=mild symptoms, 2=moderate, 3=severe
If you do not have any symptoms, leave the box blank.

Illustration 10. Beth's Premenstrual Daily Symptoms Rating Chart

had difficulty sleeping. She suffered from poor concentration and inevitably broke dishes or appliances because her coordination was impaired. Additionally, she complained of bloating, breast tenderness, and headaches.

Brenda's husband had reached the point of desperation with these overwhelming outbursts. He even took the children and checked into a hotel for several days each month just to get away from the tension. But within days of her menstrual flow, Brenda started to feel the symptoms subside and disappear. She and her husband were frantic. "You've got to do something to help me!" she cried.

Although from the beginning of the consultation it seemed clear that Brenda had severe PMDD, I needed to confirm the diagnosis. Brenda had experienced depression after the birth of her second child but had been feeling well since then, so why was she having such a difficult time now? I needed to establish that no other medical problems were contributing to these symptoms. In addition, I wanted to know if any new life stresses were pushing her biochemical fault line. Brenda felt that things were good at home other than the problems with her premenstrual personality change, when, as she put it, "I become the Wicked Witch of the East."

Brenda was thirty-eight, and I wondered if early perimenopausal changes were causing the dysregulation of Brenda's neurotransmitters. And so we reviewed some expectable perimenopausal symptoms. Did Brenda have any hot flashes at other times of the month, any night sweats? Had there been evidence of irregular menstrual cycles, which would be a sign that her ovaries' responses were slowing down? To all these questions, Brenda responded negatively.

To complete Brenda's evaluation I ordered the usual blood work but also included thyroid, blood sugar, and urine tests. We checked her pituitary hormones, FSH, LH, and prolactin levels to see if there was evidence of early menopause.

Brenda documented her mood symptoms and menstrual cycle on the daily symptom chart. She had recently had a gynecological examination, and everything was fine. Without this exam I would have encouraged her to have a complete physical so that we could have information about her whole body and its functioning. All systems are interconnected, and we need all the puzzle pieces to construct the total picture.

Two months later Brenda came back for a follow-up appointment. Her blood values had all been normal. Her charts showed that she spiraled downward with mood and behavioral changes after the nine-teenth day of her menstrual cycle. This information indicated that her limbic-brain chemistry was exquisitely sensitive to the changing hormonal milieu of her menstrual cycle.

From this we knew that Brenda's biochemical fault line was vulnerable to hormonal changes. When she enters the perimenopausal phase of her reproductive life, her brain may have difficulty adapting to the reduction in estrogen. We would need to be on alert for future problems.

I drew a diagram showing Brenda how the hormonal fluctuations during her menstrual cycle, particularly the estrogen withdrawal, cause changes at the serotonin receptors, which in turn can short-circuit the entire neurotransmitter system, resulting in mood dysregulation and irritability.

Brenda expressed relief in knowing that there was a reason for how she felt. "I seem to spend almost two weeks in a state of crazed fury," she said.

"There is a reason for that," I said. "Watch what happens at ovulation when your estrogen levels dip. For women in your situation, symptoms start here. As a result of your postpartum depression— when your brain learned the pattern of dysregulation—your unique biochemistry is likely to be more sensitive to this small withdrawal of estrogen affecting the serotonin pathway. The effects of altered serotonin can be devastating, as you have experienced. Some of our patients say they feel a bit shaky, anxious, and tearful at ovulation. For them, it seems to pass, but then the symptoms return the week before menstruation. Others report a few days of poorer sleep, which also passes."

Brenda's treatment plan would be designed for her unique symptoms. We established that she would follow a diet rich in cereal grains, low-fat dairy, no red meat, and plenty of fresh fruits and vegetables. I advised her of the other elements of the NURSE Program and encouraged her to record her daily mood changes, watching for progress. In addition to the NURSE Program, I suggested medications to correct the neurochemical dysregulation that occurred within her menstrual cycle. Brenda's symptoms were too disruptive to her life for us to postpone treatment with antidepressants.

Using Antidepressants for Severe PMDD

Most of the research now indicates that serotonin dysregulation is involved in PMDD. Currently at least twenty published studies consistently show that the newer class of antidepressant medications, known as selective serotonin-reuptake inhibitors or SSRI agents (such as Prozac), are effective treatments for the kind of severe PMDD symptoms that Brenda was having. In fact, as we have seen, a significant number of premenstrual symptoms actually look like depression.

The SSRI medications work by increasing the amount of serotonin available within the mood pathways. For instance, Prozac "holds" the amount of serotonin in the limbic pathways stable even as the female hormones fluctuate so that the pathways are more resilient in face of hormonal ebb and flow. Consequently symptoms disappear, and women feel balanced and whole.

You might think of the SSRI medications as reinforcement to your own serotonin pathways. They simply enable your brain to do what it might have done on its own, had it maintained its usual capacity to self-regulate.

Prozac was the first SSRI agent to become available in North America. Other SSRI agents have been shown to be effective in the treatment of PMDD. These currently include Zoloft, Luvox, Paxil, and Anafranil.[3] Another medication we have found consistently effective is Effexor.[4] In addition to enhancing serotonin levels, Effexor also maintains the balance of the norepinephrine pathway. When serotonin medications cannot be tolerated, Effexor is a good next choice. A new SSRI available in the United States, Celexa, is also likely to be effective for PMDD.[5]

Many women express concern about taking antidepressants to treat PMDD, but a preponderance of evidence now shows that serotonin dysregulation is the likely brain-chemical problem underlying it. When the SSRI medications were developed to specifically target the serotonin pathways, it turns out that they were also tailor-made for the treatment of PMDD.

Each woman is different, and what works for one might not work for another. We encourage you to work with your doctor and/or nurse practitioner to find the right dose for you. Don't compare your dose requirements with those of other patients. You are an individual, and your needs reflect your chemistry and nobody else's.

Usually we start our patients on a daily dose of antidepressant. We encourage them to continue charting their symptoms for a few months so we can evaluate the medication's effectiveness. When the symptoms subside and our patients are feeling better consistently for a few menstrual cycles, they may be able to limit the medication to the last two weeks of their cycle, as several studies have indicated.

However, in some women the first estrogen drop after ovulation may sensitize the firing of limbic nerve cells and receptors, setting the stage for a longer bout of PMDD. If the third week in the cycle is not covered with medication, these patients may still have symptoms during the last week. We would recommend that such patients take the medication on a daily basis. We watch how they respond and adjust the dosage accordingly.

To date, Prozac is the only medication in this class of SSRI agents that stays in the system for a long time. This unique quality may allow it to be used for just the last two weeks of the menstrual cycle. Even in the intervening weeks, a good blood level of the medication will remain from the previous dose. All the other SSRI agents have a short acting life, from twenty-four hours to a few days, requiring daily dosing. That's why Prozac may be the first choice. However, if for any reason you cannot tolerate it, you should feel quite confident about the other SSRI agents, which you may also try in the last two weeks of the cycle.

In general, SSRIs will not affect your normal menstrual cycle; it will continue as usual, but without the premenstrual exacerbation of mood and anxiety symptoms. However, there can be some mild side effects, such as the jitteriness you might feel if you've had too much caffeine. Sometimes headaches occur in the first few days, and some people experience a loss of sexual desire. Overall, however, Prozac and the other SSRI medications are very well tolerated.

But it is important to remember that these medications don't work instantly. This is not like taking an aspirin and expecting your headache to go away within an hour. It can take several weeks or months for the proper blood levels to be established so that SSRIs can exert maximum effects on the neurotransmitters. It is easy to get discouraged, but you should persist, even if you don't feel better for the first few weeks. It may take two, three, or even four menstrual cycles to experience the full effect of the medication. It is also certainly possible that the NURSE Program can make a difference in how much medication you need to take. With severe PMDD, the NURSE Program is an adjunct to medication and may enable you to reduce your medication dosages at a later date.

The most important part of the treatment is that any medication, however prescribed, should be given with care and with detailed knowledge about your particular needs. Your response to treatment should be carefully monitored, and adequate follow-up care should be provided.

What About Progesterone?

You might have read about the use of progesterone to treat PMDD. It was in vogue some years ago, but today progesterone is considered inferior to antidepressant medications. Although there have been some anecdotal reports of "miracle cures" and progesterone gained a worldwide following for some time, no research has proven it to be effective except in very mild cases. In reality, there are few brain effects that would make progesterone a likely candidate for the treatment of PMDD.

Dr. Ellen Freeman, a psychiatric researcher in Philadelphia, conducted an excellent study on the efficacy of progesterone. She showed definitively that progesterone had absolutely no effect on PMDD symptoms. The doses in her study were large and provided the women with good blood levels of progesterone, yet their symptoms did not improve. Other studies have shown that progesterone actually worsened physical symptoms in some women. And some studies indicated that progesterone was no more effective than a placebo.

Progesterone can act on the GABA receptors in the brain, which enhance the brain's natural braking capabilities. But the GABA receptors appear to be more involved in braking anxiety symptoms than the depressive ones characteristic of PMDD. Progesterone has some sedating properties and has been used with other agents to achieve a better anesthetic effect in surgery. It is possible that for women whose PMDD symptoms include anxiety, irritability, and restlessness, progesterone may bring some relief. But as a treatment for true PMDD, it does little.

In fact, the use of progesterone might worsen mood symptoms premenstrually. We have seen some women respond quite adversely to its use, sometimes even becoming suicidal.

What About Estrogen Treatments?

Since the drop in estrogen during the menstrual cycle triggers PMDD, it might seem logical to treat PMDD symptoms with extra doses of estrogen. The theory behind using this treatment comes from the fact that estrogen relieves the hot flashes, irritability, sleep disturbances, and difficulties in concentration experienced by many women during menopause.

Dr. John Studd and his colleagues undertook this approach in London. When they used estrogen to treat PMDD, the extra estrogen rendered the overall hormone levels too high to sustain ovulation and the menstrual cycle. This prevented the hypothalamus from participating in a dialogue between the brain and the ovary. PMDD does not occur without ovulation, so of course there were no symptoms.

There are risks to this treatment, however. For one thing, additional estrogen can overstimulate the growth of the uterine lining. That creates a risk of tissue overgrowth and heavy bleeding. Because this is an important concern, progesterone should be given for a week to ten days along with the estrogen, usually between days nineteen and twenty-six, so that the lining of the uterus is sloughed off and the buildup of tissue does not occur. Unfortunately, the addition of the progesterone can produce the return of PMDD or depressive symptoms.

We believe that because SSRI medications have no effect on tissue growth in the uterus and usually do not disrupt normal hormonal events, they are a much better choice for treating PMDD.

Because PMDD is associated with ovulation, the use of oral contraceptives to stop ovulation is also an option for treatment. However, results vary. While some women experience relief, others (like me!) find that their PMDD worsens. It is our belief that those whose symptoms worsen have a history of depression and have not been fully evaluated for this.

Dire Cases

Occasionally women in our practice have severe side effects from SSRIs and have tried most of the other treatment regimens to little avail. And there are a small number who have such extreme symptoms that they entertain suicidal thoughts or have actually attempted suicide.

In these dire situations we have found it helpful to stop the cycling of the ovarian hormones altogether. In collaboration with their gynecologists, we recommend putting these patients into a menopausal state using medications that switch off the "conversation" between the pituitary, the hypothalamus, and the ovaries.[6] When the cycle has stopped, the brain pathways are no longer subjected to fluctuations across the normal menstrual cycle and the distressing PMDD symptoms no longer occur.

In most women who try this therapy the results are excellent, and most of the symptoms disappear. But there are drawbacks. Over time, the low levels of estrogen can produce bone loss and increase cholesterol levels—highly undesirable outcomes. Estrogen must slowly be reintroduced (with progesterone, to protect the lining of the uterus from overgrowing), but this can lead to heavy bleeding, reemergence of the PMDD, and depression symptoms.

Ultimately the problem with this treatment is that if we stop the medication and the woman starts to ovulate again, severe PMDD symptoms frequently return. It is not a simple process. However, women can remain on this regime as long as they are taking replacement estrogen and progesterone.

How Brenda Fared

We started Brenda on a small dose of Prozac daily. Her symptoms settled, and she had an excellent response. She also attended meditation classes and found that the techniques she learned were helpful in managing the daily stress of life. After four months she was able to reduce her medication from daily to her two "sensitive" weeks per month—from midcycle to the onset of bleeding. She continued to experience relief from her premenstrual symptoms. I advised her to remain on this regimen for at least a year, and then we would re-evaluate her situation.

Brenda had experienced symptoms of PMDD for only two to three years, so it is possible that her moods could right themselves. But given her history of postpartum depression and PMDD, her risk for perimenopausal mood symptoms is high. She might need to remain on Prozac at least until she completes the menopause process, when the dialogue between the brain and the ovary subside.

Susan, Beth, and Brenda all had PMDD, but at differing levels of severity. There are, however, mood and anxiety disorders that mimic PMDD, and their treatments are usually quite different. We will cover these in the next chapter.

Chapter 9

THE MIMICS OF PMDD

Consider what might happen if you complained of chest pains and your clinician examined only your heart and lungs because that's the only area you indicated was hurting. The pain can have many sources. If the examination is limited to just the chest area, the diagnosis may be missed. Your clinician must determine and treat the cause of the pain in relation to your whole body. To do this, he or she must ask many questions and examine you fully.

The same can be true with the diagnosis of PMDD. Although you may identify bothersome symptoms at a specific time in your menstrual cycle, these may reflect something other than just "premenstrual syndrome." Physical symptoms such as headaches, palpitations, tremulousness, dizziness, hot flashes, nausea, light-headedness, and abdominal cramps can occur with PMDD but may also indicate numerous other physical and mental problems. When there are many physical complaints, you may need other medical tests to rule out thyroid disorders, migraines, gastrointestinal disturbances, seizures, or other medical problems.

We can easily be fooled. Consequently, one of the first questions we ask ourselves when a woman complains of PMS is "Is this PMDD, or is this something that mimics PMDD?"

Your symptoms must be understood within the context of your life—genetics, stressful experiences, and other hormonal impacts—

in order for an accurate and objective diagnosis to be made. Although you may be certain that you have PMDD, it makes no sense for a clinician to accept this diagnosis a priori until he or she has confirmed it with other tests and assessments.

It can be a tedious process of elimination to arrive at a PMDD diagnosis, but the consequences of not doing so can be disastrous. Specific treatments are required for other mood problems. If your disorder is misdiagnosed, you might start on the wrong medication that might not provide any relief at all or even produce adverse reactions. Collecting as much information as possible about your life can help avoid this problem.

When Depression Masquerades as PMDD

One of the most important distinctions to be made is whether you are suffering from depression that worsens before menstruation, and therefore looks like PMDD, or whether you have pure PMDD. This was the question we had to resolve when Joan came to the Hestia Institute.

Joan was a thirty-year-old single woman who reported that she felt okay during the first two weeks of her cycle but became increasingly restless, sad, and lethargic at ovulation. She complained of headaches and backaches and being highly overreactive. She became impatient with other drivers and swore at them for simply changing lanes. If a co-worker even looked at her, she felt like "scratching her eyes out." She had gained twenty-five pounds over the last six months and couldn't control her craving for sweets.

She also told us that sometimes, premenstrually, she had begun to have thoughts of killing herself, but she had no real plan for doing so. She believed she was "in the clutches of this bad mood that will never leave." It seemed to her that a few days after her period began, she felt less agitated, but if she really thought about her mood, it was never really great. "In fact," she confided, "I haven't felt myself for the last nine months."

Joan saw her internist, who, after completing a full physical, told her, "There is nothing wrong with you. Just a little PMS. Why don't you change your diet and get more exercise."

"I wanted to do this," Joan told us, "but somehow I couldn't get up the energy to exercise or eat in a healthy way. There must be something physically wrong with me to be feeling like this."

Joan was right. There was something chemically wrong in her limbic brain, which is not easily measurable in her blood. Based on Joan's symptoms, it seemed that she had a major depressive problem with a predominance of irritability and rage that worsened during her premenstrual weeks.

When we shared this information with her, Joan said that she didn't want to start on medication right away. It was hard for her to accept the diagnosis of major depression after being convinced for so long that she had PMDD. Sadly, in our culture, we accept premenstrual symptoms as almost normal, while a diagnosis of major depression still brings with it stigma and shame. However, Joan was keen to chart her symptoms for a month to see what was really happening.

When she returned a month later with her chart, Joan could now see how her mood was fairly low for most of the month and that her energy level was always down. She also felt hostile and rageful most of the time. Her appetite had generally increased, and her sleep was disrupted all month long but much more so premenstrually. It became evident to all of us that her symptoms were present most of the time but that they worsened premenstrually. (See Illustration 11.)

Joan's diagnosis was indisputable: major depressive disorder that intensified during the third, or luteal, phase of her cycle. She needed antidepressant medication.

Once Joan accepted that she required treatment for depression, we could make a full assessment of how she came to be at this point in her life. We already knew that she had demonstrated earthquake symptoms for quite a while, so her pathways had already spent significant time learning the dysregulated way of functioning. Was this her first episode of depression? Possibly not. What was her genetic thread, her allostatic loading, her history of tremors and earthquakes? To help Joan understand the diagnosis and help her participate fully in her treatment, we would work with her to identify the fault lines in her life.

Beginning to map Joan's life involved reappraising everything with her new diagnosis in mind. In the first interview, I had asked her whether anyone had had a depressive disorder in her family. "Oh, no," she replied. "Nobody had depression." She included herself in that category.

Most clinicians might assume that this was the end of the story, but I knew to dig deeper. It is rare for a person to have a depressive disorder without a parent also suffering from a mood disturbance.

Name / Day of cycle	1	2	3	4	5	6	7	8	9	10	11	12	13	14	15	16	17	18	19	20	21	22	23	24	25	26	27	28	29	30
Date																														
Menses	M	M	M	M	M	M																								
Symptoms																														
crying, tearful												2	1				2		1		2		2	2	2	3	3	1	1	1
anxiety, restlessness	1		1	1	1	1	1					1	1				1				3		1	3	3	3	2	1	1	1
sadness														1	1								3	3	3	3	3	2	2	2
overwhelmed by things		1	1	1	1					2		2	3	2					1	1	2	2	2	3						
mood changeability	1	1	2	1	1	1	1	1		1	1	2	3	3	2	1			1	1	2				2	3	2			
anger, rage attacks			2									1	2	2	2								2	3	3	3	2		2	2
irritability	2	2		1	1		1	1				1	2	1	1						1	2	2	2			3	3		
overly sensitive																														
loss of interest					1	1						1	1			1	1			1	1	1	1	1	1	1	1		1	1
loss of enjoyment																														
feeling tired												2	2	2	2					2	2	2	2	2	2	2	2	2		
feeling guilty																														
blaming self																														
disliking self												1	1							2		2	2	2	3	3	3	3		
loss of libido																														
poor concentration	2	2		1	1		2					2	2		2						2	2	2	2	3	3	3			
confusion																								1	1	1	1			
forgetfulness													1			1				1	1		1	1	1	1	1			
social withdrawal					1	1						1	1		1	1														
appetite: incr/decr																														
suicidal thoughts/plan																					2	2	2	2	2	2	2	2	1	1
panic attacks												1	1	1																
obsessional thoughts																														
compulsive behaviors																														
avoidant behavior																														
food cravings		2	2	2	1	1	1					2	2	2							2	2	2	3	3	3	3	2	1	
sleep: incr/decr	1	1	2	1	1	1					1	1	1	1			1	1			2	2	2	2	2	1	1	1	1	1
nausea																														
abdominal bloating																														
hot flashes																														
clumsiness																														
breast swelling																														
abdominal cramps																														
headaches																														
increased energy																														
hyperactivity																														
talkative																														
start many projects																														
racing thoughts																														
buying sprees																														
elevated mood																														
euphoria																														
alcohol intake																														
medications																														
doses																														
other pertinent events																														

Scale: 1=mild symptoms, 2=moderate, 3=severe
If you do not have any symptoms, leave the box blank.

Illustration 11. Joan's Premenstrual Daily Symptoms Rating Chart

"Joan, tell me a little about your family when you were growing up. How did your mother meet your father?" I asked.

"Well, actually my mother had a somewhat tragic life," she began. "Her family was very poor, and she was the youngest of five children. She was born ten years after the fourth kid, so I guess she was a bit of a surprise. Because they were so poor, my grandparents asked their younger neighbors to care for her. As she grew up, she knew that her real family lived on the next farm over, so she must have felt awful. Her brothers and sisters were not very nice to her. She told me that she often felt as if she were an orphan and she never felt like she belonged anywhere."

Loading was certainly occurring there!

"When she was nineteen," Joan continued, "she met a boy who came to help out with the farm. They grew quite close and she married him, but I think things deteriorated when my brother and I were born."

"How so?" I asked.

"Well, all I remember about my mother is that she was in a constant rage. I could never do anything right; she criticized everything. She would throw cups of tea across the room and sometimes broke dishes on the floor. She was always angry and impatient."

"How did you feel growing up in this atmosphere?"

"I was always afraid," replied Joan, "and I worried that she would explode. I would take care of everything till it was perfect, but it still wasn't good enough. Sometimes, as I got older, I would cry and feel really bad."

"Do you recall ever having trouble sleeping or feeling hopeless?"

"Yes, often," Joan replied. "What kept me going was the thought that I would leave home as soon as I finished school."

Here it was—the history that Joan had called "no history of depression in her family." It was clear that Joan's mother had had an angry depressive disorder, which emerged, no doubt, as a result of her own pitiful and stress-laden childhood. When she had her own children, she probably became severely depressed, but it manifested more as an irritable, hostile mood.

Joan herself was subjected to a lifetime of stress-loading by a mother who was unpredictable, angry, critical, and emotionally abusive. Probably by adolescence, Joan was also depressed. However, to her this was just how life had to be—always frightening, sad, and tearful.

Now everything fell into place. Joan's dysregulated mood pathways would probably respond to antidepressant medication. But based on the degree of stress loading throughout her life, I was sure she was going to be on it for a long time. Her biochemical fault line had been altered many years ago, and it was possible her pathways would never function properly on their own. In addition to the medications, I referred Joan for psychotherapy. She needed help to process and overcome a lifetime of emotional abuse.

Joan did well on the medications and used therapy to mourn the loss of the years she had felt so miserable without knowing why. She was, in essence, now using her cortical brain to help her limbic and paralimbic brains—and then she would go on to the healing of her soul.

Many women find themselves in this situation. They finally arrive for treatment, having coped with distress for a long time. Sometimes they feel so much better on medication, they realize how bad they had felt for such a long time. Why, then, did they have to struggle for so long?

Bipolar Illness Masquerading as PMDD

Mood-swing disturbances are also frequently misdiagnosed as PMDD. Often bipolar illness is present from adolescence, affecting a woman's relationships and her life. It can manifest itself as severe irritability and mood swings premenstrually, so it is regularly mistaken for PMDD.

Kelly, whom we first introduced in Chapter 4, came to our office complaining of PMDD symptoms. She described good days in which she was full of energy and creative ideas and bad days when she would sink into a depressed, dull fatigue. Kelly had been a hyperactive, impulsive young child. After she started menstruating, her moods worsened, and she became angry and irritable premenstrually. She became depressed immediately after starting birth-control pills but felt better within a few days of stopping them.

During her upswings, Kelly had periods of elevated mood—she felt great, had lots of energy, needed less sleep, and was extremely talkative. These lasted for three to four days at a time and were usually followed by a more depressed phase, when Kelly needed more sleep, lost interest in her usual activities, and found it hard to get going. Premenstrually, Kelly did poorly, with a swing into an irritable, angry, volatile state, and once she started menstruating, she lapsed into depression. Because these mood swings had existed for much of her life, she thought they were normal and believed that she only needed help with her premenstrual symptoms.

Kelly has what is known as bipolar 2, or soft bipolar disorder. Bipolar illness was a difficult diagnosis for Kelly to accept, as it is for most women in this situation. It is quite one thing to be evaluated for PMDD, but it's altogether another to be told that you have a mood-swing problem. This is not a welcome piece of news. However, it is empowering to recognize that you have this problem, because doing so will help you learn as much as you can about your neurobiology and how the symptoms occur at the chemical level.

As we studied Kelly's history carefully, she was able to identify her periods of increased energy, when she became unable to hold on to and use information, and her more depressed emotional states. She was also able to recognize her father's mood swings—his unbridled rages and physical abuse when he was out of control. His alcoholism worsened his disorder. In fact, we discussed how her father had probably tried to self-medicate his condition using alcohol.

The abuse and fear inherent in Kelly's childhood had severely traumatized her. She realized she didn't trust men but gravitated toward those who related to her as her father did. She expected little for herself. So much of her life had been spent just mobilizing herself to get through the day that she had hardly paid any attention to the future. Although she fantasized about a good relationship with a man, she had no idea how to accomplish this. Certainly we had to deal with Kelly's mood problem, but she experienced many levels of difficulty that required attention.

Treating Bipolar Disorder

Kelly's treatment would require attention to her biochemical, cognitive, and psychological status. By virtue of her father's history, Kelly's genetic biochemical fault line was already ratcheted up a notch. Her dad's abusive behavior and alcoholism pushed her stress line up a few levels, leading to tremors. When Kelly's symptoms worsened after puberty, it became clear that her moods destabilized significantly in the luteal phase. Her exquisite sensitivity to fluctuations in estrogen levels was further evident in her unmistakable reaction to birth-control pills.

Medication would help to balance the mood swings. Using drawings of her brain structure, neurotransmitter pathways, reproductive hormones, and menstrual cycle, we talked about how her moods reacted to menstruation.

Paying attention to her brain would ultimately render Kelly much healthier and happier. She needed a personalized NURSE Program to give her brain the food, rest, and spirituality that it missed. We also would slowly teach her about the impact of hormones and life events on her brain so that she could become aware of periods in the future when she would be more sensitive to hormonal fluctuations. Psychotherapy and medications together would help her brain to regain balance in her mood state as she progressed.

Getting the Biology Out of the Way

Because Kelly had bipolar 2 illness, just paying attention to her premenstrual symptoms would be of little value. Our first priority was to stabilize her mood swings medically so she could achieve some balance for all the days of her cycle. Lithium and Depakote are first-line medications in the treatment of bipolar disorders and are excellent mood stabilizers. (Depakote is also an antiseizure medication.) Most people tolerate these medications well, although they can have side effects, as can any medication.

We decided to try lithium, primarily because Kelly was familiar with it—a good friend also was on this medication. It was important to include Kelly in the decision-making process. If she were only a passive participant in her own treatment, she would be less likely to care for herself.

Before she began the medication, we took some blood tests to establish a baseline of data as well as to ascertain if Kelly had any other medical problems. And after she'd spent a few weeks on lithium,[1] we found that she tolerated the medication quite well. Her mood swings and violent outbursts abated, and she no longer dreaded becoming depressed. For the most part, her premenstrual symptoms stopped, too, although she would occasionally become irritable at that time. This was puzzling. Our goal was to balance Kelly throughout the month.

To account for Kelly's inconsistent response, we looked at the levels of lithium in her blood several times during her cycle. We wanted to know if they changed in response to her metabolism.[2] We discovered that although Kelly hadn't altered dosages, the level of lithium in her blood was lower premenstrually than it was during the rest of the month. This suggested that Kelly's body did not sustain a uniform level of this medication throughout her cycle.

The solution was to increase the lithium by small doses[3] in the last ten days of her menstrual cycle to smooth out this drop. Once we did, Kelly's premenstrual irritability settled.

This uneven response to psychotropic medications is another example of how a woman's reproductive-hormonal cycling can affect biochemistry. If these changes are unaccounted for, mood destabilization can recur monthly, without anyone's understanding why.

Only after Kelly's mood had stabilized did we address the next level of treatment—psychotherapy. We cannot stress this point enough. With bipolar illness, if you do not effectively deal with the chemical and brain biology first, psychotherapy will be ineffective, because the brain will always be consumed with its own unstable mood. In our practice we call it "getting the biology out of the way."

Psychotherapy would help Kelly make sense of her childhood and life responses and grow with healthier relationships. Therapy is another way of caring for the brain. When life brings you more of what is good for you, the benefits abound.

Kelly's sessions centered on examining her low self-esteem and her attraction to destructive relationships. Her childhood learning (imprinted in the paralimbic cortex) had unconsciously reinforced her gravitation to men who treated her poorly. Now she had to unlearn these old behaviors and start using her cortex to analyze, observe, and understand her choices. With help, she would make better decisions for herself, not only with men but also in friendships with women. She would also examine how her father's alcoholism had been his way of medicating himself but had created such a source of misery for the family.

This was going to require a few years of work. But healing would now be possible, because Kelly no longer had to struggle daily with her fluctuating mental state.

As one woman with bipolar illness told us, "Now that I'm thirty, I need more equilibrium in my life. I have responsibilities that I can't just push away when I'm up or down. I need to function and be happy." With proper diagnosis and treatment, she can.

Part III

PREGNANCY

Chapter 10

"HOW DID THIS HAPPEN?" DEPRESSION

IN PREGNANCY

From the moment you find yourself pregnant, your life is forever transformed. Whatever your age, whether the pregnancy is planned or unexpected and whether it ends in the delivery of a premature or full-term infant, your psyche will be altered. Moreover, even if you give up the child for adoption, decide to terminate the pregnancy, or suffer a miscarriage, you will never again view the world in quite the same way.

Even when the pregnancy goes well, you still face the enormous task of motherhood—a major life adjustment that entails moving into a new stage from which there is no return.

Many women negotiate this period quite well. But there are also many who find themselves caught in the grip of a mood disturbance at this time. In fact, Dr. Channi Kumar, a world-renowned researcher at the Institute of Psychiatry in London, reports[1] that 10 percent of women become depressed at some point during pregnancy, and many experience a flare-up of the disturbance during the first twelve weeks.

This translates into enormous numbers of depressed pregnant women who are unable to summon their usual coping skills to master and enjoy this wondrous experience. Indeed, for millions, pregnancy can be a period of profound distress.

The notion that depression can occur at this time seems incomprehensible to most of us. Yet just as any illness can strike during pregnancy, so can mood disorders. The symptoms occur not because you are "bad" or because "you don't really want the baby" but rather in response to an underlying brain state in which specific areas of biochemistry are struggling to function. If you are depressed at this time in your life, your brain is telling you that its capacity to feel joy is undermined.

Depression can occur for the first time during a pregnancy, or it can recur if you have had a previous history. In most cases there are clues that tell us about your risk of mood states. When you examine past and present life events, genetics, and hormonal impacts, you can gain a fairly clear idea about the biochemical state of your brain as you move into and through a pregnancy. With the ability to map your fault lines, you can anticipate what constitutes a risk and proactively implement protective measures to prevent or diminish the severity of an anticipated depressive episode.

Sadly, most obstetric caregivers buy into the myth of the joyous pregnancy and don't appreciate just how much psychological distress can exist at this time in a woman's life, often misconstruing depressive illness as merely an "adjustment to motherhood." They frequently fail to recognize that their patient is having a serious but treatable problem. An untreated mood disorder during pregnancy can result in premature labor and delivery, low-birth-weight babies, and other complications. Moreover, depression in pregnancy can grow into a serious depression after birth that may jeopardize the important attachment relationship between mother and baby.

Emotional health during pregnancy is not a luxury. It is essential to your well-being and your baby's. If you are experiencing depressive symptoms at this time, your psychological concerns must be investigated.

Pregnancy and Your Brain

A full-term pregnancy is calculated to be forty weeks long, give or take a week or two. These forty weeks are divided into three trimesters:

- *the first trimester:* from the day that your last menstrual period began till twelve weeks[2]
- *the second trimester:* from twelve to twenty-four weeks
- *the third trimester:* from twenty-four to forty weeks

Pregnancy is a time of enormous hormonal shifts, during which your body and brain are challenged as at no other point in your life. As your brain pumps great volumes of hormones to support the developing fetus and ready you for the task of delivering and feeding the infant, it is stressed to its maximum. Pregnancy is a period of brain strain, but with care, the brain can perform its functions well.

Estrogen levels rise rapidly in the early weeks of pregnancy, and that can affect mood stability. In fact, by the sixth week estrogen levels are already three times higher than at the highest point of the menstrual cycle! In Chapter 3, we discussed how profoundly estrogen alters the functioning of the limbic neurotransmitters in the serotonin, dopamine, and norepinephrine pathways, which can contribute to at least part of the dysregulation process of depression.

If the mood pathways have experienced a dysregulated state earlier, they remember it vividly and react quickly to the steep rise in estrogen. When a woman describes how her mood deteriorates in the early weeks of pregnancy, this may be why it worsens rapidly.

The rise of progesterone, the hormone responsible for keeping the pregnancy viable until the placenta takes over, may also contribute to depression. As we said in Chapter 5, progesterone is secreted by the corpus luteum—the cells of the empty follicle. Its levels also increase quickly in the first few weeks of pregnancy. We know that progesterone can induce depressive symptoms, although we are not sure of the mechanism. It is likely to be the culprit behind the distressing mood states induced by oral contraceptives and hormone-replacement therapy.

Prolactin, the hormone responsible for milk production, rises progressively throughout the pregnancy, too. Elevated prolactin levels at other times in a woman's life (with tumors or other endocrine syndromes) are associated with irritability and anger.

The rapid rise of the stress hormone cortisol may also drive the onset of depression in early pregnancy. Within the first trimester, cortisol levels double, continuing to rise until the third trimester, when they are three times normal. Elevated cortisol levels are often found in depressed patients, reflecting disruption in the important hypothalamic-pituitary-adrenal circuit (HPA). (See Chapter 3.) In fact, a naturally induced state of HPA dysregulation occurs during pregnancy because of the unusually high levels of cortisol.[3]

If the brain can accommodate these increases in hormones via its own self-regulating mechanisms, a woman may find that after initial mood problems during the first trimester, she will feel better starting around the second trimester. The receptors and pathways settle down, possibly basking in the luxury of all the extra (antidepressant) estrogen circulating in the blood. These high levels may even contribute to the sense of euphoria that many pregnant women experience.

Interestingly, some women with histories of mood and anxiety disorders have told us that pregnancy agrees with them. In fact, several women we know have had five and more pregnancies just to reexperience the sense of wellness that this state induced. Unfortunately, they lose this effect after they deliver their babies.

From about thirty-four weeks on, hormonal changes take place to prepare the uterus for labor. Estrogen stimulates the rise of oxytocin, the hormone that promotes the uterine contractions of labor and aids the passage of milk down the milk ducts for breast-feeding. Preliminary research indicates that oxytocin plays a vital role in the initiation of instinctive maternal behavior. Estrogen helps the oxytocin receptors function properly to promote attachment to the infant. How this occurs is not yet clear.

It is possible that high levels of oxytocin at the time of labor diminish the stressful effects on the brain of the painful birth process, so that you don't come out of labor traumatized for life! Because oxytocin is a hormone that also promotes amnesia, when we ask women if they recall how painful labor was, they usually remember, but with a detached quality. It certainly does not prevent them from embarking on another pregnancy!

Considering the effects that estrogen, progesterone, prolactin, oxytocin, and cortisol have on the brain, you can see how there are plenty of hormonal reasons that women may experience an acute, early onset of mood disturbance, particularly if the pathways have already been sensitized. Depression can occur abruptly, within a few weeks of conception, or more gradually over the course of a pregnancy. Although the exact mechanisms of how this happens are yet to be fully explained, no pattern of depressive illness is benign, and mood symptoms should never be ignored.

Paying Attention to Depression Early in Pregnancy

All too often women are misinformed that emotional changes in early pregnancy will disappear after the birth of their babies. In fact, if you experience depressive symptoms early in pregnancy, there is a greater likelihood that they will worsen postpartum. We believe that an early episode heralds what's to come later.

Mood disturbances that occur early in a pregnancy and then disappear in the second or third trimester tell us that your brain has the capacity to dysregulate in reaction to hormonal changes. It is as if the brain opens and then quickly closes an important observation window into its biochemical responses. This cannot be ignored.

Consider the issue from another perspective. If you had been diagnosed with epilepsy prior to the contemplation of a pregnancy, yet your health provider did not address the continued use of antiseizure medication, this would constitute negligent care. Most of these medications are associated with an increased risk of birth defects. If your clinician ignored a history of high blood pressure, this, too, would be negligence, because blood-pressure control is vital for the health of the pregnancy.

How is it, then, that with large percentages of women suffering from depression and other mood symptoms during pregnancy, so little attention is being paid to their situation? Numerous studies consistently show that prenatal care is the most important factor in ensuring a good outcome. Yet we still rarely consider the mother's emotional health, even though it is pivotal to a healthy start in her infant's life.

When a depressed pregnant woman is not eating or sleeping and becomes progressively anxious and agitated, she could and often does experience premature labor and delivery. Yet few clinicians ask about or connect emotional state with what may be going wrong in the pregnancy. Our high-tech Western culture just does not seem to grasp the concept that the state of our mind affects our body. A woman's brain counts!

The Adverse Effects of Stress During Pregnancy

Experiments with rats and monkeys show that when a pregnant female is distressed,[4] her fetus receives less oxygen, leading to lower fetal heart rate and blood pressure. In fact, in one study the fetus's heart rate dropped so low that the researchers thought death was imminent. In other studies confirming these findings, it appears that sleep and rest reverse the ill effects in the pregnant monkey and her fetus.[5]

More recent human studies indicate that untreated depression and anxiety are detrimental to the well-being of the baby. For instance, when Dr. Morten Hedegaard investigated the emotional health of 8,719 pregnant women in Denmark, he found that psychological distress in pregnancy, particularly if it occurred after the twenty-eighth week, correlated with premature labor.[6] Other studies have shown that if depression and adverse life stresses are present during a pregnancy, mothers are more likely to deliver low-birth-weight or premature babies.[7]

It is not our intention to scare you about the effects of mood and anxiety on your baby, but to emphasize how important it is for your emotional state to be taken into consideration. Remember, depression cannot be diagnosed from your external appearance. Most women who are depressed look quite normal. They have come into our offices well dressed and groomed; they converse rationally. But the facade falls apart when we ask the right questions, uncover their problems, and they finally feel heard and validated. Although you may hope that your doctor or midwife notices something in your face, he or she may not. Don't wait for a question or for someone to just somehow "know" that something is wrong. Speak up if you are feeling emotionally unwell. Early treatment can save you and your family much heartache.

Kayla Fights Depression

When a woman calls for help during pregnancy, it's usually because a serious situation has arisen. Kayla's call came in late one afternoon. "I need help desperately," she said. "Something is very wrong. I feel awful. I can't go through a pregnancy like this. I'm almost at the point that I could terminate this pregnancy."

Kayla was a thirty-eight-year-old mother pregnant for the second time who found herself in crisis early in her first trimester. She was unable to sleep, hadn't eaten much for a week, felt restless, and experienced a complete loss of interest in her work and her life. The world had become "black, desolate," and she felt there was no point in living. She couldn't even derive joy from little Johnny. In fact, she felt as if she were a burden to him and her husband.

This was not a new experience. Kayla had suffered from postpartum depression after Johnny's birth but was successfully treated with Prozac at that time. She and her husband had been advised to wait four years before conceiving another child, presumably to avoid the risk of a second depression.

They had received incorrect information. Extending the interval between pregnancies does not protect against another depressive episode. This is especially true since Kayla had already endured some depressive episodes earlier in her life, though she had not deemed these "depression."

Kayla's father had been an alcoholic, and she carried the ravages of growing up in a family fraught with unpredictability. She described times when she felt quite overwhelmed and had to push herself to get out of bed in the morning. She always linked these episodes to the sleepless nights she spent in fear of her father and his angry outbursts when he was drinking. In fact, her brain was telling her that it was in distress, unable to regulate itself sufficiently to control the sleep cycle.

As children, she and her sisters would sit at the top of the stairs and listen carefully for the sounds of their father's drunkenness, worrying about their mom. There they sat, these three little mites, shivering, hearts pounding, every muscle tensed and ready to go. But to do what? Who were they against their father's wrath and power? These nights of apprehension became a regular part of their life experience. Home did not bring safety and comfort, but vigilance, fear, and anxiety. The sadness was to come later.

Imagine how Kayla's young brain reacted during these circumstances. It mobilized to be in a constant state of alertness, aware of danger all the time, especially at home. In this situation her stress circuits were pushed to their limits. Kayla's home life was a war zone.

As a young adult Kayla had sought psychotherapy to help disentangle herself from her complicated, chaotic family. She very much wanted to develop a spirit of trust in her marriage and other relationships, so that she could articulate her needs more clearly. Locked into a heightened sense of responsibility for everyone around her, Kayla also needed to learn how to care for herself. Through therapy, she became more effective at accomplishing these goals, but she and her therapist had never addressed the biochemical underpinnings of her periods of depression.

Most psychiatric clinicians have been taught that when a person has adequately resolved her conflicts, the depressive periods pass. Neither Kayla nor her therapist realized how Kayla's previous life experiences, coupled with her genetic heritage, had already primed her brain for dysregulation.

When I asked whether she had had a previous psychiatric history prior to her postpartum episode, Kayla answered no. Regarding herself as very functional, she noted that she had coped with life's distresses resiliently until now. But not without a cost to the brain. Kayla's short-lived episodes of depression in the past, on top of a childhood fraught with stress, had slowly taken a toll on her brain. This ultimately led to the most severe episode of depression—the earthquake—after Johnny's birth.

In the light of Kayla's life history, it was likely that she would experience depressive symptoms again after she stopped taking Prozac when her son was three. Although she had no overt depressive symptoms, she began experiencing premenstrual mood changes at that time. She became irritable, anxious, and tearful, and her mood worsened to the point that she had to push herself to accomplish her daily tasks.

She used a small dose of Ativan, an antianxiety agent, to help her calm the irritability and sleep through the night. Although she thought that she did better after her period started, she acknowledged that sometimes she did not feel as well for a while longer. This led me to suspect that this epidsode had been more than just PMDD.

In time the depressive disturbance extended to the entire month. The emotional crisis brought on by her second pregnancy was not surprising in this context. It had nothing to do with conflicts about the new baby or her family. Rather it was simply her brain reacting to the hormonal challenge, telling her it was in trouble. Her biological symptoms needed urgent treatment.

Depression and Abortion

If Kayla went untreated, it was entirely possible that she would terminate the pregnancy. That might leave her feeling distraught and devastated. Thoughts about terminating a pregnancy are common among women who become depressed at this time. When they feel unheard and are unaware of the biology of depression, they may make an impulsive decision and then suffer the consequences for the rest of their lives. Yet for a woman in the throes of an acute biologically driven depression, the contrast between life and the pregnancy feels black and white—it's an all-or-nothing proposition. As Kayla said, "It's either me or the baby." We believe that whatever decision a woman makes, whether to continue or abort the pregnancy, would best be made when her neurotransmitters are in better balance.

Women who have reached this point need to know that treatment can be instituted and will be effective. Within their darkness they must find hope. They may also be at risk for suicide. When caught in the grip of such dismal feelings, the link to life can be tenuous. Support and encouragement about the positive effect of treatment are crucial.

Medical Treatments for Depression During Pregnancy

Although the ideal is to be medication-free throughout pregnancy, this may be unrealistic or even unsafe for many. A number of studies suggest that Prozac is relatively safe to use, even in the first trimester of pregnancy.

Eli Lilly, the company that manufactures Prozac, has collected information on more than fifteen hundred women who have taken this medication through their pregnancies. Their research and that of other scientists confirm that there is no evidence of increased birth defects, miscarriages, or premature labor and deliveries in these women when compared to the general public.[8] Although this is a relatively small number of pregnancies, these findings are somewhat reassuring, and other studies have confirmed them.[9] We believe it is unjustified to withhold this medication from pregnant women suffering from depression, given the possibility of other complications.

Those with depressive disorders require thoughtful management through pregnancy, just as women with diabetes do. With diabetes, elevated blood sugars lead to complications in the baby's development and the mother's health. The same holds true when a pregnant woman is depressed. Often, careful management requires that antidepressants be used to control the severity of the symptoms. Every woman's situation is unique and requires a careful assessment of the risks and benefits of medical treatment.

Preliminary results from Dr. Gideon Koren, who leads a world-renowned research group at the Motherisk Program at the University of Toronto, suggest that Paxil, Luvox, and Zoloft (also selective serotonin-reuptake inhibitors like Prozac) seem not to be associated with birth defects or major problems during pregnancy.[10] Although this research is still preliminary, it does begin to alleviate our concerns about whether these medications can be used safely. More information will be welcome.

Prozac doesn't appear to have an adverse effect on the delivery or the newborn. Only one report told of a baby who experienced some transient jitteriness and rapid heartbeat after delivery when his pregnant mother had taken the antidepressant. In a few days, however, these symptoms settled. This is likely to be an uncommon occurrence.

Many women worry that antidepressants may have a lasting effect on their fetus's brain, which could influence the baby's future behavior or development. A recent study conducted by Irina Nulman, another researcher at the Motherisk Program, compared children of women who had received Prozac during their pregnancies with those who had received older antidepressants. The children's ages ranged from eighteen to thirty months. The study found that there was no effect on language development and intelligence at this point. Although this information is comforting, it still does not tell us whether there could be other effects on development and behavior at a later stage in the children's lives.

We discussed this information with Kayla, and she decided to start medication. Her husband understood that she needed this treatment and was supportive, saying, "You have to be well to carry this baby and be there for Johnny." Within two weeks, Kayla reported that she was sleeping better and feeling less agitated during the day. The deep blackness was starting to lift. "It feels like there are more grays than blacks," she told me. "I feel a sense of light returning to my soul." Soon her appetite returned, and the desperate suicidal mood lifted completely. She was on her way, and the thoughts about terminating the pregnancy disappeared.

Kayla continued on her medication throughout the pregnancy. She delivered a healthy baby boy and did well through the postpartum period. We didn't lower her Prozac dose at the end of pregnancy because we knew she was at increased risk for worsening depression in the postpartum period. We wanted to avert this and maintain her mood health, so she could enjoy her growing family without a daily struggle for well-being.

Using the NURSE Program for Depression During Pregancy

Many women experience the onset of depressive symptoms in pregnancy with less vehemence than Kayla did. In fact, depression during pregnancy doesn't always require medication.

Diana, whom we met in Chapter 4, became anxious and depressed early in her pregnancy after a move from the New York. Her husband's immersion in his new position left her feeling lonely and disconnected. He was a quiet man, and she feared that he didn't care about her or the baby.

Diana reluctantly acknowledged family problems but felt that she had emerged fairly intact. "My Dad was an irritable and violent workaholic, and my mother always covered for him. She worked hard to see that everything in the house was perfect so he had less to complain about when he came home. My brother and I generally stayed out of his way. My mother has always been a worrier. She used to have stomach problems with cramps, and episodes of diarrhea. She took Valium occasionally, prescribed by her internist." Here were the red flags from her history.

As Jeanne discussed with Diana her fault lines, Diana began to understand how she came into her childbearing years biochemically challenged and ready to develop depression. The diagram Jeanne drew showed clearly how a difficult childhood coupled with the stress of the move and the biochemical effects of her pregnancy had tipped the balance. Armed with explanations about her biochemical status, Diana felt more in control of the situation. Once her symptoms made sense, she could become an active participant in her treatment.

Jeanne and Diana applied the NURSE Program to develop some helpful strategies. Assessing Diana's food intake and sleep disturbance, Jeanne determined that she was doing well nutritionally, but she wasn't getting enough rest and relaxation. They planned to monitor Diana's sleep patterns, and Jeanne prescribed a short-acting antianxiety medication at night to allow Diana's brain biochemistry to reregulate during a good night's sleep.

Jeanne also recommended psychotherapy to engage the reasoning capacity of Diana's cortical brain in quieting her limbic brain by validating the realities of her sad childhood.

Diana realized that she had a long way to go in therapy to resolve many of her childhood feelings and fears, and that this was not going to be achieved within this pregnancy. She and Jeanne talked about her relationship with Carl and her need to feel that he was an active partner in the pregnancy. She desperately wanted emotional reconnection with him, but she didn't know how to speak honestly with him, or he with her.

Since Diana had had little experience in sharing her authentic feelings and thoughts without fear of retaliation, she needed help learning and practicing these skills. Jeanne suggested couples' therapy for Diana and Carl to focus on their relationship and find more effective ways of communicating. This would certainly be necessary after the baby was born.

Pregnancy can precipitate a sense of neediness and a search for confirmation about oneself. Support and connection with significant people in your life is a fundamental part of emotional well-being at this time. In fact, pregnancy is a physiological state in which dependence and regression are normal. When accomplished women experience these emotions, it often reminds them of dependent feelings they might have worked hard to overcome. They can feel frightened and confused at the reemergence of such feelings. Psychotherapy would help Diana accept her renewed need for dependence. Sometimes establishing a good, trusting bond with a caregiver who encourages you to talk effectively, identify your problems, and communicate your needs can be very helpful in alleviating some of the depressive symptoms.

But Jeanne felt they were treading a fine line. Diana definitely had symptoms of anxiety and major depression, and Jeanne wanted to avoid premature labor and delivery. They would remain vigilant of her response to the NURSE Program, assessing her sleep, agitation, and irritability, mindful that this might not be sufficient to bolster her biology. Jeanne set a target date to reassess Diana's symptoms. If her moods didn't shift within two weeks, they would discuss the introduction of an antidepressant into her care plan.

At the two-week checkpoint Diana reported some improvement. She was beginning to feel less anxious, and her mood seemed better. In psychotherapy she was learning that her emotions were normal, given the changes in her life, and that there were ways for her to assert her needs and feel more connected. As she and Carl were able to exchange their feelings about how they both missed their families, he admitted how much he worried about providing for them adequately. This revelation made them feel more like a team.

Diana could respond that she was feeling insecure about being a mother. She had never realized she could be open and honest and say what was on her mind. This couple had begun the process of listening to each other and communicating—the process of healing.

Diana began labor at thirty-six weeks and delivered her daughter earlier than expected. Jeanne wondered if the depression had played a role in the slightly premature labor. Was the baby trying to escape a uterine environment that was incompatible with its growth? Perhaps she was saying, in effect, "I gotta get out of here!" Fortunately, the infant was relatively well, and after a few days of difficulty maintaining her temperature and blood sugar, she had no further trouble.

By eight weeks Diana, her husband, and their baby were doing well. She had no depressive symptoms and felt good on her NURSE Program. We continued to see her in our practice until her baby was almost two.

Every Woman Is Unique

The severity of your symptoms will determine the form of treatment instituted. Sometimes just having someone listen and validate what you are feeling can be enough to decrease the symptoms of depression. This might be accomplished by having a group of women with whom you talk, or by consulting a therapist or a counselor. We encourage you to use psychotherapy, since it provides a place to be heard, valued, and connected and to learn about yourself. It affects the nerve pathways and can reregulate the aspects of their functioning that can be altered.

While using your cortical skills in psychotherapy can alleviate distress, in women whose loading is high and who are clearly experiencing significant depression, the best result comes with a combination of therapy and medications. We must treat the depression so that further alterations in the brain chemistry do not occur.

Planning a Pregnancy When There's a History of Depression

If you have a history of depression, it is preferable to plan your pregnancy with your doctor so you don't have to make hasty decisions to get off medication, which may heighten your risk of relapse. Depending on your particular history, the medications you're taking, and your fault lines, you may or may not decide to taper the medications prior to pregnancy. This is a critical decision to make with your clinician, since not all medications are safe in pregnancy, nor do we have research data on all of them. If you do decide to taper your medications, do so slowly to avoid withdrawal symptoms.

The NURSE Program will serve you well.

- *Nourishment and Needs:* Establish a well-balanced diet. Be sure you're getting sufficient stores of calcium, protein, and folic acid. You'll need more of these nutrients during pregnancy.
- *Understanding:* Unearth the origins of your depression. Evaluate the fault lines that might have lead to this earthquake. Seek psychotherapy if you need help sorting through confusing emotions. Analyze your needs and situation. Recognize what is stressful and what relaxes you. Avoid the situations that make life more difficult. Know what is important for your and your unborn baby's health.
- *Rest and Relaxation:* Make sure to get enough rest. Sleep about eight hours a night, or find time during the day to nap or put your feet up for an hour. Learn relaxation techniques. Enroll in a meditation or relaxation program. Many of our patients have found these helpful.
- *Spirituality:* Find the time to appreciate the spirituality inherent in pregnancy. This is a very special period in your life, but it is fleeting. You will deliver your baby before you know it. Keep a journal of your feelings and experiences during your pregnancy. It's wonderful to share it with your child when he or she is older.
- *Exercise:* It's a great way to reduce stress. But this is not the time to start climbing mountains. Swimming is the best! Stretching and yoga are also excellent techniques to keep your muscles supple, but check with your obstetrician about your particular limits.

If you are unable to taper off all your medication using relaxation techniques and other strategies and find that uncomfortable symptoms have recurred, you may have a more severe symptom pattern. This just means that your brain needs extra help in regulating itself, and you may need the biochemical help of medication. Or perhaps the antidepressant effect of estrogen in pregnancy has not overcome dysregulation in the mood pathways.

If you are on medication in the third trimester, don't try to cut back before you deliver. You are entering a high-risk period—the early postpartum period—when we frequently see worsening of depression. If your symptoms have been absent during pregnancy, they may return soon after you've given birth, concurrent with the rapid loss of estrogen and progesterone.

Because antidepressant medications can occasionally produce some withdrawal symptoms in newborns, it's wise to discuss your medications with the pediatrician who will be caring for your baby. These symptoms are usually transient, and most babies fare very well.

Seeing a therapist through the pregnancy is helpful in getting support. If symptoms return or worsen and you need medication, this is not a failure. Many brain-biochemical mechanisms are associated with mood disorders, and we actually know little about how pregnancy may influence them.

Every woman is an individual, and you need to participate in the treatment that works for you—not some rigid philosophy or a program that another woman used. The important goal is for you to remain well and deliver a healthy baby. This means weighing the risks and benefits of various approaches with your doctor, paying close attention to your symptoms, and taking your personal needs seriously.

Depression and Infertility Treatments

Millions of women are unable to conceive without the help of medications that stimulate the production of eggs, and many others need surgical intervention to place the egg and sperm together. Most programs that treat fertility problems offer psychological counseling and evaluation.

But while infertility can be a stressful experience, consideration is rarely given to women who enter programs with a mood disorder and find themselves worsening during treatment. In fact, it is rarely mentioned that most of the medications used to augment hormone levels or to stimulate egg production generate mood swings and depressive symptoms.

Fertility medications like Clomid, Pergonal, and Metrodin act in the limbic brain—in the very areas responsible for mood stability. They can produce quite severe depressive and unstable moods with tearfulness, uncomfortable physical symptoms, and sleep disruption. Some women also complain that their ability to pay attention and remember is quite impaired while they are on these drugs. If you experience significant reactions to these medications, it is important to evaluate whether you have an underlying condition that predisposes you to a mood problem.

Remember, too, that progesterone can worsen mood problems, particularly if you have a history of mood disturbance (see Chapter 8).

Yet progesterone is frequently prescribed to help a pregnancy become established once the egg is successfully fertilized.

Moreover, by the time you are involved in a fertility program, you may have also undergone a significant period of stress in trying to become pregnant. And you may be facing more stress as a result of the treatments. It can be difficult to sort out which came first, the chicken or the egg! Therefore, it is always important to establish your baseline and to evaluate the quality of your life before and during these procedures.

Be sure to discuss with your practitioner any previous mood or anxiety disturbances you are aware of so that this can be taken into account as infertility treatments are planned and progress. You can tailor the NURSE Program to help address the mood swings and depression you might feel when taking these drugs. Pay attention to what your brain is telling you. Your moods and how you think, recall, and behave will clue you in to what is happening. Care for your brain while undertaking these programs.

Domestic Violence in Pregnancy

We would be remiss if we did not discuss physical and verbal abuse before we end this chapter. Sadly, domestic violence is prevalent in our society. According to recent statistics, about 2.5 million cases of battering occur in the United States each year.[11] In 1993, Canadian statistics showed that one in six women report spousal abuse and that at least a third of these reports involved severe aggression by choking, kicking, beating, or using a weapon.

Dr. Donna Stewart, a physician-researcher at St. Michael's Hospital in Toronto, recently reported that physical violence in a relationship increases during pregnancy and that miscarriage, alcohol, and drug use among the victims are frequent outcomes of these pregnancies.[12] Dr. Stewart notes that although women are frequently struck on their abdomen during pregnancy, fewer than 3 percent report the abuse to their doctors, even when their injuries are visible. This suggests, too, that they are seldom questioned about the nature of the injuries. If abuse has occurred during pregnancy, it generally escalates during the postpartum period.

Recently there has been an increase in public awareness regarding domestic violence and what women can do. Today most clinicians will ask screening questions to ascertain if there is any hitting, slapping, pushing, shoving, or verbal harassment going on in their patient's home. If this is happening to you, it is critical that you tell your caregivers, so they can help you find safety and support.

A woman I treated revealed to me the degree to which women are ashamed about the abuse and will not divulge the information. I had been treating her for postpartum depression after the birth of her first baby. I felt I had a very good relationship with her and that her progress was excellent.

However, when her baby was nine months old, Trisha called to tell me that she would be missing her appointment that week. "I'm leaving the state to stay with relatives," she explained. Severe physical abuse had occurred for the duration of the pregnancy—all through the time that she was seeing me. I was horrified and anguished.

If Trisha could not divulge what was going on, especially within the safety of a good therapeutic relationship, to whom could she have turned? I was angry with myself for not asking. I had fallen into the trap of expecting that there would be no domestic violence in a middle-class, highly educated patient, or rather expecting that she would tell me if there were. This revelation changed our assessment practices; we do not take anything for granted anymore.

This incident was another reminder that pregnancy is a time of multiple stressors, both physical and emotional. These stressors can start to tug at your soul and your brain chemistry. Emotional symptoms during pregnancy can be as serious as medical complications. Your emotional well-being throughout pregnancy is as important as your physiological status and your unborn baby's growth and development. Never let yourself come second in your pregnancy.

Chapter 11

"IS IT SAFE FOR ME TO GET PREGNANT?"
BIPOLAR DISORDER AND PREGNANCY

For many women, mood-swing disorders first emerge during adolescence or early adulthood. Often the disturbance looks more like irritability, impulsivity, and rage, with periods of low mood, than outright depression. The fact that these women often function quite well (especially when in a hypomanic state) often disguises the mood problem.

It is clear, however, that the hormonal shifts of pregnancy also affect bipolar disorders. A woman with diagnosed or undiagnosed bipolar disorder is at risk for a worsening of the illness during pregnancy. The good news is that careful planning will help her remain well during her pregnancy and ensure that she delivers a healthy infant.

Diagnosing Bipolar 2 Disorder
Bipolar 2 disorder is probably the most undiagnosed and undertreated of all types of mood disorders. During the reproductive years, women with this condition often react adversely to birth-control pills and fertility medications. They may develop serious depression during pregnancy and can become quite ill after their baby is born, especially if the diagnosis is missed.

Beatrice, a single, twenty-one-year-old college student, was unaware that she was suffering from bipolar 2 disorder when she noticed that her period was late. She was unconcerned at first, as this had happened before during times of stress. However, when she began to experience nausea and light-headedness, she knew that something was different—she was pregnant.

Scared at the prospect of an unplanned pregnancy, she tried to push away the impulsive feelings of irritability and anger that grew out of her anxiety. But soon she felt she couldn't leave her dorm room to attend class for fear of screaming or "losing it" with someone. She felt as if she were going to jump out of her skin.

She called the therapist with whom she had been working for several years. The therapist tried to help Beatrice understand her sudden and severe downturn of mood based on the unplanned pregnancy. But the experience of hurtling this much out of control was alien to Beatrice. There had been times when she felt up and down, but she had never felt quite like this. She could not believe that her intense irritability had anything to do with the pregnancy.

When she called her parents, they were supportive and helpful initially but then became impatient with her reactive behaviors. They told her, "Pull yourself together and make some decisions."

"I wish I could," she lamented. "Something is very wrong. I just don't have control over this!"

Beatrice then paid an urgent visit to her primary-care doctor. Her pregnancy test was positive, and his response was terse and unhelpful: "Either pull yourself together or terminate the pregnancy," he said. When she shared his response with her parents, they were taken aback. Surely such early adverse reactions to pregnancy must be well known in the medical community. Although they would be supportive if Beatrice chose to terminate the pregnancy, they felt there must be other alternatives to explore. They made some phone calls and finally contacted us. We asked the family to come in immediately.

When Beatrice arrived at our office, she was tearful, restless, and irritable. We took a full history. Beatrice had been an active child, often described as "high-strung and emotional." When her parents put her to bed, she wouldn't quiet down, and she would sometimes awaken through the night. She was even irascible in the morning. When she was upset, she became quite overwrought, unable to wind herself down. She reacted with intense, impulsive emotion to all experiences. Sometimes she felt unable to contain her feelings; an interaction with another person or an event would generate exuberance or misery.

After menstruation began, Beatrice noticed that sometimes she felt quite down and distressed. However, these episodes would pass, and she would just go on. At other times she felt elated, creative, and energetic, staying up late into the night to write poetry. The good periods lasted a day or two and occasionally a bit longer. Then the irritability would reappear.

This experience is fairly typical for a young woman with bipolar illness. Unfortunately, parents and health-care providers often attribute these swings to the moodiness of adolescence.

At the age of seventeen Beatrice began psychotherapy to help her negotiate these periods. Both she and her therapist believed that as she matured, gained a greater sense of control, and worked out her conflicts, the emotional storms would dissipate. But although she was now a college senior, she had not noticed much improvement. The mood changes coinciding with the pregnancy were the worst she had ever felt. And they were compounded by the unrelenting nausea of early pregnancy, a symptom of her body's response to the rapid increase of hormones.

We asked some questions about Beatrice's hormonal history. She told us that she had had a severe reaction to birth-control pills, becoming quite depressed within a few weeks, so she stopped them. She also described "wicked PMS."

"About a week before my period is due," she said, "I find myself getting irritable and short-tempered with everyone around me. I crave chocolate, find myself unattractive, and feel overwhelmed by the slightest little demand. I don't sleep well, and I'm generally more anxious. I have thrown things across the room, broken vases—that sort of thing.

"This isn't a pretty picture, and I am not proud of my behavior. But when this anger gets hold of me, I can't let things go. It just pummels my mind. When my period starts, I feel so much better. I actually feel like something demonic inside me is melting away."

Beatrice went on to talk about her family. Her father's brother had had mood swings, and the family suspected he had untreated manic-depressive illness. He often drank alcohol, but she did not know much more about his life. Over time, they had lost contact with him.

Her father sometimes stayed in his bedroom for days, calling in sick to work. When he retreated to his room, the family just left him alone. They thought that he got overwhelmed with his life, but nobody ever spoke about it. It never occurred to them that this was a facet of depression. When he came out, everybody knew that Dad was back!

Given her family history, Beatrice came into life with fairly substantial genetic loading for mood disturbance. Her reactions and "high-strung" demeanor were not just phases she would outgrow. Rather, they gave us information about the biochemical hardwiring in her brain. Her periods of depression and elevated mood made it clear that she had bipolar 2 disorder. She had been struggling with this condition for a long time. The rapid depression she experienced when on birth-control pills and her "wicked PMS" were other clues that her brain mood pathways responded unfavorably to hormonal shifts. This susceptible brain biochemistry had been primed and ready for a major hormonal event—a first pregnancy.

Being able to negotiate school and now college while managing the difficult emotional roller coaster within was a testament to Beatrice's survival skills and her ability to withstand discomfort. But with this pregnancy she was unable to summon the inner fortitude that had allowed her to push against the driving forces in her brain.

Until her dysregulated biology was treated, Beatrice would be unable to effectively use her therapy and other techniques like visualization, meditation, or journaling. She required medical treatment quickly, so that her symptoms would quiet and she could direct her energies toward the decisions she needed to make regarding this unplanned pregnancy.

Whether or not Beatrice chose to continue the pregnancy, she would require a NURSE Program that would help her through her life psychologically and physiologically. It would include medication, emotional support, and education for both her and her family.

Because her predominant mood was depression, a low dose of Prozac[1] would enable Beatrice to function, eat properly, get to her prenatal appointments, and feel capable of undertaking the psychological work ahead. We started carefully, mindful that we didn't want to push her into a hyperactive state, and she responded well.

Beatrice would be in a high-risk group for severe postpartum depression or even psychosis if she carried the pregnancy to term, and she would need to take precautions against another earthquake. The medication Depakote or lithium would help to maintain her mood health at that time and help her to summon the coping skills necessary to negotiate single motherhood. She continued the pregnancy, remaining well throughout. With ongoing treatment, she has done well, and her baby is thriving.

From our clinical experience with more than a hundred women with bipolar illness, it is clear that some women who have bipolar 2 disorder can do well during pregnancy and can remain off mood-stabilizing medication. They are, however, at risk for exacerbation of their symptoms in the postpartum period.

Treating Bipolar Disorder While You're Pregnant

Although we had recommended small doses of Prozac for Beatrice during her pregnancy, most often bipolar disorders require treatment with mood-stabilizing medications such as lithium, Depakote, or Tegretol. If you have been diagnosed and treated for one of these disorders and come into the childbearing years already on medication, you will need to discuss the management of your medications even before you conceive. That's because some of these drugs have the potential for creating birth defects.

Lithium, one of the mainstays of treatment for the last thirty years, has allowed thousands of people with bipolar disorder to live normal and productive lives. For women, this has also meant being able to give birth to and raise children. And the good news is that women can take lithium through a pregnancy.

As recently as 1993 clinicians believed that lithium was toxic and produced a serious heart defect[2] in the growing fetus at a significant rate. However, some researchers believed the peril to be overstated. Given the large numbers of women who take lithium for bipolar disorder and their high risk of becoming ill without the medication, it was important to properly assess the real danger of staying on lithium during pregnancy.

In 1993 Dr. Lee Cohen at Massachusetts General Hospital found that if a woman took lithium in the first twelve weeks of pregnancy, the risk of having a baby with this heart defect was one in a thousand, rather than one in four hundred, as previously believed.[3] Although these data still tell us that lithium can cause the heart defect, the risk is far lower than previously calculated.

Based on these new data, you can anticipate remaining on lithium during pregnancy if your risk of becoming ill without the medication is high. But, as always, your situation should be assessed according to your needs and safety.

Do children whose mothers take lithium through their pregnancies show normal development later in life? One study of sixty children up to five years of age found that when these youngsters were compared to those whose mothers had taken no medications in their pregnancies, there were no differences in their development.[4]

Many women with bipolar illness are treated today with the anticonvulsant medications Depakote and Tegretol. Both drugs, however, carry potential risks of spinal-column, facial, limb, and intellectual abnormalities. We avoid using these drugs during pregnancy at all costs and, if possible, switch our patients back to lithium. If that's unfeasible, we prefer Tegretol to Depakote. All women on these medications must take 1 milligram of supplemental folic acid daily, since stores of this nutrient can deplete as a result of taking these medications.

On a preventive note, every woman treated with anticonvulsant medications should take 4 milligrams of supplemental folic acid for three months prior to conception and then continue on 1 milligram daily after conception and beyond. Adequate levels of folic acid can reduce the risks of spinal-cord birth defects.

The development of numerous new antiseizure medications, which are being used to treat bipolar disorder—such as Neurontin, Lamictal, and Topamax—raises both new hope and new questions. At the moment there is little information about the new medications and their risks, especially as regards protecting a woman and her baby through pregnancy.

Very preliminary evidence suggests that large doses of alpha-omega-3 fatty acids can enhance mood stability in bipolar patients. Studies remain to be done to clarify whether fatty acids can enhance mood during pregnancy, thereby allowing a woman to remain medication-free or reduce the dosages of medications required.

Heather Wants to Get Pregnant

Heather and her husband came to the office for a consultation. "We have been married for four years, and we really want to have children," she told Jeanne. "But I have bipolar one disorder. I had mood swings during my teenage years and was diagnosed when I was twenty. That's when I had my most severe manic episode and was hospitalized. The doctors treated me with lithium, and I've more or less remained on the medication ever since.

"I had a very hard time with this diagnosis," Heather continued. "I was glad I was doing well on lithium, but I was also very angry, although I didn't know at whom. I wanted to test how I would do off lithium. I also missed the feeling of being 'up' and energetic and having lots of creative thoughts. So I stopped taking it. Six months later I became manic again and was put back on lithium.

"I was pretty bad at remembering to take it every day. I stopped the lithium again after four or five years, believing I was 'cured.' Of course, I got sick again."

Heather's experience is quite common. It's hard at any age to accept that you have a chronic condition that will require medication for the rest of your life. Many young patients with bipolar disorder interrupt or play around with their medications to test what their doctor has told them. Also they may feel so well on lithium, they believe they are "cured."

"I'm currently taking lithium,"[5] Heather continued, "and the doctors told me that it can result in birth defects if I stay on it while I'm pregnant. But recently I've heard differently. What are the real risks?"

Jeanne apprised Heather about the new, revised risks of the medication, but then Heather expressed concern about the dosages. "Will I need more if I get pregnant?"

"There doesn't appear to be a significant need to increase or lower the dose in early pregnancy," Jeanne responded. "Sometimes doses can be divided and taken more frequently during the day."

"What might I expect in the first weeks?"

"You may experience more mood shakiness," Jeanne explained. "You could feel more depressed or have some difficulty sleeping. You may feel a little racy or irritable, but it is hard to predict which symptom, if any, will occur. Early pregnancy is a time of rapid hormonal change, so whatever you experience premenstrually, you might also encounter during the first trimester. But it's likely that the changes will only last a few weeks.

"We could also give you small doses of Ativan, a short-acting anti-anxiety medication," Jeanne continued. "It would help if the irritability becomes uncomfortable."

"Is it possible that I will do better during the pregnancy and not need lithium at all?" Heather asked wistfully.

"I would love to say yes, but in reality you would be courting another manic episode. There is no evidence that pregnancy prevents mania or depression in women with bipolar one disorder. Unfortunately, discontinuing lithium would leave you open to a relapse."

"Even if the chances of a heart defect in the baby are lower, how will I know if our baby has a problem?" Heather pressed on. "I can't imagine having to wait the entire pregnancy to find out. I think I would be a nervous wreck."

"We wouldn't subject you to that," Jeanne replied. "We would advise you to take a high-resolution ultrasound around the sixteenth or eighteenth week of the pregnancy. This new test gives a more accurate picture of the fetus's heart chambers and other organs. At that point you would know if there are any problems to be concerned about."

Heather's husband, Tim, joined their conversation. "So are you saying that we should just go ahead and try to conceive?" he asked.

"Yes, that is what I would suggest."

Heather conceived within four months, and her pregnancy went extremely well. She remained on her usual dose of lithium throughout. But because lithium levels in a pregnant woman's blood are an unreliable measure of her condition, we generally assess how the mother-to-be is doing by her outward symptoms: sleep, appetite, behavior, and mood.

Heather experienced a little mood changeability and restlessness in her first few weeks, so Jeanne prescribed small doses of Ativan, as needed. As Heather neared her twelfth week, she started feeling better. The ultrasound examination showed the baby to be completely normal. Again around twenty-four weeks Heather started having problems sleeping. Jeanne prescribed Ativan for a few weeks, just at night, and this settled.

As Heather entered her thirty-sixth week, she continued to do well. She had a great deal of support from her husband and family. Now it was time to discuss her approaching labor and delivery—especially how Jeanne would manage her medication, given the sleep deprivation she was likely to encounter after the baby was born. The latter is an important issue, since lack of sleep can trigger manic symptoms.

The first four to eight weeks after delivery are the most critical; this is when new mothers with bipolar disorder are likely to become ill. The most successful management of this illness at this juncture takes into account blood levels of lithium immediately before and after delivery and over the first two weeks postpartum.

Typically, clinicians recommend the dose of lithium be reduced by 300 milligrams the week prior to labor,[6] to allow for the rapid loss of water and salts that occurs with the delivery of the placenta. When these are lost so quickly, it can push up the lithium levels in the blood. Nevertheless, during the first postpartum week, it is important that levels of lithium stay in the highest therapeutic range, since lower levels would leave one open to breakthrough symptoms.

Even with these maximum levels, we still sometimes see the emergence of irritability, restlessness, and racy thoughts during the first week. We may prescribe short-term antianxiety medication to settle some of these symptoms.

Heather delivered a healthy baby boy and experienced no problems with mood changes. Her husband and mother took the nighttime feedings for the first three weeks so she could catch up on her sleep. We gradually adjusted her dose of lithium back to what it had been prior to pregnancy, and she remained well.

Managing and accommodating your life to remain well during pregnancy, within the constraints that bipolar illness poses, is a priority. It's crucial to adjust your lifestyle to include healthy eating, exercise, rest, and time to connect with meaningful activities. Taking yourself seriously and knowing what you can do to promote better stability in your brain goes a long way toward enhancing your adjustment to this illness. This speaks to the need for a good relationship between you and your health-care provider. You have an important role to play in living with bipolar disorder.

Chapter 12

ANXIETY DISORDERS IN PREGNANCY

Mood disorders are not the only emotional-health concerns that can arise during pregnancy. Anxiety disorders are distressing for those who suffer from them and, if untreated, may also make it profoundly difficult to function. Yet we believe that obstetric-care providers have not fully appreciated how serious the effects of untreated anxiety can be on a pregnant woman.

For instance, when Eliza complained to her obstetrical provider, "I'm not sleeping, and I feel really anxious all the time. My heart races, and I'm out of breath," he simply replied, "Oh, many pregnant women feel like that. It will go away after you have the baby."

This is not so. Many pregnant women *do not* feel so anxious, and Eliza's situation was only likely to worsen after delivery—not improve. Her brain was telling her loudly and clearly that it was unable to contain the anxiety response. Indeed, because her clinician did not appreciate the seriousness of Eliza's anxiety symptoms and take appropriate preventive steps, her condition worsened after the birth of the baby. Eliza was hospitalized for severe anxiety and depression— an expensive proposition and a tragic one, since she lost valuable early opportunities to bond with her newborn. Yet this misfortune was so unnecessary.

The Perils of Untreated Anxiety During Pregnancy

Eliza's situation is not unusual. Women with a history of panic attacks prior to pregnancy are at great risk for postpartum depression.

Anxiety, whether mild or severe, can also harm the fetus. Research in animals has shown that chronic anxiety can increase the rate of stillbirths, retard fetal growth, and alter the placenta's functioning. In 1996 Dr. Vivette Glover, a physician-researcher at Queen Charlotte's Hospital in London, described preliminary results from her study investigating the effects of mood and anxiety on the unborn baby. She showed that blood flow to the fetus is reduced when mothers experience high anxiety, because the uterine arteries constrict. Since this blood is the only way oxygen and nutrition get to the fetus, anxiety (much like stress and depression) may lead to premature births, inadequate nutrition, low birth weight, or other complications.

Mary, a thirty-two-year-old nurse, found herself in a dangerous situation due to her panic attacks. She had complained of increasing anxiety throughout her pregnancy, suffering daily bouts of indigestion, headaches, and diarrhea. She also felt intermittently breathless. These symptoms made it difficult for her to sleep. She underwent numerous tests, all of which were normal. She continued to feel anxious and also told her care provider that her thinking was clouded.

"All of these symptoms come from the pregnancy," her obstetrician replied. "They'll go away after the baby is born."

When Mary was thirty-three weeks pregnant, her labor started unexpectedly with sudden hemorrhaging from her vagina. She and her husband raced to the emergency room, where the physician on duty told them, "Your placenta has torn off the uterine wall; we only hear a faint heartbeat from your baby. We have to do an emergency cesarean section. Prepare yourselves. The baby might not make it!" The infant survived, but only barely. She spent four weeks in the neonatal intensive-care unit until her lungs matured.

Mary's untreated panic symptoms were induced by a flood of stress hormones into the bloodstream. These stress hormones also coursed through the placenta, causing the blood vessels in the placenta to contract so strenuously that they actually pulled it away from the uterine wall.

After her baby was born, Mary felt more anxious than ever. She had constant diarrhea and could not think clearly. When her baby came home, she fell apart. She could neither eat nor sleep. She became highly agitated and was unable to care for herself or her infant. Eventually Mary became quite depressed, and we were called in to help her.

Mary's life picture gave us clues that she would experience an earthquake during a pregnancy. She had lived with mild anxiety symptoms since childhood, when she experienced stomachaches, dizziness, and chest tightness. As an adolescent she developed symptoms of "irritable bowel syndrome" with pain, diarrhea, and constipation. She always had difficulty beginning a new school year. When she left home for college, she suffered a period of depression, which resolved itself over time.

Mary's anxiety always increased prior to her period, showing a hormonal connection. Indeed, her symptoms had worsened throughout the pregnancy. If they had been recognized and treated, her difficulties might well have been avoided.

Anxiety During Pregnancy

As you can see, untreated anxiety is not a benign condition. Aside from the damage it can do to mother and fetus, we know that other psychiatric problems can also arise from it, such as alcohol addiction and even suicide. Women suffer disproportionately more than men. Symptoms often emerge after puberty and are sometimes exacerbated during the premenstrual phase and at other reproductive events like pregnancy, postpartum, or menopause.

Panic attacks are biochemical, and they do not go away on their own. One theory, put forward by a world leader in anxiety research, Dr. Jack Gorman at Columbia University, suggests that they are triggered by abnormal firing in the old parts of the brain in the locus ceruleus. This brain structure is the main depot for the neurotransmitter norepinephrine, which activates a cascade of reactions that eventually trigger the fight-or-flight stress response.

Also, since individuals with panic disorder appear to be sensitive to carbon-dioxide levels in the blood, and it is thought that carbon dioxide can trigger firing of the locus ceruleus, this may then set off a domino effect on the other limbic structures involved. For reasons we do not yet understand, during panic attacks discharges are fired randomly to prepare you for fight or flight, although there is no danger or threat.

There are still many unanswered questions when it comes to anx-

iety disorders during pregnancy. For instance, we don't know how all
of these neural firings in the brain relate to the hormonal flux that
occurs during pregnancy. We're also unsure whether pregnancy triggers anxiety attacks as it can depression.

To Panic or Not to Panic?

Although Mary and Eliza experienced worsening panic attacks during
their pregnancies, it is common to hear of women whose panic attacks
subside during pregnancy. For instance, Drs. Donald Klein, Deborah
Cowley, and Peter Roy Byrne found in three separate studies that
women who experience panic attacks prior to pregnancy frequently
report improvement in their symptoms when they are pregnant.[1]

Progesterone may have something to do with this. Donald Klein
suggests that because the high levels of progesterone in pregnancy
augment the breathing rate, there is more oxygen and less carbon
dioxide in the blood, so the locus ceruleus receives less stimulation.
Another possibility is that the high levels of progesterone attach to
the GABA receptors, thus acting as a brake on firing activity, leading
to a reduction of anxiety symptoms.

The symptoms may also decrease as a result of the higher levels
of circulating estrogen during pregnancy. This enhances serotonin
levels and other transmitters in the mood pathways. In fact, it is
entirely possible that all of these hormonal mechanisms are working
to some degree to reduce or stop the symptoms of panic in pregnancy.

Although it is difficult to predict who will improve during pregnancy, who will remain somewhat symptomatic, and who will worsen,
Dr. Klein's data indicate that if a woman has not had active panic
attacks in the few months before conception, she will do relatively
well through the pregnancy. If, on the other hand, there is evidence
of symptoms, then it is likely they will persist through pregnancy and
will require treatment, either with medications or behavior therapy.

Identifying Panic Disorder in Pregnancy

In our practice we have identified many women who have had panic
attacks prior to pregnancy but who did not know what these strange
physical sensations were. Many women term their experiences "attacks" or "episodes," or as one woman whom we saw called them,
"dizzy spells."

When Nina developed dizziness, confusion, and nausea, she received high-technology medicine at its best. Although tests revealed nothing abnormal, thousands of dollars later she was told (by a process of elimination) that she might have a problem with the balance apparatus in her inner ear. When she became pregnant, these episodes went away. She thought that finally the dizziness had cleared. She was wrong.

When the "dizzy" spells returned in her third trimester, Nina went into premature labor and delivered a baby at thirty-two weeks. Her infant spent six weeks in the ICU before he could go home. In the meantime, her "dizzy" spells worsened, the fogginess continued for much of the day, and her mood state deteriorated. In desperation, Nina's obstetrician referred her to us for an evaluation.

Within the first ten minutes of our interview the diagnosis became apparent. Nina had a panic disorder and had followed the path we see so often. She had developed panic attacks about three years earlier, although symptoms were limited to the dizziness, confusion, and nausea. When she became pregnant, the symptoms disappeared in the first two trimesters.

Nina's panic symptoms returned in the third trimester and possibly contributed to the premature labor and delivery. If she had been treated for these symptoms, she might have avoided this as well as the six weeks of intensive-care for her infant.

Five years later Nina became pregnant again, but now she was treated with small doses of Klonopin, an antianxiety medication, throughout. She delivered a thirty-eight-week baby who did extremely well. Proper management during pregnancy goes far in preventing the traumatic complications of premature labor and delivery, not to mention saving hundreds of thousands of dollars.

Panic in the ER

Some years ago an emergency-room physician called to review a case of a forty-two-year-old pregnant woman with a "serious psychiatric problem." Sally had arrived in the ER with an increased heart rate, difficulty breathing, choking sensations, sweating, and feeling faint. She was thirty-three weeks pregnant and acknowledged that the symptoms had gradually worsened over the last twelve weeks. Now she could no longer sleep.

The hospital staff had run many tests, but all the results were normal. Baffled, they had begun to entertain the notion that these

were panic symptoms. Unfamiliar with the appearance of panic disorder during pregnancy, the resident told Sally that there must be
something about this pregnancy that frightened her. Sally disagreed.
"I tried to get pregnant for five years, and until now everything was
fine," she protested.

Sally refused to leave the emergency room until the staff gave her
something to help her sleep. That's when the resident called me. I
recommended that Sally go home with a prescription for a small dose
of Klonopin and that she call for an appointment the next morning.

Sally turned out to be a petite, feisty, striking woman, who was by
this time quite amused at the interaction in the emergency room.
"You should have seen them, Dr. Sichel," she said with a grin. "They
were so scared of me. They were tiptoeing around, making these
ridiculous suggestions. They seemed not to understand the difficulties
I was having. One suggested taking the antihistamine Benadryl to
help me sleep. Another said I should try hot milk and honey.

"I told them, 'If it were that simple, I wouldn't be in the ER!' I
don't think they realized what it means to have a panic attack while
you're pregnant. If I weren't pregnant, they probably would have han-
dled it better."

I learned that Sally had experienced mild panic attacks in the past,
but they had been short-lived and she was usually able to use
breathing techniques to get through them. Her mother had also experienced anxiety problems and "rage attacks," in which she would
scream, smash things, and sometimes hit Sally. I would bet that
Sally's mother had an untreated depressive or anxiety disorder.

Not surprisingly, Sally left home feeling pretty bad about herself
and spent thousands in psychotherapy to reclaim her emotional balance. She believed that her anxiety and panic attacks occurred in
response to unearthing and reexperiencing the pain of her childhood—especially now that she was pregnant. She felt that once these
issues were resolved, the attacks would go away.

I did not agree. I knew that panic attacks tend to be a long-term
biochemical problem. As a result of her living with the stress of her
childhood experiences, Sally's brain biochemistry was loaded. Given
her mother's history, Sally might have had a genetic predisposition to
panic disorder. Besides, she was having more panic attacks of longer
duration and greater intensity than ever before. This indicated that
the structures in her brain that set off these attacks were in tumult.

Sally had arrived at pregnancy with a genetic history and life stressors that put her at a higher risk. Her anxiety and mild panic attacks constituted what we call tremors, and these had now worsened in pregnancy. This information gave us some idea of how the rest of her pregnancy and postpartum might proceed. She would need medical intervention to quell the symptoms of her attacks, especially since panic symptoms and sleep disruption could jeopardize her pregnancy by precipitating premature labor.

Sally agreed that she could not go on like this, so we continued the low dose of Klonopin that she had started in the emergency room.[2] Her sleep patterns returned to normal, and the anxiety lifted as her delivery date drew near. But anticipation of the pending labor brought out Sally's fears that she would panic during labor. "What would I do then?" she wanted to know. We shared with her the fact that none of our patients had ever experienced a panic attack at that time, but she was still dubious. "I think you'd better come to the labor, so that if I do have an attack, you can stop it!"

"One of us will come if that would reassure you," I replied, "but it will not happen."

As it turned out, Sally's labor experience went well; as we predicted, no panic attacks occurred. Sally gave birth to a beautiful son, with no complications resulting from the use of Klonopin in the pregnancy.

Antianxiety Medications While You're Pregnant

If you have a history of panic attacks and you are on antianxiety medications, some guidelines can help you manage them during pregnancy. Most women treated for panic disorder are taking benzodiazepine medications such as Klonopin, Ativan, Xanax, or Serax. Others may be taking selective serotonin-reuptake inhibitors (SSRIs) like Prozac, Zoloft, and Paxil. Another antidepressant, Effexor, has also been effective for panic attacks. Of the older antidepressants, the tricyclics (imipramine, desipramine, and nortriptyline) work, too.

Klonopin, Ativan, Serax, and Valium slightly increase the possibility of giving birth to a child with a cleft lip or palate if a pregnant mother takes them in the first trimester. But the danger is minimal. Dr. Lori Altshuler, a psychiatrist at the University of California, Los Angeles, evaluated all the studies available for benzodiazepine medications and found that it appeared that the risk for this birth defect goes from 6 in 10,000 cases in the general population to 7 in 1,000 cases in women taking these medications, which is a very small relative risk.

It is also possible that Klonopin or other benzodiazepine medications taken in pregnancy can give rise to minor problems in the newborn. These may include temporary breathing difficulties, sleepiness, lethargy, or slow suckling. But these symptoms clear in a few days, and there do not appear to be any problems after that.

It is important to weigh the risks of using the medication in the first trimester and later. If you have severe panic attacks and have been unsuccessful in tapering medications in the past, then you might decide to remain on your medications through the pregnancy. If you do need to stay on the benzodiazepines, try to keep the doses low. If these low dosages do not alleviate the symptoms, you might switch to an antidepressant medication—one that is effective in controlling the panic symptoms and has good research data supporting its use with pregnancy.

For instance, Dr. Lori Altshuler[3] used the tricyclic antidepressant nortriptyline to control panic symptoms in a pregnant patient without antianxiety agents like Klonopin. Although the patient was on a steady regimen of nortriptyline, Dr. Altshuler gave her an extra dose of the medication when the patient felt as if she was about to have another panic attack. This technique was very effective.

Because we have so much more data on the use of Prozac and the older tricyclic medications during pregnancy, you might consider switching from the benzodiazepines to an effective antidepressant prior to conception, with the expectation that you might remain on the antidepressant during the pregnancy.

In our practice we carefully evaluate how a woman taking medication for anxiety disorder is doing after the first trimester. If she is doing well, then we might try to taper medications in the second trimester. It may be possible to lower the dose or discontinue medications completely. This strategy can be attempted as late as the third trimester. However, in our experience, if a woman cannot comfortably taper the medications in the second trimester (when she may be getting the most systemic benefits from the estrogen, progesterone, and lowered carbon dioxide), then it is unlikely she will be able to taper later.

Untreated panic attacks in pregnancy are a risk factor for postpartum depression. Because of this, even if our patients manage to make it through the pregnancy without medical treatment, we recommend beginning medication as soon as their baby is born to prevent the worsening of panic symptoms and the onset of depression.

Obsessive-Compulsive Disorder During Pregnancy

About 3 percent of the population has obsessive-compulsive disorder (OCD). Many thousands of people don't realize that there is a name for the repetitive behaviors and thoughts that they have experienced for years. Or they just think all this checking, repeating, and washing is part of their personality. People also don't realize that there are effective treatments for the symptoms they experience. They may have learned to live with and around them until the day their lives are disrupted by them.

The symptoms of obsessive-compulsive disorder often begin when women are in their twenties. In periods of increased stress and when hormones fluctuate, symptoms can worsen. Thus, many women who have OCD find that their symptoms and distress increase premenstrually, during pregnancy, postpartum, and sometimes during the perimenopausal period.

Because many women choose to bear children in the years when symptoms become more apparent and because these disorders can worsen significantly in pregnancy and in the postpartum period, knowing how they are going to fare and getting help for the disorder during pregnancy is very important.

OCD, Pregnancy, and Your Brain

Slowly, researchers are learning about which brain-chemical pathways are involved in the symptoms of OCD. Although the onset of symptoms can coincide with pregnancy, there is still little information about what the triggers may be. Traditionally, psychiatry has explained OCD symptoms as relating to conflicts in a woman's life. However, while a trigger can be psychological, the actual symptoms reflect a purely biological process. A particular stressor that occurred during the pregnancy may have tripped this biological response.

You might think of the process as an electrical circuit that does not yet have an on-off switch. The circuitry is there but requires the switch to activate it. We're still unsure what that mechanism is.

But our understanding of OCD took a giant leap when researchers discovered that the newer SSRI antidepressants (Prozac, Zoloft, Paxil, and Luvox) are the most effective in treating its symptoms. An older tricylic antidepressant, Anafranil, is also useful, since it is more active in the serotonin pathways than the other tricyclics. It is fascinating how we learn about the brain from side effects or positive effects of different medications! The effectiveness of these medications indicates that serotonin pathways are more involved in OCD symptoms than are other neurotransmitters and their pathways.

Since we know that estrogen can have a profound effect within the serotonin pathways, it makes sense that all of the naturally occurring hormonal changes during the childbearing years can put women at risk for OCD or for a worsening of their preexisting symptoms. Even if they choose not to have children, they will be subject to the hormonal changes that occur across the menstrual cycle and before menopause.

The effects of hormonal change on women who have OCD are largely unknown and as yet unresearched. Because of this, what we describe here is the result of our clinical findings and observations.

When Trauma Triggers the Onset of OCD

Doctors advised Elizabeth, a Catholic woman pregnant with four fetuses after the use of fertility medications, to reduce the pregnancy to just two babies so that at least two would have a good chance of survival. Terrified that she would jeopardize all the babies if she did not take action, she followed this advice but was filled with remorse immediately after the procedure.

Soon Elizabeth started obsessing about her "terrible deed." She believed that anything she touched was a potential poison to the remaining babies, and so she washed her hands thirty times a day. She even required her husband to wash his hands constantly, but still she could not seem to get rid of the "contamination" surrounding her. Eventually she was housebound, fearing contagion from the outside world. Her waking hours became a nightmare of germs and washing.

Although Elizabeth had had no prior history of OCD, the enormous stress of aborting two fetuses, so contrary to her belief system, represented a noxious threat to her innermost views about the sanctity of life. We might understand it as a terrible blow to her soul—a blow that switched on the OCD symptoms. "I don't think I can live with myself," she told us. "The joy of my twins will always remind me of what I did. I feel sorrow and pain—even grief. Sometimes I am completely overwhelmed. I pray that I can be forgiven."

We speculated that Elizabeth must have had a genetically determined vulnerable chemistry waiting for something to push it over the edge. And we were right. As it turned out, her mother had had panic attacks. The psychically toxic event of aborting two fetuses triggered an already susceptible brain biochemistry.

Elizabeth required Prozac to help her cope with her condition and cooperate with her medical team. Although the medication would likely minimize her OCD symptoms, the act of terminating those two lives could haunt her for the remainder of her life if she did not deal with it. Consequently, she also needed long-term intense psychotherapy to grieve for the babies who did not come to fruition, in the service of life for the others.

Psychotherapy relied on Elizabeth's strong beliefs to help her with the grieving process. Out of loss could come life. Out of sacrifice could come hope. With hope, in time, she could heal and move on.

Lisa Uses the NURSE Program for OCD

Lisa, a thirty-five-year-old married woman, came for help when she was thirty weeks into her first pregnancy. "I'm in a constant state of anxiety and panic," she told us. "Everything is wrong. I'm convinced that pesticides have hurt the baby, and I'm sure that some of the workmen repairing our house have contaminated my sheets and linens with the AIDS virus."

Lisa went on to describe that she could not get these thoughts of contamination out of her head. "I just don't have any control over them. At first, when they started, I could push them away, but now it is impossible. Nothing I do can get my kitchen clean enough. Now I only stay in my bedroom and no other room in the house. I haven't been into the kitchen for weeks."

Lisa had gained only seventeen pounds by this late date in her pregnancy. She was ill with anxiety and was not eating well at all. She had been told that many women become anxious during their pregnancies.

Lisa had no "history" of any psychiatric illness. Nor had she ever been in therapy or counseling. Yet she had always been an anxious person who worried about her health. "I always dwell on potential disasters," she told us. "I try to anticipate every possibility so I can avoid it. For example, I don't like being closed up or riding in elevators for fear of being trapped if there were an accident."

When we asked about her menstrual cycle and her moods, Lisa replied, "I've always been very jumpy before my period. I worry more and dwell on things more than at other times. I think this has been happening since I was thirteen. Then, when I menstruate, I go back to the usual worrying I normally have."

Lisa's resilience was striking. She had survived most of her life with anxiety and fear, but she had managed. In her family you just did not talk about how you were feeling.

Lisa's grandmother had always had "anxiety," and as she got older, she didn't like to leave the house. She was always cleaning and concerned about germs. Lisa's mother was a "stickler for cleanliness," too. Her mother and grandmother had incorporated these symptoms into their lifestyles so that they appeared not to interfere drastically with their lives. Lisa had a genetic predisposition to OCD, but she didn't know that these behaviors had a name. Although this was the first time Lisa had sought help, she carried many familial and hormonal risk factors for the worsening of her obsessional symptoms during pregnancy and in the postpartum period.

We explained to Lisa her fault lines and the emergence of the earthquake at this time. "Now, you are having severe symptoms of OCD as well as a depression," I noted. "We need to think about beginning medications today because you haven't gained enough weight, and the extent of your worrying may compromise your baby's health." Lisa voiced her concerns about starting treatment, but she also knew that she was not well and felt she didn't have much choice but to try medication.

Her husband agreed. "I've never seen her like this," he confided.

Lisa felt much more comfortable about beginning medications after we discussed their relative safety and how we weigh the risks and benefits. She began on a small dose of Prozac each morning,[4] to be increased gradually, if necessary, to stop the OCD and depressive symptoms. We also started her on Klonopin twice a day[5] to relieve her agitation and panic attacks until the Prozac began to work.

Lisa and her husband returned the next week. She was already much improved. She was sleeping through the night, her appetite had picked up, and she had gained four pounds in one week. Her anxiety had significantly decreased, but she continued to have obsessions about contamination and was still worried that her fetus was infected with AIDS.

Five weeks later, despite the initiation of treatment, Lisa went into premature labor and delivered a four-pound baby girl. Lisa had suffered significantly during her pregnancy, and paltry weight gain might have contributed to this outcome. Lisa was fortunate, though, that her baby did quite well. She had no breathing problems and started gaining weight readily. After four weeks in the ICU the baby went home.

Lisa remained on her medications for the next year. She was a wonderful mother. She always brought her baby to our visits and beamed at her child's every accomplishment. The depression that had occurred in her pregnancy had not returned, and her OCD symptoms were in remission. She actually laughed when we talked about her worry that the linens and the kitchen had been contaminated with the AIDS virus. Those concerns had melted away with the medication.

Loving motherhood and undaunted by her first pregnancy, Lisa soon started to talk about having another baby. But a second pregnancy would require advance planning.

In view of Lisa's improved condition, we decided to taper her medications as much as possible over a three-month period prior to conception to see if symptoms would recur. We would try to take her through this next pregnancy on as few medications as possible. However, we warned Lisa that in view of the previous severe episode, her OCD symptoms and the depression might return, which would mean we would consider using medications again.

A short while after Lisa discontinued Prozac, she became edgier, more anxious, and more restless at night. Since she was showing some symptoms of early relapse, we decided to use the NURSE Program to contain her symptoms. Lisa started relaxation exercises but worried that this would be insufficient to rein in any recurrence of anxiety symptoms. "I'm worried that this anxiety is going to trigger more severe symptoms," she told me, but she was adamant about staying off the medications. "I just want to give myself the chance to be well in this pregnancy."

Slowly, Lisa was able to induce a deep state of relaxation using her exercises. She took care of her nutritional needs and focused on her capacity for wellness through the pregnancy. She put all unnecessary tasks on hold and made arrangements to walk four times a week with a friend. By implementing these important aspects of the NURSE Program, she was in a state of excellent brain health when she became pregnant.

We met frequently through the pregnancy and found no recurrence of her OCD symptoms or depression. She would often say, "This NURSE Program is my lifeline. You've given me the courage to try this again. I really don't feel concerned this time, because I know that if anything starts to happen, it will be treated."

Often the relationship a woman develops with her treating clinician through the pregnancy prevents anxiety and the flare-up of severe symptoms. It creates a vital support system during a potentially high-risk period.

This speaks to the power of psychotherapy, which in some instances works like medication in the brain. In the same way that stress can undo biochemistry and drive it to dysregulate, a supportive and caring therapeutic relationship can confer a soothing regulation of the neurochemistry and perhaps decrease the firing from neurons in the brain stem and limbic area. With proper support, your emotional state can remain stable, even in a high-risk situation.

Lisa went through each trimester with ease and at thirty-eight weeks delivered a beautiful, healthy son. She chose not to breast-feed. We restarted Prozac after Lisa delivered, since the risks are substantial for the worsening of OCD in the postpartum period.

Lisa did well, and at one year postpartum we discontinued her Prozac. So far there has been no relapse of OCD. She knows that she could experience the reemergence of these symptoms at any time. They are just dormant at the moment. Still, her brain is regulating itself, and she and her growing family are happy.

If You Think You May Have OCD . . .

If you think you may have OCD but have never been diagnosed, it would be important for you to put in place a support network before you become pregnant. That means finding a clinician who can prescribe medications and/or a good therapist. We feel strongly about anticipatory planning and education. You'll want to develop strategies with your health-care team to work with whatever might occur.

Make the time to interview and find the right match between you and a therapist *before* you have a crisis, as we know that the disorder tends to exacerbate in pregnancy and after the birth of your baby. Interview a psychiatrist as part of your treatment team. You will need to have a therapeutic relationship with someone familiar with OCD during pregnancy.

In addition, you may find it useful to join a cognitive-behavioral group to learn strategies to help you cope with obsessive thoughts and compulsive behaviors. Ask your health-care provider for a referral, or contact the Anxiety Disorders Association of American at (301) 231-9350 or the Obsessive-Compulsive Foundation at (203) 874-3843. You'll also want to identify friends with whom you can share your struggles and family members who would be willing to help.

If you have already been diagnosed with OCD and are receiving treatment, discuss a medication-tapering plan with your doctor or nurse practitioner. If you are unable to taper off medication completely, be aware of which medications can be safely used through the pregnancy.

The postpartum period can be a time of worsening for a substantial number of women who have OCD. Talk with your doctor about which medications you might use after you deliver. We have found that many women with OCD experience the added symptoms of depression for the first time during the postpartum period. The SSRI class of antidepressants is highly effective in the treatment of both disorders, so you need not despair. With the NURSE Program and with proper support and medication, you, too, can do well during this exciting time in your life.

Part IV

POSTPARTUM:
A VULNERABLE TIME

Chapter 13

POSTPARTUM DEPRESSION: THERE IS A LIGHT AT THE END OF THE PAINFUL JOURNEY

The postpartum period is a time of unique and immense hormonal shifts, psychological impacts, and developmental demands—all of which can impinge on your brain simultaneously. Even the ancient Greek physician Hippocrates recognized the special vulnerability of this period. There's no other point in your life in which all the relevant risk factors coincide quite like this, so we should not be surprised that this is a period of high risk for the emergence or worsening of a preexisting emotional problem.

Postpartum mood and anxiety disorders strike one in ten women who give birth, and recent studies suggest that this may even underestimate the real figures. In a landmark 1987 study Dr. R. E. Kendell[1] cross-referenced more than fifty thousand deliveries with psychiatric admissions over a twenty-year period. He found that the first three months after the birth of a baby were the highest time of risk for psychiatric illness, particularly for psychosis, in a woman's life. It is not an exaggeration to say that postpartum mood and anxiety disorders are the biggest complication of birth today. Yet despite the epidemic proportions of such illnesses, they fail to receive the attention they deserve.

For many women and their families, these disorders are unexpected and devastating, plundering the anticipated joy of parenthood. Although in most countries the focus has been on depression, several anxiety disorders can emerge at this time, as well as the depressive stage of soft bipolar disorder and, as we've mentioned, psychosis.

As with all types of emotional disorders, the illnesses can range from mild to severe. Sometimes symptoms are so difficult that women—despairing and hopeless that recovery will ever occur—take their own lives. This is a needlessly tragic occurrence, since effective help is available today.

Psychiatrists in the later part of the nineteenth century and the first third of the twentieth century believed that childbirth somehow served as a trigger for changes in the brain, which accounted for severe emotional problems in women who had previously been well. Unfortunately, the wisdom of their observations was swept away in the avalanche of analysis-based psychiatry that overtook the practice and theory of psychiatry in the ensuing years. As a consequence, the biological and hormonal components' contribution became obscured. But the time has come to reassert the influence of biology in the evolution of these disorders.

A Time of Dependence

Sadly, in our culture women are often ignored when they cry for help, particularly around the care of an infant. There is a subtle feeling that they are just "hysterical or crazy" if they are struggling. Much of our culture is based on the masculine principles of mastery, independence, and separation. But separation and mastery don't lead to success in childbirth. The feminine principles of connection, care, concern, and community must prevail. The postpartum period is an inherently regressive time, when a woman needs to depend on others for care, food, and safety. She must be able to relinquish her assertive role and allow others to care for her so she is freed to care for her baby.

The most primary relationship a human being has is the attachment to mother. Caring and nurturing blossom within this primal bond. Could this be why women seem to have developed different brains, driven by the important activities of nurturing, emotional connection, and attachment?

In the following chapters we will show you how postpartum emotional disorders emerge in a number of women. We have selected cases that illustrate the range of illnesses you may encounter at this fragile period of your life. Through our patients' stories we will describe identifying markers present at the first prenatal visit, how to distinguish between the different types of disorders, and effective treatment strategies. Using your understanding of these cases and the guidelines we suggest, we urge you to seek appropriate help and discuss treatment strategies with your caregivers should you suffer from a postpartum disturbance yourself. There is no need to suffer in silence.

The Princess's Plight

In a televised interview with Barbara Walters the late Princess Diana spoke of her experience with "postnatal depression." We learned that she had suffered from depression as well as an eating disorder. Additionally, she revealed that she had tried to harm herself by throwing herself down the stairs during the early stages of her first pregnancy.

Diana's courageous disclosures gave women who have suffered similar experiences in silence the impetus to speak up. One participant in a Depression After Delivery support group told us that she wrote a thank-you note to Diana. She was grateful that the princess had shared her story and had provided a brief window of opportunity to validate that depression after the birth of a baby is an equal-opportunity disorder. There is little protection from these problems— even if you are the Princess of Wales.

Postpartum depression is a real emotional disorder that arises after the birth of a child. It manifests itself as an array of depressive feelings, physiological changes, and behaviors such as sadness, loss of interest and enjoyment in life, irritability, feeling overwhelmed, sleep and appetite disturbances, and altered and negative views of oneself. Anxiety and agitation, rather than a sad, withdrawn demeanor, often characterize it. These symptoms may impair your ability to participate fully in your life and in the care of your newborn. As with depression at any other time, symptoms can range from mild to quite severe.

The illness often begins in the first two to three weeks after delivery, but sometimes women come for treatment only many months later. They have used all the coping strategies they could muster just to survive. Or the depression may have a more insidious onset, some months after childbirth, after the stresses of the new experience cumulatively affect the brain. Some women experience mild to moderate symptoms for several months, and then life reverts to normal. In others, symptoms will not resolve and may worsen. But depending on

the stressful situations they face and their brain-chemistry vulnerabilities, all these women are at risk for other bouts of depression after
subsequent deliveries and at other times in their lives.

Usually an episode of depression after giving birth will be the most
severe a woman has ever experienced. In fact, this is what brings
many to psychiatric care for the first time. This is a fragile time for
the self-esteem of the ablest of women and is made much worse by
the occurrence of a depression. You can easily feel that you are failing
at the most "fundamental of tasks"—being a mother.

But where is it written that motherhood is an easy job, or better
yet, one that comes naturally? New mothers are rarely told that this
will be the hardest career they will have and that they will need
significant help.

As you will see, there are several compelling reasons to intervene
early and treat the illness thoroughly.

Proper Diagnosis Is Important for Everyone

It is not uncommon for us to see women around the ninth month
postpartum. They often walk into our offices quite beautifully
dressed, with their faces made up and nails manicured. Sometimes
they maintain such a high degree of care around their infants that
their true state of despair is not readily apparent to outsiders. But
when we talk with them, we discover that they are suicidal—hanging
on to life by a thread. When they describe how difficult the previous
months have been, we wonder how they coped at all!

It's even more distressing to ascertain why they have remained silent about their suffering. Sometimes they "mentioned not feeling
well" to their obstetrician, pediatrician, or primary health-care provider, but because they looked so good, the clinicians assumed that
"not feeling well" was really "not much of a problem," and there was
no further probing. Or they were told that "the blues" were temporary
and would pass.

But as we have seen, when mood pathways spend any amount of
time dysregulated, the brain can learn and incorporate this altered
state. If you have been hanging on by a thread for months, your
biochemistry is "frayed." It may take longer for antidepressants to
work. It can also require more therapy time, because you may have
developed maladaptive coping strategies, which are now restricting
your life.

Waiting so long to seek treatment also poses an increased risk for future episodes of depression. The neural pathways may dysregulate spontaneously, leading to a recurrent depressive condition that may be more difficult to treat. Besides, depression in a postpartum woman usually doesn't "just pass." Although at times the condition may abate on its own within six to twelve months, more typically it lingers and worsens.

Whereas women with postpartum depression can preserve a certain degree of functioning, particularly around their infant, if the depression becomes severe enough, they can withdraw from society. Relationships shut down, and in the context of continuing losses, the sense of failure compounds, often leading to suicidal thoughts and plans. Indeed, Professor Louis Appleby at the University of Manchester in the UK reported in 1998[2] that the postpartum period may be a time of increased risk for suicide, often by violent means. The suicide attempts we see in these women are frequently quite serious, indicating that there is a real intention to die.

Postpartum depression can also have adverse consequences on the family's stability and development. Unfortunately, when it is unrecognized, family ties may rupture. Marital difficulties or divorce often date back to the birth of a baby and an unidentified, untreated mood disorder.

A depressed new mother, although continuing to care physically for her child, may find herself unable to participate with joy in her baby's early development. A great deal of important early interaction with the baby can be lost. Mothers may superficially function, making it look as if they are coping, but the infant can pick up on their demeanor.

Infants need animated facial expressions, soothing words, and confident physical holding to relieve their distress. As a result of these important interactions, their brains make myriad important connections that will affect their mood health and normal emotional development. These may be compromised if you are suffering from a mood disorder that influences the way in which you relate to and handle your child.

What Causes Postpartum Depression?

The risk factors for postpartum depressive illness frequently are present even before pregnancy. In fact, most of the time, if a comprehensive prepregnancy assessment is done, we can predict who might become ill postpartum. As you saw in earlier chapters, childhood and adolescence carry the keys to current biochemical events. Many women who become ill postpartum have come into adulthood with an already vulnerable brain biochemistry, pushed into dysregulation by childbirth's many impacts. Let's look at some of these risk factors more closely.

PREVIOUS EPISODES OF DEPRESSION

Although many studies suggest that postpartum depression emerges for the first time after delivery, we have found this situation to be rare. Instead, we have learned that if we ask the right questions, a woman will reveal that she has experienced mood disturbances before.

Unfortunately, often women don't know that they have a history of clinical depression because they don't recognize their symptoms as such. They use their own descriptions for how they have felt, such as "emotional distress," "struggling to survive," "periods of sadness," "floundering," "going crazy," "immersed in darkness," "living in a cloud," "overwhelming exhaustion," " numbness," or "overly sensitive." Frequently these don't tally with the more formal way that mental-health clinicians ask about depression.

Shirley, a thirty-two-year-old woman who came for help postpartum, told us that this was the first time she had experienced such tearfulness, inability to sleep, loss of confidence, difficulty concentrating, and overwhelming despair. After several sessions of psychotherapy, she realized that the periods of lethargy, oversleeping, overeating, and low self-esteem she had suffered earlier in her life were in fact depression. Because she had pushed herself to function at college and work, however, she had not thought of herself as having a mood disorder. Now she understood that this postpartum depression was a reemergence and worsening of a preexisting problem.

A recent investigation by Kenneth Kendler, a psychiatric epidemiologist at the Medical College of Virginia, Richmond, reveals that twelve is the average age for the onset of depression, but that through adolescence and early adulthood a person may experience only limited symptoms. The most common are sleep disturbances, fatigue, and thoughts of suicide. Other symptoms include appetite alterations, low self-esteem, malaise, and irritability. As you can see, sadness or even the loss of interest in activities, so typical of depression, are not necessarily prominent at this time.

In fact, even mild depressive disturbances that last for less than two weeks hold a significant risk for a more severe episode later in life. In women this more severe episode often occurs postpartum. So the fact that a new mother has not experienced all the symptoms of depression does not rule out previous, albeit milder episodes.

Interestingly, eating disorders—anorexia and bulimia—have a similar risk value. In these situations the HPA axis is also dysregulated (see Chapter 3), just as happens in recurring depressive illness, rendering the brain vulnerable to future depressive illness.

Some women who have been in therapy for depression feel that they have already effectively dealt with their earlier life concerns and are surprised at the recurrence of the illness postpartum. But even though they might have made significant strides in understanding the issues of their family of origin, their biology may already be altered at an intracellular level.

A HISTORY OF DIFFICULT LIFE EVENTS

Women who have been exposed to abuse—physical, emotional, or sexual—often on an ongoing basis, come into their adult years with stressed brain biochemistry. Trauma of any kind significantly induces dysregulation within the stress and mood pathways. These changes in brain chemistry are slightly different from those present in depression, but depression often accompanies the symptoms of trauma. Women with histories of trauma and mood disorder are at risk for worsening of their depressive symptoms during pregnancy and postpartum.

A FAMILY HISTORY OF PSYCHIATRIC DISORDER

Most women who experience a postpartum psychiatric problem have a family member with a mood or anxiety disturbance. Many of our patients tell us that they know their parents had depressive problems but never dreamt of getting help. Others report alcoholism or drug abuse in a parent and/or grandparent. In many instances it is clear that these individuals had been treating their own mood problems with drugs and alcohol.

THE UNIQUE LIFE STRESS OF HAVING A BABY

Pregnancy and postpartum can thrust you into a vulnerable situation, both emotionally and physically. Little in life prepares you for this experience. Becoming a mother is one of the few "jobs" in our society for which there is no orientation program or probationary period. We don't know of any other business that throws you into the water and says, "Well, there you go—sink or swim. We'll see you in eighteen years. No problem, right?" That company would be bankrupt in a flash! Yet that's what happens with postpartum women daily.

Whether or not you're aware of it, "on the job" motherhood training is a crash course in confronting your past, present, and future. Life experience becomes your primary teacher. Even the education provided in birthing groups doesn't come close to readying most women for how they feel after delivery. They often lose confidence and are overwhelmed, needy, exhausted, and fearful. Many require deep stores of emotional support.

Most new mothers describe a staggering sense of having lost control of their lives. This is normal. Your life *is* literally out of control—your baby's needs are in charge! Infants don't wear watches, nor do they carry day planners. They are narcissistic, needy, demanding beings, intolerant of frustration. They have to be totally self-focused; the drive to survive consumes them. You need patience, knowledge, support, and stable brain biochemistry to help you through this developmental process. A lot of good humor wouldn't hurt either!

Regardless of your biochemical status, intrinsic to new motherhood is an exhausting, roller-coaster ride of emotions. This is a time of role change and conflict. Relationships shift, and you must renegotiate your place in the world. You may also be at the mercy of your own unrealistic expectations.

For instance, one woman, trying hard to be an attentive mother and a "good wife," returned to work soon after the birth of her baby, putting in long hours. But between the new baby's demands and her own need to please everyone, Fran got little sleep. Instead of seeing how much she was accomplishing, she began ruminating on her shortcomings. In Fran's mind every other mother seemed to balance family and work without difficulty. Her expectations for what she thought she ought to achieve in this phase of her life were unrealistic. In response to these distorted expectations she began to see herself as a "failure."

Fran began to feel desperate, discouraged, and defeated. She stopped sleeping and eating. When she finally came to see us, she was exhausted and weighed even less than she did before she became pregnant.

When you feel out of control, alone, and unsupported, these feelings may constitute so significant a stress on the brain as to precipitate depression. Perhaps, too, the vast hormonal shifts occurring at this time may render you less able to withstand the effects of emotional stress.

Illnesses in your infant or complicated medical and obstetric situations can intensify apprehension. A family move, a secure job unexpectedly lost, or financial problems can also destabilize your life. Your own parents may be ill or dependent, further stressing you.

Difficulties with your partner related to communication or child care during the postpartum period can also affect your brain. In fact, any situation that increases unrelenting strain on the brain's biology during this vulnerable time can cause it to tip out of regulation and precipitate a depression.

Caring for a new baby requires a high level of mental and physical well-being in addition to a lot of support. If you bring into your postpartum experience a fragile, vulnerable biochemical system, you and your infant may be at risk.

THE MASSIVE HORMONAL SHIFT

Colossal hormonal changes are considered normal during and after the birth of your baby. Yet even though the process is "normal," it impinges on your brain and can alter biochemical pathways, just as we demonstrated (in Chapter 5) can happen during the "normal" hormonal fluctuations of the menstrual cycle.

Estrogen and progesterone levels are at their highest at the end of your pregnancy. As soon as the placenta is delivered, hormone levels drop precipitously. In fact, your estrogen level reaches that of a normal menstrual cycle within twenty-four hours! Recall the vast number of estrogen receptors in the limbic brain. If this hormone contributes to mood stability, imagine how profoundly its rapid removal can impair mood health in vulnerable women.

After the initial drop, estrogen levels remain somewhat low until the pituitary gland and ovaries resume the menstrual cycle. How long these organs are quiet can vary. If you are not breast-feeding, some activity can begin within two to four weeks of the birth of your baby. If you are breast-feeding, the hormones of lactation often suppress pituitary functioning; it may take months for your menstrual cycle to reestablish itself.

Although there have been no formal studies of this phenomenon, it is possible that in some women this prolonged period of low estrogen may contribute to depressive symptoms. It also appears that estrogen may be a factor in enabling antidepressants to work effectively. Perhaps early onset postpartum depressions are harder to treat due to these lower levels. When we have added estrogen to the antidepressants we give to patients with early postpartum depression, we have had some good responses, although we can't be sure exactly what caused the improvement—the estrogen, the antidepressant, their combination, or the placebo effect!

Prolactin, the hormone that enables milk production, increases rapidly as estrogen levels drop, and this may also contribute to irritability and sensitivity early in the postpartum. Milk production depends on a hormonal environment of low estrogen and progesterone and high prolactin.

Progesterone takes a few days to "normalize" after delivery. Its rapid unbinding from the GABA receptors in the brain may add to anxiety. This is why a woman may say, "I feel as though I am jumping out of my skin."

Katherine Dalton, a physician in England, popularized progesterone treatment for postpartum depression. But there is no clear evidence that it is effective, since there is no mechanism by which we can understand how it might work. Indeed, progesterone often exacerbates depression, so it could precipitate or even worsen depressive symptoms in some women. We do not recommend progesterone treatment for PMDD (see Chapter 8) or for postpartum depression.

The shifts that occur in thyroid-hormone activity after childbirth may also be part of a postpartum depressive illness. From 5 to 9 percent of women have abnormal thyroid levels postpartum, and some of them are depressed as well. Usually thyroid medication rectifies the problem, but the depression must be treated in addition to the thyroid. *Measurement of thyroid levels is an imperative part of treatment for postpartum depression and in any other type of depression situation.* If these levels are abnormal, treatment for depression can be compromised.

The Varying Shades of Blue

The "baby blues," also known as "maternity blues," are a transitory, mild episode of mood instability that affects from 50 to 80 percent of new mothers. These women typically describe feeling tearful, sad, anxious, irritable, edgy, and fatigued shortly after they have delivered. Some even have sleep problems. Usually the baby blues last from between seventy-two hours to about twenty-one days. If your symptoms persist after twenty-one days or if they suddenly appear after several months, you should consider the possibility of depression. Also, if the intensity of your symptoms gets in the way of your daily life, this may not be the blues but depression.

Maternity blues fall within the realm of a normal reaction to the physiological changes that occur after childbirth. But the blues are not always self-limiting. Michael O'Hara, a research psychologist at the University of Iowa, has shown that 25 percent of women who have had maternity blues go on to develop postpartum depression. This makes perfect sense. The baby blues are actually a mild form of depression. The brain experiences some degree of dysregulation in its pathways, but in this case it is able to right itself quickly.

Unfortunately, with the shortening of hospital stays to forty-eight hours or less after delivery, today you may experience baby blues once you arrive home, where you may find yourself at the mercy of limited resources beyond those you and your partner can pull together. In addition, in today's mobile society you may have few contacts with female relatives or other experienced mothers in your community from whom you can derive support and validation of your emotions and new experiences.

In fact, while in the throes of the baby blues, you may feel that your emotions don't make sense. Believing that you should be happy, you may think that something is wrong with you. Or you can feel ashamed that you are not coping the way you think you should. If you continue to ruminate on negative thoughts, this may well indicate a progression of the blues into depression.

Coping with Maternity Blues

Given the statistics, it's useful to anticipate that you are likely to encounter the baby blues. This is a critical time to take care of your brain. The blues should be treated with reassurance, education, support, and family involvement. As a new mother, *you* need to be mothered. Turn to others who feel comfortable to you. Ask them to shop for food, prepare your family's meals, or do the laundry. You need nourishment, support, understanding, time to rest, and mentoring. Offers of help should be gladly accepted. The magic of a new baby is intrinsically spiritual, but it will elude you if you are totally exhausted.

Set up a strategic care plan that will help you take care of your brain. This should ideally continue for at least six weeks postpartum and preferably longer. Implementing the NURSE Program has never been more necessary and potentially effective.

Since sleep is essential for the brain to reregulate itself biochemically, we encourage an environment that enables you to get adequate rest. Keep your baby in the room with you so you can easily pull him or her into bed with you for nighttime feedings. (But if your newborn sleeps noisily, move the baby to another room, so you can get your rest.) If you are bottle-feeding, prepare bottles ahead of time and have your partner do one of the middle-of-the-night feedings. Rest periods are mandatory, so be sure to follow the traditional advice to sleep when your baby sleeps.

The Complicated Blues

Occasionally the maternity blues will continue into the fourth and fifth weeks postpartum. Clinically speaking, this is no longer a classic case of the blues, but a form of what we call "complicated blues," which verges on postpartum depression. If this happens to you, we encourage you to seek an evaluation from a mental-health professional to rule out a depressive disorder and also to implement strategies to prevent the worsening of the symptoms.

Samantha called our offices at four weeks postpartum, referred by her obstetrician. In a phone conversation with Jeanne, she described that she had been unable to sleep since her son David was born. She quickly added that David had been admitted to the hospital for a fever of unknown origin when he was four days old. "He had a spinal tap, a bladder tap—it was horrible," she explained. "I thought maybe he was dehydrated because my milk had not come in, but they couldn't find anything wrong. We stayed in the hospital for twenty-four hours. And now I can't sleep. I'm so anxious, all I do is cry." She complained of stomachaches, diarrhea, and overwhelming worry about her son.

As Jeanne listened, she thought that this was a traumatic way to become a new mother—a sick baby and fear that her milk was insufficient. She also detected a sense of guilt. Samantha seemed to believe that her son's illness was somehow her fault. This innate sense of maternal responsibility is common in the early days of new motherhood because of the intense vulnerability that women have in connection to their newborns.

In addition to the "normal" stresses of labor, delivery, and postpartum, Samantha had experienced the acute stressor of her baby's hospitalization. Mired in that trauma, she was no longer able to accept reassurances about David. Jeanne took this new mother's concerns seriously.

Samantha came into the office accompanied by her husband, Zack, and David. She appeared overwhelmed and spoke rapidly while twisting a tear-dampened tissue in her nervous hands. Zack was conscious of David's every murmur and took him out of the infant seat as soon as they entered the office. He cuddled David while rubbing Samantha's arm. Initially they talked about how scary and emotionally exhausting their most recent experience had been, validating that this was indeed a pretty terrible way to become parents.

Jeanne then moved on to Samantha's menstrual history. Her periods had been irregular most of her life, and in order to conceive she had used the fertility drug Clomid, which had caused mood changes. "I felt irritated and exhausted," Samantha explained. "I was so glad the drug worked in the first cycle. I'm not sure I could have lived with those symptoms for too long. The pregnancy, however, was wonderful. We were so happy."

Samantha denied any history of mood disorder, but her father, though in recovery for many years, had been an alcoholic. She thought her mother was fine. Although Samantha couldn't remember childhood feelings of moodiness or depression, Jeanne wondered how Samantha had felt coping with an alcoholic father.

Jeanne made some immediate brain-care recommendations. Samantha's many symptoms were getting in the way of her everyday living. Targeting them would help her restore her biochemistry, not only from the crisis of her son's hospitalization but also from the stresses of her infertility treatment, her pregnancy, and delivery.

The earthquake model helped this couple understand the reasons for Samantha's symptoms and for the treatment suggestions. After they'd charted Samantha's fault lines together, Jeanne began to review each of the aspects of the NURSE Program with this young family. As a lactating woman, Samantha had to pay careful attention to her nutrition and fluid intake. She needed to eat small, frequent, healthful meals and drink eight to ten glasses of water daily. Zack promised to have healthy food and water readily available. He had another two weeks of paternity leave coming and wanted to help out in any way possible.

Rest and sleep would facilitate the healing of Samantha's dysregulated biology. Jeanne also knew that the stressors of the past few weeks, the insomnia, and Samantha's anxiety had probably affected her milk supply. Since David had already sampled infant formula at the hospital, Jeanne suggested that Zack take over one of the night feedings with a bottle of formula. That would allow Samantha to sleep deeply for a longer stretch.

Upon wakening, Samantha could resume her breast-feeding schedule until the last feeding in the evening. If Samantha could sleep in a room where she might not hear David cry, that would help, too. As a former lactation consultant, Jeanne was anxious that Samantha maintain the breast-feeding relationship.

Samantha was concerned about her milk supply. Jeanne discussed the physiology of milk-making and milk-giving and its relationship to sleep and anxiety. Prolactin (which helps create the milk) and oxytocin (which promotes its ejection from the breast) are also affected by stress. Jeanne reminded Samantha that they would evaluate her NURSE Program closely. "This is not going to go on forever," Jeanne reassured Samantha. "As soon as you begin to feel better, you can take back the night feedings. You don't need to pump to increase your milk supply. Just nurse David frequently during the day."

They also discussed the need for daytime rest periods. Jeanne encouraged Samantha to use some of the breathing techniques she had learned in childbirth classes to promote the relaxation response. She prescribed a small dose of Klonopin for Samantha to take at the last evening feeding. The medicine would help decrease her anxiety by treating the biology of the stress reaction. Jeanne hoped that the Klonopin would allow Samantha to get into a deep, undisturbed sleep.

In addressing spirituality, Jeanne explained how important it was for Samantha to take time for herself. She encouraged her to appreciate the process of becoming a mother as a spiritual evolution of great stature. It was also important that she focus on the moment and not on the "what ifs" that were beyond her control. Jeanne suggested that Samantha keep a journal. This is often quite helpful for new mothers. You can write letters to your new baby to share with him or her later.

They looked for a way for the whole family to get out of the house to get some exercise, fresh air, and sunlight. Jeanne suggested they take David for a daily walk. That would give the couple time to chat, as well as get the mood-lifting endorphins flowing.

Jeanne also suggested that they meet for a number of crisis intervention sessions to ensure that as a family they were experiencing some immediate relief. For now her goal was to provide a place for Samantha to develop a trusting relationship, retell the story of the past few weeks, and use her cortical skills to make sense of the experience. After that, they could evaluate whether Samantha wished to continue in psychotherapy. Samantha left the session with tremendous faith that she would feel better.

Three days later Samantha called as planned. "I feel so much better, I can't believe it," she exclaimed. She was less anxious and had slept through the three previous nights. Ready to resume the nighttime feedings, she would try that night and check in with Jeanne the next day.

Everything from that point forward went well. Jeanne saw Samantha for a total of six visits, at which time she spoke about her burgeoning confidence. After reviewing the stress and fear engendered by David's hospitalization, she was able to move beyond this experience. She now understood how she needed to take care of her brain so that she would be available to her son and confident in her mothering abilities.

As you can see, the NURSE Program is constructed with simple, easily achievable goals. Through the course of Jeanne's therapeutic relationship with this family, they would continue to build, enlarge, change, and adjust the plan to work for Samantha, bringing her cortical skills to bear on her biochemistry. At a six-month check, Samantha, Zack, and David were still doing well, evolving as a family.

Samantha had had the complicated blues, compounded by the trauma of her son's hospitalization. With early intervention, however, we were able to prevent further biochemical loading and keep her symptoms at the level of a tremor. If she were to become pregnant again, we would initiate the NURSE Program once more to protect her brain.

A Tragedy Averted

Karen, a thirty-seven-year-old first-time mother, and her three-month-old baby arrived at our office for a follow-up appointment. While supporting Jennie over her shoulder, she beamed at us, "Hi, Deb. Hi, Jeanne." At the sound of our voices, Jennie turned her head, and we were treated to her gorgeous, glowing smile. "Isn't she wonderful?" Karen cooed, proudly turning her baby to face us more directly. We listened for a few more minutes to Karen's animated revelations of her infant's progress.

A few weeks earlier Karen had been severely depressed. She had even contemplated suicide, but now her mood was vastly improved.

Unfortunately, wellness during pregnancy does not predict how a woman will fare postpartum. All too often she can be radiant while pregnant, but her mood can go downhill very quickly after the baby's birth if she carries the pertinent risks. Although well during her pregnancy, Karen, like many women who find themselves in severe emotional distress after delivering a baby, carried one high-risk factor that would have predicted a depression. Her brother, Brian, had killed himself a few years earlier when in the throes of a serious depression.

The suicide of a family member indicates the presence of severe depressive disorder, which other close relatives may carry genetically. Moreover, a death in the family by any means is in and of itself a significant life stressor that will strain the brain's biology.

Karen had told us that after Brian's death she was tearful for quite a while, but she had no one with whom to share her sorrow. Her mother's usual coping style was to deny that anything was wrong and just move on. Karen knew that her mother had experienced depressive episodes at various times but had never gone for help. She would withdraw, wait it out, and then act as if nothing had happened. When Brian died, her mother followed this pattern. The family was uncomfortable talking about his death, so they simply avoided the subject. But Karen was bursting to share her grief and feelings of loss.

Tragic events take their toll in any family, but suicide does not occur in a family where everything is "fine." The silence after Brian's death reflected the family's general inability to discuss distressing topics. They did not have the language with which to speak about their individual pain, or to ask for help. When a family can find the language of loss, they may use it to lower barriers, bear a little of each other's load, and open the door to healing.

Although Karen had denied any personal episodes of depression before the birth of her first child, she knew she was in trouble within days of the delivery. She felt hopeless, believed she was worthless, and thought her family would be better off without her. Everything looked dark within her world. She had no wish to get up in the morning. Dealing with each day was more than she could manage.

When she appreciated what Brian must have gone through, it made things even worse for her. How had it happened that he'd had nobody to confide in about how bad he'd felt? How had the walls between her family members become so high? How could her family move through life in the silence of each other's pain?

I remember sitting with Karen in Jeanne's office. Every movement of her body reflected her desperation. Her face was anguished, creased, and tear-streaked, her head bowed. "Will I ever feel better? All I can think about is what my brother must have felt like when he killed himself. He must have been so alone—like I am now. I'm almost in physical pain, and I'm afraid I'll never be well again." This is a common fear among postpartum women with severe depression, reflecting their hopelessness about their plight. Unfortunately, when women are alone in their illness, they can make serious attempts to harm themselves.

We reassured Karen that we would not abandon her and that we would find a medication regime that would work. We ascertained that she had support at home. Even though her mother could not talk easily about how she felt, she was readily available to help. And her husband assured us that he would take over the care of their infant.

We encouraged Karen to call us day or night. We would see her three times a week until her recovery was in progress. Then we would reduce the visits to once a week, but more could be added if needed. On the days that she did not come to the office, we would speak with her on the phone to provide support and care. We knew that the frequent contact would be needed to bridge the time before the medications kicked in.

It took four weeks for Karen to respond to ample doses of the antidepressant Zoloft. But when this happened, she did well, going on to a full recovery.

Now she was taking great pleasure in her baby's development. "She found her thumb this week!" she told us excitedly. Oh, what a heartening step that is; only a mother knows its significance. This "surprise" has the potential to grow into a wonderful self-soothing measure for the baby when she rouses and can suck herself contentedly back to sleep. No more getting out of bed four times a night to put the pacifier back into her mouth!

Karen was responding to treatment, and we were out of the woods. It sounds a little odd to include ourselves in the ordeal, but that's how it feels. This is a team effort. It is not only us, as the treating clinicians, prescribing and providing care and concern, but the active partnership with our patient in each move along her healing trajectory that makes the difference. In the beginning we take the lead, making the treatment decisions, but as the recovery progresses, women become active in their own healing, and it's wonderful to see.

A mother's smile and joy at her baby's development following a severe depressive illness is one of the thrills we get in the practice of psychiatric medicine and nursing. It reminds us again of the spiritual rewards inherent in our work. We have spent much time on the phone, pulling a family through the dark pit of postpartum mood disorders. There is light at the end of the painful journey—you must remember this.

Antidepressants for Postpartum Depression

Once upon a time, family practitioners prescribed "uppers" for women who complained of postpartum fatigue and then sleeping pills to counteract the stimulating effects of the uppers. They simply did not understand what was happening for these new mothers! Of course, today we have superior antidepressant medications to help women recover from depression. (We discuss them in detail in Chapter 10.)

A woman with severe postpartum depression often needs these antidepressants to help reregulate her brain biochemistry. Jane was just such a patient. "My stomach is in knots. I don't know what I'm afraid of, but I can't make it through the day," she told me. "I had to call my husband home. Something is wrong." Jane was describing exactly how it feels to have an acute onset of depression. She didn't complain of sadness but rather of anxiety and physical symptoms. Her limbic brain was signaling how dysregulated it was.

A slim, intense woman, Jane sat on the edge of my couch, glancing nervously at the baby in the infant seat at her feet. Jane was four weeks postpartum. It had been a planned pregnancy. Thirty years old, she'd had a "completely normal existence" prior to this. Now, however, she had difficulty concentrating and intense anxiety. "I can't eat.

I've lost thirty pounds. I'm terrified. I wake up at four or five in the morning and have such stomachaches and diarrhea, I feel as if I'm going to die.

"This is the worst thing that has ever happened to me. I can't focus, I can't even cry anymore. I don't want to do anything. I feel like I'm going crazy; my brain is mush. At night I'm a bit better, but I'm afraid to go to sleep because I know I'll wake up and have those horrible feelings again."

After taking a history and constructing with Jane her fault lines, it was clear that she had a severe case of postpartum depression. As I discussed the diagnosis with her and her husband, I reassured them that there was every reason to believe she would get better. Jane worried about what she could do to help herself. Unfortunately, her condition was not entirely under her control.

Ken just sat there looking dazed and frazzled. "We'll do whatever we have to," he offered. "I just want my wife back." Ken's response revealed his coping style. He wanted instructions to follow to ensure that all would be well. He never considered that there might be no finite directions, or that recovery might not follow a predetermined path. This is a very scary time in the lives of new parents, and they are desperate to feel better.

We decided that Jane needed to start medication right away. Until we got the biology under control, she would find motherhood difficult. Her symptoms were interfering with her development and her attachment to her infant.

To alleviate the anxiety symptoms she was experiencing, I considered using antianxiety medication along with an antidepressant from the class of selective serotonin-reuptake inhibitors (SSRIs). We talked about how we would gradually increase the dosage of the antidepressants and that we would be collaborating closely on that process.

It often takes three to four weeks for an antidepressant to work. During this time Jane would need much reassurance and support. In our society, we're so used to the "quick fix." Have a headache? Take a pill and it will go away! But these medications must accumulate in the system and take time to work. Paradoxically, this requires a high degree of trust in a care provider whom a woman may have just met.

Jane went home that day feeling devastated. She still did not accept that this was happening to her. At her next visit a week later, she admitted that she had stopped the medication because she had severe diarrhea and just felt "horrible." Her reason for not calling? "I didn't want to bother you."

Sadly, this is not uncommon. Many women have internalized the idea that they don't deserve to be cared for, that others' needs are more important, or that they will just muddle through because that's what they've always done. Imagine how difficult it is for such a woman to live with an illness that demands a different set of responses.

Reinforcing the fact that I was here to help her during this difficult time, I reminded Jane that she had permission to call me whenever she needed. Given the side effects of the first medication we had tried, we switched to another one that was kinder to her digestive tract. We planned a telephone check-in time, so I could support her through the acute stage of the illness, and we also set up another time to meet.

Jane tolerated the new medication well, so we gradually increased the dosage to a therapeutic level. She began feeling better by the end of the second week. But we were now on alert for any exacerbation of symptoms as she approached her menstrual period, which replicates a part of the postpartum hormonal shift. As the hormone levels change premenstrually, they may again deplete serotonin levels, worsening depression symptoms. Within the fragile state of healing, the brain receptors can react to the impact of the normal cycling. Jane did have some mild depressive symptoms, but it was unnecessary to adjust her medication.

Nine months later, still doing beautifully and feeling well, Jane was eager to discontinue the medications. "I am fine now," she said. "All this is behind me." This is a common request when women feel normal again, but I was a bit hesitant. Although the postpartum ordeal was over, it was possible that her mood pathways would not function on their own without the help of the antidepressant, at least at this early phase.

Jane had had a severe depressive episode, and we feel strongly about keeping women in this situation on their medications for longer than a year because of the pathways' long-lived capacity to function in a dysregulated state. In fact, depending on how well they have recovered, sometimes we keep our patients on medications for a few years.

Jane found this hard to digest. She could not accept that she might need the medication for any longer. "How can you tell if my symptoms will return if I stop the medication?" she demanded. We would only know by trial and error. If we weaned her from the medications and she reexperienced the symptoms, that would tell us she needed to take them for a while longer. I was concerned whether she was emotionally prepared for that eventuality.

Jane wanted to try, so over the next few months she slowly came off the antidepressants. But after three months she called to say that the old anxiety and fear were beginning to return, especially prior to her period. Reassuring her that it was not her fault, I said, "This simply tells us that your mood pathways have not yet resumed their ability to function without medication. This is biology and just the way things are, at least for now."

Because we are dealing with the brain and medications, all too often it is harder to accept that some mood disturbances are not under our control and that we can't merely will them away by feeling "strong."

Jane's next piece of psychological work came in accepting this new reality and integrating it into her life. "How many more surprises are in store for me?" she wondered. "All I did was have a baby, and my entire life has turned upside down. Now that I'm over postpartum depression, I may still have an ongoing depressive illness. It just never seems to stop! Are there other women like me?"

Of course there are. Many are in the same situation. But given Jane's difficult family history and her severe postpartum depression, it was likely that she would need antidepressants for some time. We just didn't know for how long.

A year after Jane resumed the antidepressants, she wanted to have another child. We decided that she would phase out the medication prior to conception. However, we were also acutely aware that she could relapse and might need to resume medications based on the intensity of her symptoms. But Jane was now much more prepared for these possibilities.

She became pregnant, and things went well until about twenty weeks, when her symptoms returned. Her appetite fell off, and she found it increasingly difficult to sleep. Worried that she would worsen, Jane decided to take antidepressants again. Responding well to her medications, she gave birth to a healthy son. Jane maintained her medication levels, and this time she had a normal postpartum experience.

If a woman has a history of depression before she conceives (or if she has had a previous postpartum depression) but does well during pregnancy, we usually resume antidepressants postpartum to prevent a relapse.[3]

Medications and Breast-feeding

Many women who must take antidepressants because of postpartum depression worry that the medication will find its way into their breast milk and affect their babies. This is a valid concern, but one that need not impinge on the medication schedule.

Zoloft, for instance, is a short-acting SSRI antidepressant that accumulates at a very low level in an infant's blood, despite fairly significant levels present in breast milk. Dr. Zachary Stowe, a research psychiatrist at Emory University in Atlanta, has reported[4] that when mothers took doses of between 25 and 50 milligrams of Zoloft, no detectable levels of medication were found in their babies. When they took higher doses (100 and 150 milligrams), their infants had minuscule amounts of Zoloft in their blood[5] but might have higher levels of the active breakdown metabolites of Zoloft. Although we're uncertain of the impact of those active metabolites, it is possible that they may influence the baby's brain chemistry.

Stowe cautions that several different factors can determine how much Zoloft will be present in an infant's blood. These include the mother's daily dose, the peak time when Zoloft is transported into the milk, how often the baby feeds, and whether he or she empties the entire breast. You can, however, reduce your infant's intake of medication if you pump and discard the milk present in the breast seven to eight hours after you've taken the medication. This is the time that Zoloft is most likely to be transported into the milk from your blood.

Dr. Katherine Wisner at Case Western Reserve University addresses the dilemma that so many women face when they need to take an antidepressant and want very much to breast-feed. Her findings echo those of Zachary Stowe. She also found that all the babies in her study were thriving and developing normally.

Dr. Wisner and her colleagues feel that the use of Zoloft while breast-feeding is acceptable, but she cautions that "a safe level of exposure to any agent is difficult to establish. Although all the infants are thriving, chronic exposure to very low doses of antidepressants could affect the normal neurological development in ways we do not know about at this time."

Antidepressants from the tricyclic class that have been studied in breast-feeding include imipramine, desipramine, nortriptiline and clomipramine. Negligible amounts of these agents accumulate in the infant's blood, so they are a good alternative to the short-acting SSRI medications.

Prozac may accumulate in the infant's blood due to the long time it takes to be fully metabolized.

Clearly, you and your doctor must discuss which antidepressant to use if you're breast-feeding and its effect on your infant. This dialogue will help you weigh the pros and cons of breast-feeding while taking medications. Your NURSE Program could include breast-feeding as well as pumping (and discarding the milk for one feeding) to limit your baby's exposure to the peak of drug secretion into breast milk.

Some of the other SSRIs appear to parallel the results of Zoloft (Paxil, Luvox, Celexa). But the studies are small, so we can't be 100-percent sure about safety. This is an individual decision to be made with your caregiver. It is certainly important to consider the effects of medication on the breast-fed infant. But you do have options. And it is equally important that you, as your baby's mother, feel the physical and emotional stability necessary to your own and your baby's health and security.

Taking care of your brain in the postpartum period makes good physiological and emotional sense. Because the hormonal and psychological onslaught on the brain is so significant, periods of sound sleep, good nutrition, exercise, and a minimum of demands can go a long way in enabling your brain to reset itself and promote its usual coping abilities over the initial weeks. And when necessary, appropriate medications can lift you from depression and restore the joy inherent in this important time of your life.

Chapter 14

THE POSTPARTUM-DEPRESSION IMPOSTOR:
BIPOLAR 2 DISORDER

Another form of postpartum depression often goes unrecognized for many months—and sometimes even years. Women can travel from doctor to doctor, trying to discern what's ailing them and why they aren't responding to any of the treatments prescribed. But although they seem to be suffering from a profoundly serious and treatment-resistant depression, in actuality they are dealing with undiagnosed bipolar 2 disorder.

Dr. Hagop Akiskal, a professor of psychiatry at the International Mood Center at the University of California, San Diego, suggests that 4 percent of the U.S. population experiences this form of mood-swing problem. Because women's brains contend with the fluctuating effects of estrogen and other important hormones, those with bipolar 2 disorder are especially vulnerable to severe depressive symptoms during the postpartum period.

Any evaluation of postpartum illness should rule out this diagnosis as part of determining the correct treatment plan and preventive measures.

Predictable Patterns

We have learned that new mothers with bipolar 2 disorder often follow a predictable course in the days and early weeks after delivery.

They experience a hypomanic phase (in which they are full of energy and require little sleep) immediately after the birth. This is followed by a severe depression two to three weeks later.

If you have suffered from depression after the birth of a baby, it is critical to determine whether you have experienced these variations in mood. If your health-care provider fails to recognize the elevated mood of the first few weeks, then the incorrect diagnosis can be made and the wrong treatment begun. This may not only lead to treatment failures but might even worsen your mood problems, causing further self-disparagement.

The Dangers of an Unrecognized Bipolar 2 Illness

Over the years we have seen many women in our practice in whom the diagnosis of bipolar 2 disorder was missed. Sometimes their mood-swings were ascribed to PMDD, or sometimes, if the clinician failed to ask about hypomanic mood during pregnancy and immediately after delivery, the more common type of postpartum depression was diagnosed.

Proper diagnosis is essential, since as a consequence of her increased emotionality, a woman with bipolar 2 will often experience disruptions in her personal and professional life. In fact, we believe that many of the women who attempt or commit suicide in the postpartum period suffer from an undiagnosed bipolar disorder.

It is unclear why so many women with this illness are suicidal. Perhaps the mood disturbance becomes severe so suddenly that these mothers harm themselves before they or their loved ones can mobilize to get help. Or perhaps the hypomanic phase of the bipolar disorder was missed, and the illness was misdiagnosed (as pure postpartum depression) and mistreated, allowing symptoms to worsen and the sense of hopelessness to become overwhelming.

We see the most profound and severe depressions in women who have this diagnosis, but we must be constantly vigilant to differentiate women with bipolar 2 disorder from those with pure postpartum depression, because treatment is quite different for the two conditions.

When used without other mood-stabilizing medications such as lithium or Depakote, antidepressants are usually ineffective for bipolar illness. In fact, they can even worsen the condition. Over time this can lead to an illness that does not readily respond to treatment— a tragedy for all concerned.

Feeling Too Well

Melissa was a thirty-two-year-old woman who came to our office eighteen months after the birth of her first child. At that time she had fallen into a serious depression that didn't respond to any of the antidepressants she had tried. She was desperate. Struggling through each day, Melissa claimed that she was nothing like the high-functioning advertising executive she used to be before her baby was born. Moreover, she could remember little about her child's first year.

"That in itself has been a dreadful loss that still feels emotionally painful," she explained. "After Alex arrived, a cold emptiness descended into my life. There he was, out there in the light, my warm and lovely child. But we were so distant from each other, me in the cold and he in the warmth. I don't think I could bear to experience that again. Even now my thoughts can drift back to those toneless days.

"But to tell you the truth, my life still feels dulled. It has a 'so what?' quality. I can grab hold of a good feeling for a few hours; my hopes are up; maybe this thing is eventually going away. But then it dissipates. Now, eighteenth months later, here I am, with my sad and complicated stories and medications that don't work. It's really quite a mess."

This was not a good situation. Eminent doctors had seen and treated Melissa, and I was unsure I could add much. Perhaps she was one of those unfortunate women who just never reclaim their wellness after the birth of a child. But hers was a moving story. I thought perhaps I might pick up something that others had missed, so told her I would give it a try.

The first step was to establish the diagnosis. "Has anyone ever told you what type of depression you have?" I asked.

"No, I have just been called 'major depression,' " she lamented. "My name changed from Melissa to major depression! I have become a disorder! I have lost my identity in so many ways after having this baby. Why? Are there different types of mood problems?"

"Yes, and they're usually treated differently."

I proceeded to talk with Melissa about her childhood, parents, adolescence, menarche, and PMDD. It turned out that her father was moody, "but that was just who he was," Melissa explained. "We learned to live with his ups and downs."

I asked about her moods at other times, and whether she had periods of increased creativity, when she stayed up late and needed less sleep or if she ever felt confident to a point that the experience felt unreal.

Melissa acknowledged that she did have periods of elevated mood when she became highly creative and her whole world sparkled. "Well, yes, but that's just how I am. Is that abnormal? The energy comes from inside me. It's like a motor running. I could always do more than other kids at school. Actually, it was neat!"

"Did this ever change?" I wondered.

"Yes. Sometimes I felt drained. I would crash for a few days, maybe a little longer, but then get up and feel better—sort of recharged. But I always put it down to having done so much that I needed time to refuel. Sometimes I could be out of sorts, fussy, and irritated. It often seemed that I could get angry quite easily."

As we continued to talk, Melissa recalled that as a teenager and in her twenties she began to experience changes in mood before her period. She would feel quite down, edgy, and irritable. "I have a short fuse at those times," she told me. "It's not at all pleasant!" And she acknowledged that she had had significant problems with mood-swings on an oral birth-control pill years earlier. Because of those side effects she had stopped the Pill.

Melissa's description of her symptoms painted a fairly typical picture of bipolar 2 disorder. She'd had episodes of a persistently elevated, expansive, creative mood—hypomania. These were usually short-lived—only days long—and stopped spontaneously with a switch into a normal or depressed mood.

When I asked how she had fared during the pregnancy, Melissa said, "Oh, I felt extremely well. In fact, I felt as well as I did during my active periods. I never got tired, until maybe the last couple of weeks."

It seemed as though Melissa's mood during pregnancy was unusual; she had too much energy. Perhaps she was mildly hypomanic at that time, possibly as a result of the antidepressant effect of pregnancy's high levels of estrogen.

She then described exactly what I expected to hear. "During the first two weeks after Alex's birth, I felt extraordinary. I came home, cared for him, and did all the washing, cooking, cleaning, and shopping single-handedly. I had a tremendous amount of energy. I was on top of the world, managing everything. It almost seemed as if there wasn't enough to do. I couldn't understand why my friends had told me they were so tired after having their babies. I wasn't getting very much sleep, being up with the baby at night, but I wasn't tired. I didn't even need naps. I thought I was superwoman. Motherhood was just a breeze. 'Wow,' I remember saying to my husband. 'This is great! Maybe we can have another baby much sooner than we thought!'

"Then suddenly it all changed. I woke up one day feeling slow and down. I had to push myself to get out of bed. 'Oh, I've been doing too much,' I told myself. 'I probably need a day of rest to catch up.' But things got worse, and within a week I was really depressed. I lost my energy and my drive. I wanted to sleep most of the time, and I didn't feel like eating. It never went away. Days turned into weeks, and I searched for a doctor who could explain what was going on and help me.

"The psychiatrists gave me all sorts of interpretations about my family of origin, including my overdependence on my mother and father, my inability to separate, my lack of readiness to accept the new responsibility of a child in my life, and many more. But I couldn't connect to these. If they were true, how was it that I had managed my life so successfully before having Alex? It didn't make sense."

By the time Melissa came to me, she had tasted every antidepressant available. None was successful.

Unfortunately, these well-meaning clinicians had asked about past psychiatric history and depression, but no one had carefully probed Melissa's pregnancy and postpartum period, looking specifically for a period of elevated mood. And Melissa had told them that she had always been well until now. The depression had just come out of the blue. According to Melissa, she had no history of anything!

It's easy to see how the diagnosis was missed. Because an accurate, detailed history had not been taken, at first glance it appeared that Melissa had done well in her life and through the pregnancy. Then, bingo, at two weeks postpartum she had tumbled headlong into a depression that seemed to arise from nowhere. However, Melissa's depression was quite predictable, because she'd had symptoms of a bipolar 2 disorder all along.

The other doctors had only asked her, "How did you do during pregnancy?" without investigating the possibility that she'd been *too well* when she responded "Great, fine!" And in taking a postpartum history, nobody had questioned her about how she'd felt *day by day* after her delivery.

It was no wonder that the antidepressants had made little difference. Melissa needed to take mood-stabilizing medication coupled with antidepressants. She responded very well to Depakote. We cautiously added a tiny dose of the antidepressant Paxil after a few months because she experienced some depression. Twenty-one months after Alex's birth, Melissa was finally well.

Melissa Tries Again

Now Melissa wanted to have another child. I thought she might be able to go through at least part of a second pregnancy off medication, since she had done so well through the first one. Depakote causes serious birth defects (see Chapter 11), so we want our patients to be off Depakote during pregnancy.

In fact, there is a good chance that a woman with bipolar 2 disorder will remain well off medication, especially through the first twelve weeks of pregnancy, if she has diminished her dosage step by step. We term this "buying remission time." (In contrast, a woman with bipolar 1 disorder is much less likely to remain well off medications.)

Melissa needed to taper her mood-stabilizing medications slowly over four to six weeks in order to be medication-free when she conceived. It's important to do this gradually. Anything shorter than four weeks can precipitate another severe episode of the illness. In our practice we recommend weekly visits and a custom-designed NURSE Program during this vulnerable time so that we're able to intervene if symptoms exacerbate.

After the first trimester a decision can be made to restart medications, depending on a woman's emotional wellness. Given how well she had felt during her first pregnancy, there was a good chance either that Melissa could remain well throughout this second pregnancy or that she might have mild symptoms. I would see her frequently to assess whether she was headed toward a relapse. Should she begin to have symptoms, I might start her on lithium, because it is safer for the fetus than Depakote.

It's important to note here that every woman's case is unique. Although I made these recommendations for Melissa, for other patients I might recommend different medications or none at all. There are no guarantees as to how a woman will actually fare during pregnancy. If you have this disorder and problems do arise, you and your physician must evaluate and respond to the situation within the parameters of safety for you and your fetus.

Can You Breast-feed While on Mood Stabilizers?

Melissa had wanted to breast-feed her second child, but we could not recommend it, especially because we had put her back on a mood stabilizer after her daughter's birth to prevent a relapse of her depressive symptoms.

Lithium accumulates in a baby's blood to a significant level. Since currently we have no information about the impact of lithium on a baby's developing brain, we prefer to see mothers on lithium use formula to feed their babies. Depakote does not appear to accumulate in an infant's blood, so it provides an alternative to lithium.

During the pregnancy you may have no choice but to continue on your medication, and your fetus may be exposed to it. But since an infant's brain development continues after delivery, it is just as well to stop the exposure to these medications, if possible. Forgoing breast-feeding, while certainly a loss, outweighs the potential risk of your becoming ill again. It is far more important for you to be well and capable of establishing a warm and loving relationship with your child.

Melissa's situation occurs far more frequently than we can imagine, and this is tragic. Most of the women whom we have met and diagnosed with bipolar 2 illness postpartum have described their lives prior to this episode as perfectly normal, but with the added feature of mood-swings. Like Melissa, they have always thought, "This is just who I am." They never imagined that they were at risk for a severe depression after the birth of their babies. But they were, in fact, particularly vulnerable.

Having a depression that is resistant to antidepressant medications often leaves a new mother feeling desperate and despairing. "Nothing works for me," she thinks. "I'm a hopeless failure." If you recognize yourself in Melissa's story, it's important to consider how pregnancy and postpartum will affect your brain and begin to develop regimens to help you negotiate these periods with better mood health.

Chapter 15

POSTPARTUM ANXIETY DISORDERS

Depressive disorders are not the only mood problems that can occur during the postpartum experience. The onset or exacerbation of panic or anxiety disorder is common at this time, too. If you were suffering from an anxiety disorder prior to your pregnancy, it can worsen after you deliver. Even if the disorder abated while you were pregnant, it may still recur postpartum, often accompanied by depression.

The good news is that postpartum anxiety disorders can be successfully treated with antianxiety and antidepressant medications and therapy. You will find much useful information on this kind of treatment below and in Chapter 12 on anxiety disorders during pregnancy.

The Living Nightmare of Postpartum OCD

Pamela was thirty-nine when she first became pregnant. She and her husband had delayed having children because of their careers. Then, when they were finally ready, they coped with infertility problems. After three years of trying, and with the help of reproductive technology, Pamela became pregnant. She felt emotionally well during the whole pregnancy, and although her labor was long, she delivered a healthy baby boy weighing eight pounds.

Pamela recalled the excitement that welled within her moments after her son's birth when the nurse laid him on her chest. "Nicholas was the most beautiful baby I'd ever seen," she told us. "I couldn't take my eyes off him. The whole event was unbelievable and magical." Pamela experienced an intense early bonding to her infant.

But during the first night in the hospital she began to feel restless, anxious, and tired. When the nurse brought Nicholas to her in the morning, a terrifying thought crossed her mind as she gazed on him. She envisioned how blood would pour from his head if she threw him to the floor. Horrified by this specter, she tried to push it away. What could this incomprehensible vision mean? But then another followed. "I could throw him out the window." She again saw bloody images. She quickly placed Nicholas in his bassinet and called the nurse to return him to the nursery.

She hoped she would be fine after some sleep. But when she woke the next day, the thoughts returned. She began sweating and breathing hard. Her heart pounded. She wondered how she could go home feeling like this, but decided that all she needed was sleep. Surely all mothers feel this way, and no one talks about it.

At home, gruesome irrational thoughts whirled in her mind through all her waking hours. She walked into the kitchen, saw the knives, and visualized herself stabbing Nicholas. She thought about how easy it would be to push his little face under the water when she was giving him a bath. Try as she might, she had little control over these intrusive images; they were constant. Deep within her, she knew she loved this child and would never hurt him, but self-doubt crept in as these terrifying thoughts continued, beyond her power to control them. She became anxious about being left alone with him.

Admitting to her husband that she was having "odd" thoughts about their baby, Pamela pleaded with him not to leave them alone. He couldn't understand this request, assured her she would be fine, and left for work. It was impossible for him to imagine the despair that had prompted Pamela to ask for help. Each day after he went to work at 7:00 A.M., she put the baby in his car seat and took to driving around town. Where did she go? "Anywhere. I just drove and drove. I knew that I must not be alone with this baby. I couldn't trust my mind."

By 9:00 A.M., she felt she could safely visit a friend. "This would prevent me from acting out any of these horrible thoughts toward Nicholas," she explained.

Pamela knew that her thoughts made no sense at all. She carefully asked her friends if they'd had any "funny" mental images after their babies were born. "No," they replied. "What are you talking about?" Feeling isolated and appalled at herself, she experienced an over-whelming sadness engulfing her. She lost her appetite and quickly dropped to ten pounds below her prepregnancy weight.

Pamela began to avoid Nicholas, inventing all kinds of excuses not to be alone with him. "Something is terribly wrong," she pleaded with her mother and husband. "I think I am losing my mind." She couldn't sleep, think, or plan. Although she knew that her thoughts were ir-rational, she couldn't stop them. She began to wonder if anything prevented her from becoming one of those mothers who kill their babies. "How am I any different?" she asked herself.

"My hold on sanity tenuous, I called my obstetrician," she contin-ued. "I tried to tell him about these funny thoughts, and that I wasn't coping. I was so afraid I was going to lose control."

Her doctor told her that he had never heard of this. "You sound as though you're just exhausted," he responded. "Maybe you need a vacation. Or maybe you weren't cut out to be a stay-at-home mom. Perhaps you should return to work."

Pamela couldn't accept what he was saying. "I was screaming in-side, only silently," she said. "My family didn't understand, my friends didn't understand, my doctor didn't understand—nobody was hearing me. For the first time I believed I would be better off dead. When killing myself seemed like the only way out of this ordeal, I decided to admit myself to a hospital. My husband still didn't get it, but he went along with my decision. I've never felt so alone in my life. The birth of my beloved child, planned for years, had become a living nightmare. This was my postpartum experience."

Another of our patients, Sara Kirschenbaum, described her anguish poignantly in an article published in *Mothering* magazine:

Around five weeks postpartum I began to have serious doubts that I could care for him. I scrutinized baby books—reading and rereading their single paragraph on postpartum blues. They talked about the big life changes, being emotional, crying at the drop of a hat. They em-phasized getting sleep and eating well. These words seemed frivolous and irrelevant. I envied the women for whom these words were writ-ten. They were certainly not relevant to me. . . .

. . . but the worst were the images that seemed to come from no-where into my mind and ricochet there obsessively all day and night. Images of throwing this most precious being onto the floor. Of severing his limbs. Of baking him in the oven. Of sexually abusing him. They certainly hadn't mentioned this in the chapter on the baby blues!

No "they" hadn't. And that's because neither Sara nor Pamela was suffering from the baby blues. Instead they had postpartum obsessive-compulsive disorder.

Bonding, Postpartum OCD, and Your Brain

We don't accept that the symptoms Pamela and Sara describe have anything to do with latent or hidden hostilities toward their babies. In fact, when we hear professionals suggest this analytical interpretation as a cause or explanation of postpartum OCD, we believe that it devalues and in essence victimizes mothers who suffer from this disorder. It blames them for something that's not their fault and entirely out of their control.

The old psychoanalytic explanation is based on a complete ignorance of the unique hormonal and brain-chemistry changes that occur after delivery. Nevertheless, this is still the rationale that many health-care providers offer these unfortunate moms.

In fact, the mechanisms underlying the onset of these bizarre thoughts relates intimately to the cascade of brain hormones that trigger bonding—a mother's special emotional connection to her child so vital for the infant's care and survival. The ability to attach and remain the parent-caregiver is the remarkable step that has marked our evolution from reptiles to mammals.

As Paul MacLean, an eminent neuroscientist at the National Institutes of Mental Health, proposes, family-centered behavior is established by suckling, interacting with, and playing with the infant. Mothers provide most of this care and nurturing. But appropriate maternal behavior is not learned, and it doesn't just instinctively "happen" either. Rather, it depends on a complex series of biochemical activities in the brain.

Although little is known about how maternal behavior occurs in humans, we are learning about how it works in the brains of rats. A vital location for a rat's maternal behavior is the first primitive layers of the cortex that surround the limbic brain, known as the cingulate gyrus. As you may recall from Chapter 3, this is also an area of the cortical brain involved in depression.

In 1955 Dr. John Stamm at California Institute of Technology found that when the cingulate gyrus was destroyed in pregnant rats, they lacked the necessary maternal behaviors to care for their pups, and most of their offspring died. In the 1960s Dr. Burton Slotnick, a research psychologist at the University of Illinois, confirmed these findings, showing that besides ignoring their pups after delivery, the altered rat mothers didn't prepare their nests in the last days of pregnancy. Paul MacLean's research group at the National Institute of Mental Health has corroborated that indeed the cingulate gyrus is a specific brain location where maternal behavior is activated, at least in rats.

The possession of an intact cingulate gyrus is not, however, the only important element that determines effective maternal behavior. Nurturing and attachment also depend on the operation of intact hormonal mechanisms both in the last weeks of pregnancy and after delivery. This sequence of events relies on specific estrogen levels, which in turn prepare receptors in the cingulate gyrus for the action of oxytocin.

Oxytocin is the peptide hormone that induces contractions during labor and the expulsion of milk from the breasts. In addition, it is one important biochemical means by which nurturing and attachment are initiated. Dr. Thomas Insel, a biochemist the National Institute of Mental Health, has found that the cingulate gyrus is rich with oxytocin receptors that activate the attachment process.

Not only are an intact cingulate gyrus, oxytocin, and good levels of estrogen required, but it also appears that a particular gene promoting maternal behavior must function for the full process of attachment to occur. Preliminary work by Dr. Jennifer Brown and her colleagues at Children's Hospital in Boston suggests that if this gene is inactivated in mice, they will be profoundly deficient in their ability to nurture their young. Even though nurturing behavior can also be learned, these genetically altered mice were unable to learn it when exposed to it.

It is possible that similar mechanisms constitute part of the attachment process in women. If the cascade of hormonal effects does not activate the nurturing gene, perhaps the bonding between mother and baby will be delayed. We have also seen that some mothers never attach to their children, but this may be determined by other complex factors that may be both genetic and learned.

When there is no maternal behavior in mice, the pups die. In humans, if bonding does not occur soon after delivery, babies are still cared for until maternal behavior kicks in. In most situations, learning and experience help to foster attachment.

What does all of this have to do with mothers who experience devastating irrational thoughts postpartum? Well, when you consider the characteristics of normal maternal behavior, you will note that in a paradoxical way it resembles obsession. A mother's intense preoccupation with her infant's constant needs and her hypervigilance around potential dangers begin soon after delivery. Feeding, cleaning, and continual checking ensure that this dependent little creature has the best chance of survival. At any other time in life such close attention to another's needs might be considered abnormal.

In the 1950s Dr. Donald Winnicott, a British pediatrician and psychiatrist, observed this special mother-baby connection. He coined the phrase "primary maternal preoccupation" to describe it. This is a time of intense union between mother and infant. He even went so far as to suggest that it resembled psychotic behavior—the boundaries between baby and mother are blurred, and mothers become fixated on their infants.

We know, of course, that this is not psychotic behavior but absolutely normal within the context of new motherhood. In fact, when a woman is *not* preoccupied with her newborn, it evokes concern in those who observe her detached behavior.

It is quite possible that oxytocin's kindling of this intense engrossment with the infant may have a lot to do with the obsessional nature of normal maternal behavior. But in women who experience postpartum OCD the brain may overshoot this process, resulting in terrifying fears of harm befalling the baby.

Many women state that when they first see their newborns, they are unmoved, often because they are exhausted or because the baby's appearance doesn't match their expectations. But much like Pamela, mothers with postpartum OCD often report an intense, immediate bonding with their infants. Their comments are uniformly remarkable for their passionate adoration: "He was magical" or "I had never felt so adoring of anything in my life" or "I loved her intensely from the moment I saw her" or "I couldn't bear to see him in anyone else's arms."

Mother and newborn seem to be Superglued together, but an ironic twist is about to occur. For as these moms describe their intense preoccupation and heightened vigilance about anything that could pose a potential threat, it is as if their protective antennae are up and roving, fixing on situations in which harm might befall their infants. Naturally, objects like knives, stairs, ovens, open windows, bathwater, or the infant's exposed genitalia can provoke concern about potential harm.

In normal situations the mother's identification of a threat is followed by her move to protect her newborn. In postpartum OCD, however, the thoughts regarding the danger and protection begin, but somehow they don't find their way through to their logical conclusion. For instance, the thought about the harm that can be inflicted by a knife gets biochemically stuck in a groove, much like a phonograph needle gets stuck in a scratch on an old record, repeating the same refrain endlessly. The frightening images and thoughts repetitively thunder in the mother's mind, triggering a cascade of anxiety and agitation, but because of the biochemical dysregulation she has no capacity to silence the relentless images.

These bizarre thoughts, therefore, represent an excess of a mother's normal attachment and protective instinct. Another hormonal shift after delivery may also contribute to these problems. As mood-stabilizing estrogen precipitously falls postpartum, serotonin receptors and levels may be compromised. But the full emergence of postpartum OCD is probably contingent on much more than just oxytocin and estrogen. There may well be other hormonal shifts about which we still know very little that also influence or trigger OCD symptoms.

A Widespread Problem

We are unsure exactly how many women experience mild, moderate, or severe postpartum OCD. Obsessive-compulsive disorder affects 3 percent of the general population; that's about seven to ten million people in the United States. More than half are women. Since women between the ages of eighteen and forty-four are most vulnerable to mood and anxiety disorders, probably a vast number of new mothers experience this problem. Because risk groups include women who have obsessional living styles (they worry excessively and are overly concerned with being organized, neat, and prepared), the numbers may well exceed even our most conservative estimates.

We have seen more than two hundred women with this disorder in our practice alone, so we believe that there may be many thousands of others who experience postpartum OCD but who suffer in silence or who are incorrectly diagnosed and treated.

Treatments for Postpartum OCD

Medication choices generally include one of the SSRI antidepressants or Anafranil, a particularly serotonergic tricyclic antidepressant. We usually begin at low dosages and raise the level of medication until the symptoms disappear or are minimal. Antianxiety medications such as Klonopin, Ativan, or Buspar may be needed to augment the effects of the SSRIs. We have found that group therapy for these women is also very helpful. They feel validated when they realize that other women have the same problem.

Some of the women who have endured postpartum OCD find that they are able to go off the medication after a year or so. They do, however, report occasional episodes of premenstrual anxiety and that an odd thought pops into their minds from time to time. Other women are unable to discontinue the medication therapy. Like many women with postpartum depression, they go on to have recurrent OCD. There does not appear to be any way to predict how a person will fare. It's a question of time, and we usually take a wait-and-see attitude.

OCD appears to be a recurrent problem, however, for sufferers during subsequent pregnancies and postpartum experiences. Every woman with postpartum OCD with whom we have worked has experienced a recurrence during succeeding pregnancies. As a result we recommend that you initiate preventive anti-OCD medication therapy very quickly after the birth of your next baby, without waiting to see what's going to happen. It's just too risky, and you deserve to have a balanced, relaxed postpartum experience.

We allow our patients to breast-feed their babies while taking antianxiety medications if the doses are low. Others breast-feed while taking an appropriate SSRI or tricyclic antidepressant.

If You Had OCD Before You Became Pregnant

Now thirty-two, Pauline had experienced mild OCD symptoms since she was eighteen. They took the form of her washing her hands several times a day, but she had simply worked this routine into her life. She believed that she was extremely assiduous about germs and dirt. Additionally, she checked her electrical appliances (to make sure they were off) a few times prior to leaving for work or going to bed. Also, the objects on her chest of drawers had to be lined up in a specific order before she felt enough peace of mind to fall asleep at night.

On the few occasions when she was unable to carry out her hand-washing, checking, or arranging rituals, she became distressed and anxious. She felt a tension building within her, which dissipated when she could set everything right.

During her pregnancy these mild symptoms persisted and then worsened as she neared the date of delivery. "I began to wash my hands maybe thirty or forty times a day," Pauline told us. "I was afraid that if I didn't, I would somehow contaminate the baby in my uterus. Then, after Jessica was born, when visitors came into the house, I insisted that they take off their shoes. I had them wash their hands, turn off the tap with their elbows, and then dry their hands on a fresh towel. But even this didn't reassure me about the germs." There was a direct relationship between Pauline's laundry pile and the numbers of visitors she had each week!

"I kept everybody at a distance from Jessica, fearful that they would breathe on her and contaminate her. I even went so far as to purchase surgical masks for people to fulfill this obsession.

"My husband became furious with me. He said he couldn't live like this, but truly, I couldn't help it. We were at loggerheads all the time. Then I became more and more down. I cried every day. I slept terribly, waking every hour. By four A.M., I couldn't get back to sleep, even though Jessica didn't wake up until seven. I needed help desperately. My husband imagined I was going to live that way forever and that our relationship was over."

Pauline entered her pregnancy with preexisting obsessive-compulsive disorder. When she came for help, she was unable to function normally, and she was at her wits' end.

We started Pauline on Anafranil, an antidepressant that also works well in the treatment of OCD. Beginning on a low dose, we pushed up the levels every few days until Pauline's symptoms disappeared. This physiological process took about six weeks. During that time Pauline came in for weekly therapy, and we developed and implemented her NURSE Program.

Pauline also became involved in a behavioral treatment program to augment her medication. This required that she use strategies of *thought-stopping*. That is, she would talk to herself, using her cortical brain to tell the obsessional thoughts to stop and reassuring herself that she would not act on those thoughts. She also used positive phrases such as "I will not respond to that" or "I will not pay attention to this silly idea" or "I'm having a good day; I will not allow this to interfere" to negate the thoughts when they intruded. She used a relaxation-response method (yoga) to quiet her anxiety when the thoughts came into her head. As another outlet for her emotions, she wrote in her journal when she felt anxiety building about germs and hand washing.

Slowly, Pauline began to feel better. In fact, a few months after her first visit, she came into the office and reported that she had not changed her hand towels for a week and that her washloads had become manageable. She was on the mend.

When Giving Birth Is Traumatic

We'd also like to alert you to a different type of anxiety disorder that can occur postpartum—post-traumatic stress disorder (PTSD). Sufferers experience nightmares and flashback images of whatever horror they have endured. They become fearful and vigilant and often depressed as well. Sleep is disturbed, nightmares are frequent, worries of further harm or even death continue unabated, even though the threat has disappeared. Physiological symptoms of chronic anxiety, such as headaches, stomachaches, and bowel symptoms, can also occur. People with PTSD may be unable to work or carry on any semblance of a normal life.

PTSD is usually associated with sudden catastrophic events, such as wartime experiences, devastating car accidents, rape, assault, natural disasters, or any form of sexual, physical, and/or emotional abuse, including the witnessing of a murder. It may seem odd to place the birth experience among these awful traumas, but for some women childbirth may have been so emotionally or physically painful, that the disorder can occur.

Usually when new mothers with PTSD have physically recovered from the birth experience, they try to bury the traumatic psychological wounds in the dark recesses of their minds. They want to convince themselves that how they feel is unimportant, that their only goal was to have a healthy baby. But by so doing, they don't appreciate that at the time of the traumatic event their limbic brain was thrust into a dysregulated panic/fear response. Brain strain occurs when the stress reaction causes excess norepinephrine and other steroids to circulate in the blood.

These women may find that they cannot leave their houses for fear that they will have an "attack." Indeed, flashbacks of the devastating event can constantly retraumatize them. Although during pregnancy they had planned to go back to work, they may now be unable to do so. Without treatment with antianxiety and antidepressant medications and therapy, their lives can become waking nightmares.

One of our patients, for instance, suffered PTSD after she underwent an emergency cesarean section before she was fully anesthetized. She feared that she and her baby would die. After she came home from the hospital, her family cared for her beautifully but she couldn't relax. "I feel as though I'm waiting for something terrible to happen," Linda told us. "I can't sleep. I have a recurrent nightmare in which I reexperience the searing pain from the first incision. I wake up sweating, breathless, believing I'm back in the operating room. Now, four months later, I still have severe anxiety episodes and feelings of helplessness and dread."

Linda had been through a horrific experience. Knowing that her baby was in trouble and having an emergency cesarean section would have been bad enough. But the surgery was begun prior to adequate anesthesia and completed with a general anesthetic, for which she was totally unprepared. Taken together, all of this constituted a traumatic blow to her psyche. She was now experiencing symptoms of a classic post-traumatic stress disorder, precipitated by the traumatic birth.

When natural disasters occur or people are enveloped in war situations, Critical Incident Debriefing teams (CID) with specialized training in helping victims are dispatched. These teams help victims use their cortical skills to work through the biochemical stress response. Perhaps we need to call in such teams after birth experiences like the one Linda had! This would have helped unburden her of the experience, and perhaps as a result, some of the stress response might have quieted.

Unfortunately, too few medical staff appreciate how seriously impaired patients can become after this kind of trauma. In fact, often they make matters worse by dismissing the experience—suggesting that it is all behind the victim or that no one was truly in danger—further invalidating the woman's reality.

Another patient developed PTSD the first time she visited her premature infant in the neonatal intensive-care unit. This was her second child. "When I saw my baby," Liz explained, "I felt my mouth go dry.

My legs become wobbly, and I got light-headed. I thought he looked like a chicken, but I hated myself for thinking that. I gazed at his little head, wrapped in a bandage that covered his eyes, with all the tubes in and out, the beeping monitors, and his spindly body, and I had the odd feeling that this was not really my baby. I had delivered something inhuman."

Liz became mute and unresponsive after this shock; psychologically she just "checked out." She suffered from what's called traumatic dissociation. Although she was "conscious," her mind no longer processed information or participated in the world. This was a protective move. Liz's mind was shielding itself from the fright she experienced during that first visit to the nursery.

We prescribed an antidepressant, which Liz took for a year. In psychotherapy she used her cortical skills to come to terms with how she felt about her infant's prematurity. Because she was not at great risk for relapse (since she had no genetic history of anxiety disorders) the NURSE Program helped her maintain her balance thereafter. Were she to become pregnant again, we would monitor her closely, using anticipatory therapy to work through the potential of her becoming retraumatized. However, she chose to limit her family to two children, so this was unnecessary.

Liz went on to do very well. And her son has progressed beautifully in the care of this wonderful, loving mother.

Chapter 16

AVOIDABLE TRAGEDIES: POSTPARTUM
PSYCHOSIS

Derek's call came early one morning. I remember his words clearly. "Dr. Sichel," he said urgently, "I think we have a problem. Rachel is staring blankly ahead of her and won't respond to anyone. She's just muttering nonsensical phrases. I can't believe this. She had been doing so well until now. Yesterday she was fine. It's all so sudden. It's been eight weeks since she's had the baby, and I guess I thought we were home free."

My heart skipped a beat. These were words I did not want to hear. Our efforts had failed, despite the preventive measures we had taken to avert a possible recurrence of postpartum psychosis after Rachel's second baby. We were now facing a psychiatric emergency and needed to move fast. I knew that Rachel's condition would deteriorate rapidly, resulting in more florid hallucinations and bizarre delusions if we didn't.

Several years earlier, Rachel's delight after the birth of her first child had evaporated by the third day postpartum, when she became increasingly confused. Suddenly she believed that her family was plotting her death. In her altered and delusional state, she felt she had to take the baby and escape. She became frenzied with activity, muttering incoherent phrases about plots, spies, the Holy Mother, and finding her real soul. From time to time she sighed deeply, as if woefully burdened. Derek's helpful or protective behaviors evoked only suspicion. She interpreted his every action as reinforcing her delusions.

Rachel did not feel there was anything wrong with her and resisted Derek's moves to take her to the hospital. Eventually, though, an ambulance arrived at the house. Transporting her was no easy task. She resisted the paramedics with unfathomable force, but ultimately was unable to overcome the strength of three men. Finally they hoisted her onto a stretcher, strapped her down, and drove her to the emergency room, from which she was quickly transferred to the psychiatric unit.

The family rallied around, shocked, devastated, and needing explanations. Rachel had never been emotionally ill. There was no mental illness in the family that they knew of, so what accounted for this alarming behavior? The hospital staff was of little help and gave no assurances. Rachel, they said, had deep-seated psychological difficulties, and she was unable or unprepared to take on a mothering role.

This puzzled Derek. He knew his wife too well. She was a solid citizen, accomplished in her role as an architect. There had never been even a hint of emotional instability in her life. This could not be the answer. There had to be another explanation.

After two weeks a heavily medicated Rachel was released from the hospital. At home she spent most of her time sleeping, leaving the care of the baby in the hands of the child-care helper Derek had hired. Eventually, her outpatient doctor reduced the doses of her psychosis medication. Her ramblings had cleared, as had her delusions, but now she was seriously depressed. Her outpatient doctor could provide few answers. He made no attempts to treat Rachel's depression, so she spent the remainder of the first year of her baby's life in this depressed state, struggling to cope.

In psychotherapy Rachel examined her family issues. Yes, there were ups and downs in their lives, but overall it had been a stable family. She had never been abused, she had lots of friends, and this had been a planned pregnancy. Her relationship with her husband was good. There didn't seem to be a case for family conflict. Ultimately Rachel became disillusioned with the psychotherapy and stopped going. Her depression gradually lifted, and by the time her baby was fifteen months old, she felt back to herself. There were still, however, no answers as to what had happened to her.

An inherently spiritual person, Rachel decided that she should just put her trust in God, go on with her life, and look to the future. She hoped that this bizarreness—whatever it was—would never return.

When Rachel became pregnant with her second child, she decided to see a new obstetrician in the hope of changing at least part of her previous postpartum experience. As it turned out, her new obstetrician was knowledgeable about some aspects of postpartum mental illness and referred her to our offices. When we met, Rachel said, "My obstetrician seemed to think you might know something about what happened to me after my first child."

Rachel and Derek proceeded to tell me the whole sad tale. The explanation for this episode was easy. The harder part would be preventing its recurrence.

Rachel's "Episode"

I explained to Rachel and Derek that what she'd experienced had a name—postpartum psychosis. About one to three childbearing women per thousand will encounter it. It is relatively common, although certainly not as common as postpartum depression or anxiety disorders. Nevertheless, it is a terrifyingly severe illness.

Symptoms usually show up within the first two to three weeks of giving birth, although sometimes the illness comes on more rapidly. One woman we know became violently psychotic within twenty-four hours of delivery and, to the hospital staff's terror and amazement, ripped a radiator out of the wall.

Postpartum psychosis is characterized by extreme agitation, confusion, hallucinations, delusions, and the inability to sleep, eat, or maintain a coherent conversation. Moods seesaw between euphoria and profound depression. The desperation that these women feel seems to be far more intense than at any other time of life. In fact, often they are in the grip of a suicidal depression.

In twenty years of treating this illness I have noted that when a new mother feels suicidal and acts on her thoughts, she often succeeds, because she *wants* to die. Women in the throes of postpartum psychosis use available firearms, hang themselves, or jump out of windows—all acts from which there is neither retreat nor a likelihood of rescue. Other women with suicidal intentions may take pills or cut or scratch themselves, and often they call for help immediately after the act. They are making gestures and crying out for assistance. Whatever they have done to themselves usually can be reversed with prompt medical treatment. On some level they know they do not really want to die. Not so with those who are psychotic.

When a woman with postpartum psychosis believes she must die, she can also harm or kill her infant as a result of her delusional thinking. The severity of the depression and the psychosis contribute to the urgency to hospitalize the mother and treat her illness aggressively.

What Causes Postpartum Psychosis?

Postpartum psychosis is a brain-chemical illness that we believe is initiated by a number of hormone alterations after the birth of a baby. Although the rapid drop of estrogen levels at this time is strongly implicated as a trigger to the brain events, some psychiatrists believe that altered thyroid and stress-hormone levels also contribute to the psychotic reaction.

It is possible that declining estrogen levels precipitate a cascade of biochemical events in numerous interacting pathways in the brain. It is not the actual estrogen levels in the blood that are abnormal but the impact of rapidly changing levels on the brain, which unbeknownst to a genetically vulnerable woman can play havoc with her mind.

Dr. Channi Kumar, a leading authority and researcher of postpartum illnesses at the London Institute of Psychiatry, has demonstrated that the dopamine receptors in the dopamine pathway (see Chapter 3) are more sensitive in postpartum women who become psychotic than in those who do not. Because disruptions in the neurotransmitter dopamine are involved in mood disorders and in the generation of psychosis, this research suggests that the rapid drop in estrogen may alter these receptors after delivery.

Postpartum psychosis can and often does occur in women already diagnosed with bipolar disorders. Although researchers and clinicians have stated that it often occurs "without warning" in a woman who has been otherwise well, we have begun to reevaluate this assertion. In fact, once we ask our patients about their lives in detail, we find that most who experience psychosis for the first time postpartum actually have family or personal histories that point to risk factors such as mood-swing disorders.

Indeed, in almost every situation of postpartum psychosis we've treated, we have found that a family member has depression, a bipolar mood problem, and/or alcoholism. Although the new mother may not have experienced a significant mood disturbance herself, she has a vulnerable, albeit dormant, brain neurochemistry. Perhaps because of the enormous hormonal shifts that occur after delivery, the pathways are destabilized, resulting in the emergence of illness.

Moreover, in reviewing our patients' lives we can usually uncover a personal history of mood swings prior to pregnancy. Some have had PMDD, mood changes on birth-control pills, and/or symptoms accompanying the use of fertility drugs. Sometimes a mood disturbance erupted around puberty. Indeed, we have come to believe that it is *rare* to find no evidence of previous mood shifts in women who experience an initial episode of psychosis postpartum. *The key is in taking a careful and sensitive history, so that any past disturbances can be identified.*

Rachel's History

Rachel reported no previous history of mental illness. She had never seen a mental-health clinician and considered herself emotionally stable prior to the first psychotic episode. Yet when I questioned her using the earthquake model of genetics, stress-loading as a child, and hormonal shifts from adolescence through the first pregnancy, I found exactly what I had suspected. She was indeed at high-risk.

Rachel's father had experienced untreated mood swings. It sounded as if her mother had protected the children to the best of her ability, but youngsters do not emerge from such families without some emotional scarring. It could not have been easy living with such a father. Besides, his condition alerted us that Rachel probably had a genetic predisposition to mental illness. The genetically determined hard-wiring of the brain is a powerful determinant of emotional stability.

Indeed, Rachel had experienced depression at the time of puberty, but it seemed to clear after several months. Not much notice was taken of this incident, and the family sought no treatment for her. Later, birth-control pills produced a depressive reaction and severe irritability. These clues, waiting to be uncovered, suggested that Rachel had a biochemical vulnerability, which had already given rise to tremors in response to hormonal shifts. Perhaps the massive hormonal drop at delivery had pushed this susceptible brain-chemistry into the earthquake of psychosis.

Like Rachel, many women who experience mood swings prior to a pregnancy have never sought treatment. They may have seen a therapist for counseling regarding life events or crises, but the characteristic ups and downs they live with were unidentified or unacknowledged as a sign of vulnerable brain-chemistry. Most often, as in Rachel's case, a family member has had similar problems.

Postpartum women with milder forms of mood-swing disorders (such as bipolar 2) are probably the most underdiagnosed and mistreated group. They can become flagrantly ill with psychosis in the early postpartum period. Their rapidly disintegrating mental health comes as a complete surprise, not only to them and their families but also to their health-care providers. Their capacity for mood swings is usually unrecognized, so clinicians prescribe the wrong medications, precipitating a worsening of their emotional state.

Although it is initially triggered by the birth of a baby, postpartum psychosis is chemically similar to bipolar illness. Because of this similarity, the symptoms must be treated with mood stabilizers (such as lithium or Depakote) in addition to those that control psychosis (called antipsychotics, such as Zyprexa and Risperdal), which act predominantly on the dopamine pathways. When mood stabilizers are omitted from the treatment plan, a mother is left vulnerable to ensuing mood instability (up or down), which is exactly what happened to Rachel. After her psychosis abated, she had no protection from the resulting depressive reaction and spent several months struggling to cope.

This can have tragic consequences for the infant. During the first year of life vital nerve connections are being forged in the brain, stimulated by the baby's environment and interactions with his or her mother. When a mother is seriously depressed, she is usually unable to play with and stimulate her infant adequately. This can impede the child's normal emotional and intellectual development.

My task with Rachel was to prevent this depression and psychosis from recurring after she gave birth to her second child.

Treating Rachel

In 1991 Dr. Donna Stewart, a psychiatric researcher at the University of Toronto, published a series of cases in which she sought to prevent the reemergence of postpartum psychosis in women who had already suffered one episode by giving them lithium immediately after delivery. The relapse rate with these mothers was quite low—only 10 percent, compared to the 50 to 90 percent we expect.

This was a pretty good record. In 1992 and 1995 two more studies replicated this good response. In addition to being effective, this approach was infinitely safer than other techniques, such as giving large doses of estrogen immediately after delivery (which can cause blood clots).[1]

So after Rachel delivered her second baby, I started her on lithium right away. This precluded breast-feeding. She left the hospital doing well and continued in fine spirits for the first eight weeks, until we received Derek's call. Somehow her symptoms had broken through. The psychosis appeared very suddenly and without warning. We now needed to move fast, because this illness unravels quickly.

We hospitalized Rachel and started her on an antipsychotic medication in addition to the lithium. Twenty-four hours later she was still confused, rambling, and agitated. We had to sedate her heavily while we waited for the combined medications to take their full effect. Two days later she began to menstruate with her first period after delivery. This was the answer to the acute breakthrough of symptoms.

The powerful effect of estrogen withdrawal on the brain pathways in the last week of the menstrual cycle never ceases to amaze us. When we watch how symptoms emerge so rapidly in an otherwise stable situation, we develop a healthy respect for this hormonal event. Let no one tell you that hormones have no effect on women's mental health!

Since lithium had not held Rachel through the premenstrual period, we also began a second mood-stabilizing medication—Depakote. Used for many years as an antiseizure medication, it is one of the most effective mood stabilizers available. In fact, in some situations it surpasses the effectiveness of lithium, which has been the mainstay of treatment for bipolar illness since the late fifties.

Within days of our starting Rachel on Depakote, increasing the dose as fast as she could tolerate it, the newly relapsed symptoms melted away. Her agitation cleared, her speech became more coherent, and she no longer linked rambling thoughts to random events around her. She felt well again.

Rachel would need to stay on lithium, Depakote, and the antipsychotic medication through her next few cycles, until she had no further recurrence premenstrually. This would tell me that despite the normal rises and falls of estrogen across the cycle, the mood pathways in the brain had "held" well enough to prevent reactions to the normal estrogen fluctuations. I would see her weekly to ensure her progress.

Fortunately, Rachel did very well through the next several cycles. Soon she asked if we could decrease the Depakote, since she was feeling "too medicated." I agreed, but cautioned her that we needed to do this gently so she wouldn't relapse. Slowly, over a period of three months, she was weaned off the Depakote. We also worked with her to customize a NURSE Program that might enable her brain to self-regulate. We hoped that this would help her avoid further premenstrual mood changes.

Rachel continued to do well, but she needed to remain on her lithium for at least two years. We prefer to maintain medications for longer than the usual year, because we have found that our patients maintain a higher level of mental health when we do. Also there is a good possibility that postpartum psychosis can eventually declare itself as bipolar illness, and our patients would develop symptoms unrelated to delivering a baby. In that event they would require medication over a longer term. Some women have these episodes only in the postpartum period, but others develop symptoms outside of childbearing. We have seen both situations occur.

Several years later Rachel returned to our office pregnant with her third child. Since we were fairly sure that she would encounter a relapse after this delivery, we started her on lithium and an antipsychotic medication as soon as the baby was born, and she has done wonderfully ever since.

Preventing Postpartum Psychosis

When Jeanne and I reviewed the charts of the first thirty women admitted to the mother-baby unit we helped establish in a Boston psychiatric hospital, we found that of these thirty mothers, twenty-six had clearly diagnosable problems before pregnancy but had never sought psychiatric help. There they were, in the community, going about their daily lives simply accepting that the symptoms of the mood disturbance were part of who they were.

These symptoms put them into the highest risk group for severe illness postpartum. Indeed, they could have been diagnosed quite easily during their pregnancies if someone had asked the right questions. And once they delivered their babies, a preventive treatment plan could have been instituted and the severity of the illness curtailed, avoiding hospitalization and distress to the mothers and their families.

In truth, we can predict the development of postpartum psychosis in a woman who carries risk factors. By evaluating our patients' past histories for mood swings, premenstrual symptoms, and life events that may have caused brain strain, we can develop and implement a preventive program during the acute postpartum period that includes mood stabilizers and sometimes antipsychotic medications. In the future we hope that this identification process becomes as standard as giving antibiotics to a person with pneumonia or high-blood-pressure medicine to a patient at risk for stroke.

Today we use one of two methods to prevent psychosis in women with bipolar 1 disorder as well as in those with milder forms of mood-swing illness that worsen severely after birth. Immediately after delivery of the placenta we give them lithium or Depakote. We increase the doses as fast as our patients can tolerate them. (Minimal side effects, such as nausea, vomiting, dizziness, or tremulousness, can occur. If our patients experience these side effects, we lower their dosage or keep it stable until the side effects subside. Then we continue to increase the dosage, as needed.) In most instances this is very successful.

Sometimes during the first two weeks postpartum, we supplement the mood stabilizers with one of the newer antipsychotic agents, Zyprexa (olanzapine), Risperdal (risperidone), or Seroquel (quetiapine). These medications have a superior ability to block dopamine receptors in the limbic brain. They appear to have a rapid effect in holding the receptors stable while the lithium or Depakote kicks in. We have found these methods highly effective in treating the initial onset and/or relapse of postpartum psychosis.

Avoidable Tragedies

Tragic situations occur when medical staff are unaware of the symptoms of psychosis and how dangerous they can be for a mother and her new baby. When women become psychotic, there is such a vast storm within their brains that they retain little ability to appreciate what they are doing from moment to moment. They can unwittingly kill their infants or others in a state of mental confusion and illness.

Emotional illness can be devastating to a family. When a mother harms her child while acting on delusional beliefs, many lives are changed dramatically and permanently. The ignorance of the criminal-justice system further compounds the tragedy.

The following are stories of two women who are serving long jail sentences. They have lived through the horror of untreated psychosis and its tragic consequences. These women have given us permission to use their real names and tell their stories. They desperately want their voices to be heard. The only difference between their stories and Rachel's is that they were not treated as they deserved, despite their attempts to get help.

CHRISTINA MYERS

Christina Myers is currently serving twenty-five years in prison for a conviction of manslaughter after beating her three-year-old step-daughter, Brandi, to death. Let's look closely at what happened to her.

Five days after Christina gave birth to Felicia, her husband's three-year-old child from his first marriage, Brandi, came to live with them.

As soon as she brought her baby home from the hospital, Christina started to worry constantly about everything. She became distraught about a hardened area on her baby's head, which her pediatrician told her was just a calcium deposit. This explanation did not reassure her. She began to obsess about this spot. She went to the emergency room to have it checked and was again informed that this was nothing to worry about. She saw a neurologist, who also reassured her that little was wrong with the baby. Christina, however, was becoming more and more anxious. No explanation relieved her increasing fear that something was terribly wrong.

Based on this information alone, we could say that Christina was showing signs of a postpartum illness. Obsessive worries and fears that wouldn't be calmed were a sign that she was now at risk for a rapid onset of depression. However, no intervention was initiated at this point. Her health-care providers answered her questions and responded to her concerns without putting together the whole picture. In fact, they may have considered her to be a "neurotic first-time mother." No one was paying attention to the fact that she couldn't free herself of this inappropriate and excessive worry.

Sadly, Christina's anxiety and depression worsened. You could say that her thinking was becoming irrational. Her judgment and insight were failing her. She was on a dangerous trajectory.

Christina began to believe that her baby was very ill and that no-body was telling her the truth. She prayed, "Dear God, why can't I have a healthy baby?" This delusional thinking had no basis in fact. Christina had lost touch with reality.

Then the hallucinations began. She saw Felicia's head trapped in the elevator doors. She was terrified and started to feel helpless to protect her baby. Potential danger emanated from every person and object. Within the process of her distorted thinking, she tried to find solutions. Here is what Christina wrote in recalling that time:

I was trying to be the perfect mother and wife. I thought if I planned a great Christmas for the family, this would all go away. But we didn't really have the money to do that, since my husband had just taken a new job. I got a new credit card and spent twenty-five hundred dollars on toys and clothes for the two girls. My shopping was out of control. My husband was furious and sold my car to pay off the credit card debt. I felt trapped and was more and more afraid that something terrible was going to happen to Felicia.

I told my husband and his sister about having these terrifying visions of Felicia being dead, but they just looked at me as if I was crazy, so I stopped talking. When we took the children to the doctor, I was desperate for her to ask me how I was doing or to notice that some-thing was wrong with me. She didn't.

I knew something was wrong with my baby, but they were not telling me. I knew something was wrong with me, but thought it would get bet-ter. I was so alone and terrified. Nobody noticed anything about me.

On Friday, the third of February 1989, I woke up, but I felt I was in a dream. Nothing seemed real. I was watching myself do things. I went to Felicia's room and found Brandi pulling at Felicia's feet to get her out of the crib. I just went mad. This was my biggest fear—Feli-cia's life was in danger. I had flashbacks of the sexual assaults from my father and uncle from when I was four to fourteen.

I had to protect my baby. She was already ill, I believed. Now I thought that Brandi was trying to kill her. I began to punch her as hard as I could. It was a struggle not to hit her. I pulled Brandi away and shook her again and again, punching her until she went into a coma. I had no realization of what I was doing. I was in my own desperate world of having to protect my daughter at all costs. Brandi died the next day in the hospital from the injuries I caused.

I had no idea what I was doing, yet now I am in jail for twenty-five years.

Christina had been mentally ill. She'd experienced a postpartum psychotic depression and was delusional about the health of her baby. She became paranoid, believing that everyone, including her little stepdaughter, represented a threat to her child. If anybody had asked how she was doing or had otherwise checked in with her, she could have been successfully treated and this tragedy averted.

Based on her history, Christina was at high risk for postpartum illness. When girls are sexually molested, they often develop post-traumatic stress disorder. At an early age Christina's brain biochemistry had been altered by the catastrophic trauma of sexual assault and incest. It was vulnerable and primed for an "earthquake." She became severely ill in the early postpartum period. In reading her letter, I also knew that both Christina and her family must have had a history of mood disorders. Incest and sexual abuse alone would not lead to a postpartum psychosis.

If this couple had received information about the types of emotional illnesses that can occur postpartum, they might have recognized Christina's symptoms and sought help. Only two hours of instruction at a childbirth class or in the doctor's or midwife's office would have averted this tragedy. Moreover, if the physicians she had consulted had recognized that irrational worries about a baby can signal mental illness in a mother, they might have questioned Christina about how she was doing emotionally. So little information and time would have made such a big difference.

How many lives have been affected and how much money spent on the tragic consequences? Christina's jailing costs about $35,000 a year, not to mention the expense of the trial. Her daughter, Felicia, does not have a mother—an emotional assault for a young girl. Her husband and his first wife have lost their child. At least five lives have been traumatized forever because health-care providers failed to recognize the problem.

Christina does not deserve to be in prison. She was ill. She needed medical/psychiatric care, not prosecution. Christina was a victim of the ignorance of the medical system, a victim of her illness, and a victim of the criminal-justice system, which bases its determinations on an archaic understanding of postpartum illnesses. Women in this most fragile stage of life should be supported and cared for. Instead society and our medical system abandon them.

As a society, until we start to take note of the emotional disorders that so frequently emerge through pregnancy and after delivery, we will continue to carry the burden of our sins of omission in caring adequately and compassionately for our women and their children. We will all pay dearly.

KATHERINE DILLON

When Katherine Dillon was forty-five, she discovered that she was pregnant. This was to be Katherine's first child, and she was thrilled. She was sure it would be a girl, and after an ultrasound at fifteen weeks, the gender was confirmed. She and her husband picked out the name Mylyssa Grace.

Shortly thereafter Katherine began to have severe panic attacks, but no one took much notice. By the time she was seven months pregnant, she was unable to sleep and was becoming severely emotionally ill. She became phobic about leaving her house, stopped driving the car, withdrew from life, and isolated herself. Increasingly depressed and angry, she felt like a failure but didn't understand why. She was dizzy and confused most of the time; still, no one took her complaints seriously. When she went in for her prenatal appointments, she was sure that the nurses and doctors called her "that crazy woman" and laughed at her.

Mylyssa was born by cesarean section. She had blue eyes and red hair and was beautiful. Katherine had never felt happier.

But things went downhill quickly after that. While still in the hospital, Katherine became more confused and began to hear voices. She thought that her husband and mother were conspiring to kill her and take Mylyssa away. She tried to escape from the hospital wearing just her nightgown. It took three security guards to bring her back. She was quite psychotic and delusional at this point, hearing voices and seeing people who were not there. She did not know where or who she was. Paranoid, she trusted no one. She hid from her family in the bathroom when they came to visit.

Katherine doesn't remember much more about this time. She was transferred to the psychiatric unit, where she stayed for a day and a half. Increasingly paranoid and convinced that she was being poisoned, she didn't swallow the medication they gave her there. Then she was sent home.

It's unclear how much her husband and family were told about the dangers associated with her illness, but Katherine arrived home unimproved. She tried to do the shopping and take care of the house and Mylyssa, but she didn't trust anyone. She thought the food her friends brought over was unsafe to eat. She wasn't sleeping, couldn't focus, and was still hearing voices. Katherine struggled with paranoia and depression. She felt like a failure and wanted to die. On several occasions she drove away from the house and wanted to kill herself, but she couldn't muster the nerve to do it.

One morning Mylyssa was crying and fretful. Katherine tried feeding her, but she continued to cry. In fact, she cried the entire day. Then, sometime around 4:00 P.M., something snapped in Katherine. In an effort to stop her crying, Katherine suffocated Mylyssa. Within her dazed state, she suddenly realized what had happened and tried to resuscitate her, but her six-week-old baby was dead.

Depressed, suicidal, paranoid, and delusional, Katherine had taken the life of that which was most precious to her. She left the house with her dead baby, prepared to kill herself. She thought about running herself into a gasoline tanker or driving off the road, but eventually she called her husband and the police.

Nobody wanted to believe that Katherine was ill and needed help. Katherine told us in a letter that the police treated her inhumanely, denying her clothing, water, and toilet paper. They gave her only two sanitary napkins, even though she was still bleeding vaginally after the cesarean birth. Her food was placed on the floor, and the guards made her crawl across the floor to it. Katherine was severely mentally ill, yet was treated worse than a sick animal in need of compassion.

Since Katherine, her husband, and her lawyer had no information at the time about the postpartum psychosis that afflicted her, she was pushed into a plea bargain. Because of this poor legal advice, she was unable to ask for a new trial so that the whole situation could be reappraised with enlightenment and fairness.

Postpartum psychosis is a treatable illness, but none of the doctors involved in Katherine's care appreciated the seriousness of her situation. Katherine is a victim of medical and judicial ignorance and of her brain-chemistry. Her family has also been harmed in their loss, not only of the baby but also of Katherine.

We Feel Outraged!

We receive letters all the time from women around the country who find themselves in similar situations—casualties of medical and judicial ignorance. There are hundreds of them. When is this victimization going to stop? It sometimes feels as though we are dealing with archaic belief systems. This is the same type of farcical justice that was meted out in the Salem witch trials. It's time for the United States to do better, much better.

Christina's and Katherine's lives are all the more tragic because had they received effective treatment, all of this pain could have been averted. Every day in our practice, we see women struggling with the same disorders. They receive care and compassion, just as those who now sit in prison deserved but never got. Indeed, few of these women receive adequate psychiatric care while they are incarcerated.

When mothers are convicted and sent to prison for these tragic infant deaths, they are being punished for an event that was preordained by their neurochemistry. All it took was a hormonal challenge, and their lives suddenly veered off course. It makes no sense to hold someone responsible for a neurochemical event that is out of her control. Yet in this "Decade of the Brain" (as the 1990s were declared by Congress), our society and justice system still don't want to enlighten themselves. There is a difference between a person who kills with malice and one who kills under the influence of postpartum psychosis.

Sadly, even when a woman is found to be seriously incapacitated due to a biochemical mental illness over which she had no control, she is still punished by a long jail sentence, despite the fact that these women pose no threat to society and when properly treated can lead completely normal lives, just as millions of others who have ongoing emotional illness do.

Each situation must be evaluated on its own merits. There are some women who knowingly and willingly do harm to their children. They are quite different, and we do not sanction their acts or equate them with the women whose stories we've described.

Even as we begin to contemplate the unthinkable—that many deaths attributed to sudden infant death syndrome (SIDS) may actually be mothers' deliberate acts of suffocation—we must sort out those who are ill from those who act with malevolence. Christina and Katherine were not evil; they were ill. They became the tools of the hallucinations and apparitions in their minds.

The calamities we have described highlight the disconnection in our health system among obstetrics, gynecology, psychiatry, and pediatrics. Few clinicians realize how effectively appropriate intervention can avert tragedies.

The birth of a child is romanticized in this culture, and everyone buys into it until something goes terribly wrong. But if we are going to move into the twenty-first century with any semblance of compassion, gynecologists, obstetricians, and pediatricians must pay significant attention to the mental state of their patients during pregnancy and postpartum. Mental illness is brain illness, and it is time that health-care providers as well as women, their partners, and their families began to appreciate how crucial the emotional health of the mother is to the survival and normal development of her child.

Although there is still much to learn about many of the brain mechanisms controlling these illnesses, we do have effective treatments for most women. There is absolutely no reason for new mothers to get as sick as they have. These aspects must be included in the new focus on women's health care. Without this, "women's health care" will remain a term without substance. It is imperative that the status quo change as we head into the new millennium.

Part V

NEGOTIATING MENOPAUSE

Chapter 17

MENOPAUSE: THE DIALOGUE CEASES

Until recently menopause was a phase of life that many women didn't think about because most didn't live beyond fifty-five. In fact, a mere hundred years ago the average life expectancy for a woman residing in the United States was forty-nine years of age. Today that same woman can expect to live till about seventy-nine! You can look forward to another third of your life after menopause—an average of thirty years for most of us.

Not only can you expect to live longer, you can also live better. If you're in good health, you can continue to lead an active, fulfilled life. Because of the baby boom and our longer life spans, there are more perimenopausal women in this country than ever before—forty-five to fifty million by the year 2000.

In response to these demographics, you need to be informed about how to take the best care of your brain, as well as the other parts of your body. In fact, if you take good care of your brain, in all likelihood you will automatically tend to your general health. That's because ensuring a healthy brain means addressing your diet, sleep and recreational habits, peace of mind, exercise, mood, and memory health. In other words, just as a good NURSE Program can enhance your life when you're younger, it will also promote a healthy mind, body, and soul during your menopausal years.

Health after menopause is not something that happens on its own;

you must take charge of it. That means informing yourself about what is occurring in your body and deciding how to help it and your brain be at their best. Postmenopause may prove to be the most fulfilling time of your life if you take good care of yourself.

What Is Menopause? And What Is Perimenopause?

Menopause is defined as the phase in your life when you have had no menstrual period for a year. Perimenopause is the period of years that leads to menopause. It refers to the time during which the "conversation" between your ovaries and brain gradually slows down. Perimenopause may last as long as seven to ten years, or longer. It may begin much earlier than previously believed, sometimes even in the late thirties and early forties. For some women, on the other hand, perimenopause may be quite short—only a year or two. If you are still menstruating regularly when you are fifty, this suggests that you might have a short perimenopausal phase.

Perimenopause is a term of the nineties and will be recognized in the twenty-first century as an important reproductive phase. The millions of women in the United States alone who are entering perimenopause are seeking help from their primary-care providers because they are bothered by certain symptoms prior to the menopause, *including mood and memory changes.* In fact, Dr. Raymond Burnett, author of *Menopause: All Your Questions Answered*, found that irritability, insomnia, and depressed mood rank among the most common complaints. In a consumer survey of two thousand perimenopausal women in Massachusetts, 20 percent said that their mental health was significantly worse than the year before. Contrary to popular belief, hot flashes are not the most prevalent difficulty.

In the following chapters we will explore how menopause affects your brain as well as other parts of your body. We will also pay special attention to how the hormonal readjustment during this time in your life can adversely affect your moods, memory, and sense of well-being. We hope to provide you with the tools to mitigate these changes so you can make this a most exciting time in your life.

It's About Your Brain!

When we give talks about menopause, we usually introduce the subject by telling our audience that we're going to talk about their brains. Apart from immediately attracting their attention, this brings gales of laughter, since most of us don't associate perimenopause and menopause with this organ.

But as is the case during all the other periods of your reproductive life, the relationship between your hormones and your brain is critical. Sadly, we often take the brain for granted at this time. We never consider it vulnerable to the hormonal changes associated with menopause. In fact, traditionally the focus has been on how the other organ systems slowly deteriorate with age, particularly as a result of the loss of estrogen. But your brain is a prime mover of your moods and memory/cognitive abilities and can also be adversely affected. The brain needs to continue its delicate conversation with all the other organs in your body, even though your ovaries have stopped communicating with it.

The Importance of Estrogen

Estrogen is a hormone integral to your health and brain function. Prior to menopause, estrogen had many profound ramifications in your life. It feminized important structures in your body and brain when you were just a fetus. Influenced by the hypothalamus, it set your menstrual cycle in motion at puberty. It helped to prepare you for and support your pregnancies. It promoted strong bones, maintained healthy cholesterol levels, and preserved the lining of your vagina, urethra, and bladder. It also influenced the way your serotonin and other neurotransmitter pathways reacted to normal hormonal shifts. Perhaps you experienced mood variations related to these fluctuations across your cycle.

During perimenopause your estrogen levels slowly decline. By menopause, not all of your estrogen has disappeared, but the type of estrogen circulating in your blood changes, and the levels are much lower.

There are two active forms of estrogen in your body: *estradiol* and *estrone*. Estradiol is the main (and most potent) estrogen secreted during the childbearing years. It is the final byproduct of a cascade of biochemical reactions in your body that convert a cholesterol molecule to progesterone, to testosterone, and finally to estradiol. After menopause the other form of active estrogen, estrone, circulates in your blood, but at much lower levels than before menopause. This estrogen is much weaker than estradiol. Accumulated body fat also releases the estrogen it has stored over the years, so obese women have higher levels than others and for much longer.

The Decline of Testosterone

Testosterone, a precursor of estradiol production, begins to decrease slowly before menopause and continues to decline in postmenopausal women. In fact, the level of testosterone in a woman in her forties is one third that of a woman in her twenties. Even so, after menopause the ovary remains an important source of testosterone. However, this decline may account for why some women complain of loss of libido, or sex drive, at this time. When women have their uterus and ovaries removed, an important source of testosterone is precipitously removed, which may account for the common complaint of loss of libido.

Although testosterone is a component of libido, in a Danish study 70 percent of women at age fifty-one stated that their sex drive was unchanged. Since there are so many different components to sexuality, it is hard to blame diminished sex drive on hormones alone. The role that male hormones play in women's health and well-being is still poorly understood.

As this study seems to indicate, and as you will see, the decrease in estrogen and testosterone can manifest itself as varying patterns of change for different women. Again we are reminded of the uniqueness of each woman's biochemistry and life experiences.

Your Brain-Ovary Dialogue in Menopause

The dialogue between your brain and ovaries began at puberty. This feedback system enabled your menstrual cycle to occur (see Chapter 5). As you get older, you can assume that this same conversation will now slow, become sporadic, and eventually cease. Patterns in the slowing vary significantly from woman to woman and even within one woman from month to month; there is no one way in which this process occurs.

You were born with a finite number of eggs, and the dialogue is ending because your ovaries are simply running out of them. Your hypothalamus, the area of your limbic brain responsible for secreting the hormones that stimulate your ovary to ripen a follicle and eventually release an egg, has to work harder to get the ovary, with its diminishing number of aging eggs, to respond.

The hypothalamus pumps out the stimulating hormone GnRH to trigger FSH (follicle-stimulating hormone) from the pituitary, but the follicles respond less robustly. As a consequence, estrogen doesn't quite reach the levels needed to ripen and release the remaining eggs.

This makes your pituitary gland work even harder, pumping more and more FSH, trying to get the ovaries to respond.

Eventually the brain stimulates the follicle enough to release an egg. But the levels of FSH are higher and the follicles less responsive, or sporadically so. This means that there will be times in your cycle when you don't have enough estrogen and other times when you have too much—and the follicle finally reacts. All of these permutations can occur within one cycle.

As a result, you may notice that your cycles have become irregular. Perhaps your period is delayed by some weeks, but then you bleed more heavily and have more breast tenderness. You may have some hot flashes earlier in the cycle, night sweats, or vaginal dryness during sexual intercourse that disappear once your period begins. You may miss a period for a month or two and then menstruate normally again for a while. Your cycle may shorten from twenty-eight days to twenty-five or less or even lengthen to forty-five or more, and your bleeding patterns may change. Or you may have no symptoms at all, or only one or two.

Although most women believe perimenopause to be a time when estrogen diminishes, as we noted, it can also be a time of intermittently higher levels, accounting for heavier or prolonged bleeding and increased breast size and tenderness.

How Do I Know If I'm Menopausal?

Women often want to know if a blood test can tell them whether they have reached perimenopause or menopause. There are blood tests, but due to the many fluctuations in the ovary-brain dialogue at this time, they can be unreliable in letting you know exactly where you stand.

The blood tests that are usually administered measure your follicle-stimulating hormone (FSH) and your luteinizing hormone (LH). The levels of these hormones are high only if the pituitary gland has been straining to make the ovary respond. But even if your FSH and LH levels are high one month, it's likely that they will revert to normal in subsequent cycles.[1]

A more definitive way to determine if you are approaching menopause is to count how many months have elapsed since your last period. After at least six months it is likely that you are nearing the end of this process, but you can still have an occasional period for a while. Consequently, if you do not wish to bear any more children at this time, you will still need to be careful about contraception.

Eventually your egg supply will be depleted, but the brain continues to secrete FSH and LH, still trying to make the ovary respond. FSH and LH levels increase at menopause and remain high thereafter. When there is no further response from the ovary and you have no period for twelve months, perimenopause is over and menopause has arrived.

Early Menopause?

Sometimes perimenopausal symptoms can occur years prior to any noticeable changes in the menstrual cycle. When I was forty-two, for instance, I began to have occasional hot flashes. They were not problematic for me, and I regarded them more with amusement than irritation, because I knew that this was only the beginning of a physiological process that would take a number of years to complete.

I do, however, remember mentioning my hot flashes to an internist colleague, who looked at me and scoffed that this could not be happening, as I was "much too young!" Yet I knew what I was experiencing. The hot flashes subsided for a few years and then returned, this time accompanied by alterations in my menstrual cycle.

Despite the fact that I knew what was happening to me, my colleague tried to discount my experience. It didn't fit into his view of when and how menopausal symptoms occur. How many other women are invalidated by their doctors in this way?

In fact, as a result of talking with women approaching their menopausal years, it has become clear to us that some of the physical and emotional signs associated with menopause occur far earlier than we usually expect. In our practice we frequently see women between the ages of thirty-eight and forty-five who complain of loss of well-being, mild depressive symptoms, fatigue, and sleep disturbances, along with hot flashes and changes in their menstrual cycle. Yet when they mention their symptoms to their physicians, they are often told, "Menopause doesn't start that early." Clearly something is changing, and these women know it.

We want you to notice these alterations and subtle early signs of perimenopause, because your powerful brain is once again letting you know that a new phase is being ushered in. (We have developed a Perimenopausal Rating Chart to help our patients keep track of these emerging changes. You'll find a blank rating chart in Appendix B.)

For instance, the loss of well-being may result from alterations in limbic-brain areas that are responding to varying levels of estrogen. It is important for your practitioner to hear and validate your observations and experiences, even if symptoms are not causing you too much trouble right now.

After the menstrual cycle has stopped, a number of organ systems are subject to deterioration over time without estrogen—more seriously in some women than in others—affecting the heart and blood vessels, vagina, lower urinary tract, bone, and the brain. Many authoritative texts discuss these changes in significant detail (see Bibliography). Here we will simply outline the issues that you need to bear in mind to help you assess your own needs during the peri- and postmenopausal years.

Physical Symptoms at Perimenopause and Menopause

Various physical signs and symptoms let you know that the brain-ovary conversation is coming to an end.

HOT FLASHES

Perimenopausal women often complain of hot flashes and night sweats. These can be quite irritating and disruptive. In fact, women are busy in today's world and often find that hot flashes distract their attention. Naturally they would prefer them to stop.

Hot flashes, flushes, or "power surges" as they have been called most recently, describe a sense of pervasive warmth that comes on suddenly, usually all over your face, neck, and chest. Those around you may be unaware of this symptom until you start asking whether anyone else is feeling warm! Even if you've had the tendency to be cold, you may find yourself lowering the thermostat at home in the winter and upsetting everyone else in the family or requiring your work environment to be kept cooler while your co-workers freeze.

When the flashes interfere with sleep, we call them night sweats. Sometimes a woman's only menopausal complaint is disturbed sleep, which can undermine any sense of well-being. Although sleep disruption can be related to estrogen decline, it is also a symptom of depression. That's why it's important for us to ask about other symptoms of mood and anxiety disorders to distinguish between the two.

If the sleep disturbance is due to depression, estrogen replacement won't ameliorate it.

Hot flashes are related to the fluctuations in estrogen levels, not to constant low levels, so they occur only during perimenopause, when estrogen levels are decreasing. They can last, therefore, for several months or even several years, depending on the length of your perimenopausal phase.

Researchers are not entirely clear about the intricate mechanisms within the hypothalamus that produce hot flashes. It is believed that they may be due to a hypothalamic disturbance, induced by the fluctuating levels of estrogen. Somehow the hypothalamus is tricked into believing that your body is too hot, so it responds by stimulating your intrinsic cooling mechanisms; blood is rushed to the surface of your skin to get rid of the heat and cool you down. This can cause perspiration. As a result, your body may become overcooled. To conserve heat, blood vessels then constrict, leading to a flush.

Some women have reported anxious feelings along with the sensation of heat. Depression or anxiety symptoms may worsen with the hot flash.

VAGINA AND URINARY TRACT

Estrogen also structurally supports the vaginal tissue and the lower urinary tract. When estrogen levels drop and remain low, these tissues lose their strength, elasticity, and moisture. Symptoms of vaginal-tissue changes include dryness, itching, irritation, and painful sexual intercourse due to the thinning of the vaginal lining. A need to urinate frequently, burning on urination, itching in the urethral area, and sometimes urinary-tract infections are all signs of urinary tract changes.

As time goes on, the uterus and bladder can slip from their anatomical positions due to weakening of the support ligaments. Ultimately they may require surgery to repair them. Urinary incontinence can be traced to these factors.

BONE HEALTH

Bone is dynamic tissue laid down in childhood and adolescence. During adulthood old bone is constantly being broken down and replaced with new bone tissue; this process is called *bone remodeling*. Bone remodeling continues until we're thirty-five to forty years of age, when our bone density peaks.

The depletion of estrogen alters the process of bone remodeling; calcium can leach from the bones, potentially weakening them and rendering them increasingly susceptible to fracture. Since estrogen promotes strong bones, the most rapid bone loss occurs during the first ten years of menopause.

Osteoporosis ensues when the old bone is broken down faster than new bone is made. About twenty-five million Americans suffer from this disorder, 80 percent of whom are women. However, this doesn't mean that every woman will get osteoporosis. Dr. Isaac Schiff, chief of obstetrics and gynecology at Massachusetts General Hospital, notes that three quarters of all women won't experience this condition unless they live to be very old.

Osteoporosis costs the United States about $10 billion annually and accounts for 1.5 million bone fractures yearly. Fifteen percent of those who suffer from hip fracture can actually die from complications, so this is not a disease to be taken lightly.

Estrogen deficiency is the most important cause of osteoporosis, but lack of weight-bearing exercise runs a close second. Other contributing factors include heredity, low calcium levels, smoking, medications, and chronic medical and psychiatric conditions. In a 1996 National Institute of Mental Health study, it was reported that women with histories of chronic depression had lower bone density in their hips, spines, and arm bones than those with no such histories. It was suggested that over time the hypothalamus-pituitary-adrenal imbalance and high cortisol levels in depression disorders accelerate bone loss in these women.

Since we know that women have depressive disorders long before menopause, you will need to pay close attention to the health of your bones if you have struggled with depressive disorders for many years.

HEART DISEASE

Prior to menopause the rate of heart disease in women is quite low. This rises substantially after menopause. In fact, although the general public believes that breast cancer is the number-one killer of women, heart disease holds that dubious honor, especially for those between the ages of sixty-five and seventy.[2] It is responsible for more deaths among women than any other cause. In 1991 nearly half a million women died of heart disease, compared with 242,000 from all types of cancer.

Estrogen protects women from heart disease. It helps to maintain healthy ratios of blood fats, or lipids, keeping the good cholesterol (high-density lipoproteins, or HDLs) high and bad cholesterol (low-density lipoproteins, known as the LDLs) low. When estrogen levels are depleted, this ratio slowly shifts, so that the LDLs increase and the HDLs decrease. Over time high LDL levels contribute to the process of narrowing in the coronary arteries that feed the heart muscle. The formation of plaques comprised of cholesterol, fats, and other debris eventually constricts or completely blocks the arteries, leading to chest pain and ultimately a heart attack or stroke.

Estrogen also has a direct effect on the artery walls, so that arteries are kept dilated and adequate blood can flow through them. Progesterone seems to reduce this effect slightly, so that with hormone-replacement therapy the added progesterone can reduce some of the positive effects of estrogen in the artery walls.

SKIN

The effects of menopause also become apparent in your skin. Estrogen supports the connecting tissue in the foundational levels of the skin. When estrogen declines, the skin's elasticity decreases and wrinkles develop. But remember, exposure to the sun induces far worse effects than lack of estrogen. It's important to use sunblock creams to protect your skin.

In the next chapter we will discuss more fully healing strategies for mood, memory, and the physical symptoms of the peri- and post-menopausal years.

Chapter 18

MENOPAUSE, MOODS, AND MEMORY

Millions of women find that they develop mood and sleep difficulties for the first time with the changes of perimenopause. Millions more will come to their perimenopausal years with varying degrees of depressive illness. We have found that specific groups of women carry particularly increased risk, especially those who have had anxiety or depression disturbances before. In addition, some women are particularly sensitive to the loss of estrogen.

Having said that, we must also note that once you are postmenopausal, in general you may look forward to a period of better mood stability because the hormone fluctuations have stopped.

Stella Comes for Help

Stella was a forty-six-year-old woman who had experienced periods of dysphoria—mild depression—during most of her life. Over the past six months she noticed that she felt less well generally and was pushing herself to get through each day. In fact, for some reason, now she was feeling much worse than she ever had during her previous episodes of depression.

Stella had begun to experience irregular periods, hot flashes, and drenching night sweats. She put up with these symptoms for a while, but the sleep deprivation was bothering her so much that she felt she needed some medication. When she saw her gynecologist, he pre-scribed a standard daily dose of estrogen (usually 0.5 to 0.6 milli-grams), along with progesterone to be taken between days one and fifteen of her cycle.

Gynecologists often give prescriptions for estrogen and progester-one to their perimenopausal and postmenopausal patients. This hormone-replacement therapy (HRT) can relieve the symptoms of hot flashes and night sweats, minor symptoms of loss of well-being, and insomnia, as well as many of the other physical symptoms of meno-pause outlined in Chapter 17.

You may wonder why progesterone is also prescribed if the decline in estrogen is the culprit behind many of the menopausal symptoms. Although estrogen replacement has many positive effects, it also causes the endometrium, the lining of the uterus, to grow and thicken. This has the potential of encouraging endometrial over-growth, which over time can be associated with the development of endometrial cancer. Progesterone is given to help protect the endo-metrium from such overgrowth. It causes the sloughing off of the tissue during menstrual flow, and this is precisely the desired effect. Unfortunately, as we will see, progesterone also tends to affect moods negatively.

Indeed, soon after beginning hormone replacement, Stella found that her hot flashes improved but her mood deteriorated. Her insomnia was more persistent, and she was rapidly losing interest in her usual ac-tivities. She was irritable all the time and didn't want to socialize. In fact, she felt as if she had constant PMDD (see Chapter 8).

Unfortunately, when care providers prescribe estrogen and proges-terone for hot flashes, they may not even consider or ask about other symptoms—especially those related to moods. But just as the de-cline in estrogen has a physical impact on your body, it may also af-fect your emotions and behavior. Estrogen fluctuations can alter neurotransmitter levels in the brain that may result in mood distur-bances.

Many women who have not experienced depressive symptoms be-fore find that perimenopause brings with it feelings of fatigue, a loss of well-being, difficulty sleeping, mood alterations, anxiety, poor con-centration, and changes in thinking patterns and abilities, as well as problems with memory. As you can see, many of these symptoms overlap with those of depression. Yet in most evaluations of meno-pausal symptoms, no one distinguishes between those that come from estrogen loss and those that come from depression. Unless the two are differentiated, you may receive inadequate treatment.

In cases like Stella's, it was important for us to separate the symptoms that belong to depression from those attributable to the decrease in estrogen in order for treatment to be effective. Her sleep disturbance, for instance, could be associated with night sweats or it could be part of an ongoing depressive illness. Hormone-replacement therapy will relieve the night sweats and the loss of well-being associated with sleep deprivation for many women, *but it will not alleviate the symptoms of true depression*.

Uncharted Territory

The mood and memory changes of perimenopause have been barely recognized, much less investigated. This has been a grossly underrecognized and unresearched period of life. And it's a big problem. If 45 to 50 million American women are perimenopausal at the year 2000 and 10 percent of those suffer from depression, then we can assume that 4.5 to 5 million women in this age group will have significant difficulty negotiating perimenopause. This is yet one more reason to take note of your symptoms, correlating them with your age and menstrual cycle.

You do not have to have hot flashes or night sweats or even significant changes in your periods to be flirting with menopause. Your brain may manifest only mood or memory changes as signals that the hormonal slowing of perimenopause has begun. For instance, you may find that you cannot remember names as easily as you used to, or you walk into a room and forget what you wanted!

Many women like Stella consult us because of changes in their moods or memory at this time. Some are struggling with depression symptoms for the first time at menopause, while others have had previous difficulties with mood and anxiety disorders that seem to worsen with the decline in estrogen. Women who have been taking antidepressants and doing well on them may find with the onset of perimenopause that the medications appear to have stopped working and their symptoms reemerge. Those with mood-swing disorders (bipolar 1 and 2) may destabilize at this time, despite adequate doses of medication. Other women placed on hormone-replacement therapy may be unable to tolerate the effects on mood of the progesterone component of their regimen.

When a women over the age of thirty-eight calls us for a consultation, we are always vigilant about ferreting out early symptoms of perimenopause to account for mood worsening in addition to life stress, heredity, a past history of depression, and other factors. We call this "looking for the destabilizing factor." We want to know what's happening in this patient's biochemistry to cause the change. We investigate whether she is beginning to experience the faltering of the precise dialogue between her brain and her ovaries and whether the estrogen deficiency she is experiencing may be pushing the brain-chemistry in the direction of depression.

At thirty-nine, another patient, Vicki, had been doing well on her antidepressants. Although she had missed a couple of periods, her life was stable and productive. Gradually, however, her mood seemed to worsen. We asked her gynecologist to measure her FSH and LH levels. They were elevated. Her gynecologist was astounded. Because she was only thirty-nine, he never even dreamed that Vicki's worsening mood might be related to diminishing estrogen levels. We decided to add a low dose of estrogen, since it can augment the effect of antidepressants in the brain and since her estrogen levels were low. We wanted to be sure that we addressed all the elements that might be contributing to her worsening mood. Soon her symptoms improved dramatically, much to her gynecologist's astonishment.

The hormonal fluctuations of the late thirties and early forties make the management of perimenopausal and menopausal depressive and bipolar illness more perplexing to deal with—but not impossible. More than ever, your hormones become important. It is critical to ascertain your hormonal status, including thyroid, as this information needs to be factored into the assessment of your moods.

Depression, Menopause, or Both?

Let's return to the case of Stella, whom you met earlier in this chapter. We needed to determine the source of Stella's symptoms. Was she suffering from worsening depression, from the normal discomforts of perimenopause, or from some combination of the two? To determine the answer, we questioned her about her life before perimenopause.

During her earlier periods of mild depression Stella hadn't taken antidepressants, preferring to use psychotherapy to deal with her life issues. She had never been pregnant and acknowledged that she'd always had difficulties premenstrually. She had learned to live with these monthly mood changes, taking evening primrose oil and Vitamin B_6.

Stella's mother had also had a history of mood disturbance but had never tried to get help for herself. At seventy-five years of age, she now had severe osteoporosis and got around with great difficulty. There was no history of heart problems or breast cancer in the family.

When we asked about her diet, Stella reported that it was good overall. She did, however, reveal that she occasionally binged on chocolate premenstrually. In fact, Stella's cravings for chocolate seemed to have become more frequent. In addition, her periods were lengthening and her PMS symptoms intensifying. She also noticed that she would unexpectedly drop things. When she served dinner, she would occasionally miss the plate altogether, and the food would land on the table! Sometimes this was quite funny, but at other times she just found it exasperating.

Stella's was a fairly typical picture of perimenopause. But she had other symptoms that were of concern, such as irritability, increased PMDD, cravings for sweets, and occasional eye-hand-coordination problems. Her irritability and moods were worse than ever, and her insomnia seemed unrelated to the night sweats, since estrogen replacement didn't relieve it. It looked to us as if Stella's mild, lifelong depression was worsening under the influence of estrogen's decline in the brain. Now she was coping with both perimenopause and depression.

Many scientific reports suggest that PMDD symptoms can first appear in one's forties. But it is likely that what is misconstrued as PMDD symptoms are really mood disturbances and depression associated with estrogen fluctuations during perimenopause.

Stella's history of mild depressive episodes indicated an existing problem of self-regulation in her brain. Perimenopause was further affecting her brain's ability to self-regulate. This was probably caused by the fluctuations of her hormones during this phase of life. But it was unclear whether the progesterone Stella was taking as part of her hormone-replacement therapy was also contributing to the worsening of her mood.

In order to tease out the source of Stella's symptoms, our first step was to ask her to stop taking progesterone for two months while continuing to take the estrogen. Such a short break would not cause a problem for her endometrium, and it would help us determine whether this hormone was impairing her mood health.

Women who've had mood problems in the past or who are experiencing the first onset of clinical depression at perimenopause sometimes can't tolerate the addition of progesterone to their estrogen. Physiologically, progesterone acts against estrogen in the brain. It is often thought of as the dysphoric hormone—the one that can cause mood and anxiety changes. In fact, in our practice we have found that progesterone can at times be toxic for some patients' mood states.

Stopping the progesterone made a significant difference in how Stella felt. Her irritability and moodiness partially improved, but she still was somewhat down, fatigued, and unmotivated, and she continued to complain of sleep problems. The progesterone hiatus had not fully relieved her depression, nor had the estrogen dose alone fully treated it. Because it was clear that her symptoms required more than simple hormone replacement, we recommended that she begin a low dose of antidepressant to enhance the serotonin levels in her brain.

Why not just increase the estrogen? Well, estrogen replacement constitutes a paradox when it comes to treating depression. Although it may accomplish all the tasks in the brain we might hope for in an antidepressant, it is actually ineffective in this role. Clinical depression is obviously much more complex than the mild depressive symptoms of some perimenopausal states and can't simply be treated by adding a hormone to the brain! It is likely that once the neuroreceptors and mood pathways have sustained the biochemical changes characteristic of a depression, it requires a different process to bring them back to normal—something that estrogen alone cannot do. Besides, prolonged use of high levels of unopposed estrogen can be dangerous if you are prone to breast or endometrial cancer. But estrogen will help antidepressants to work more effectively in menopause.

Stella began to take Zoloft, an SSRI antidepressant, and with a small dose found that her symptoms disappeared completely. Her sleep normalized, her energy returned, and she felt like herself again. In fact, she felt better now than she ever had in her life! For the first time she was quite joyful. She no longer walked around with the burdensome feeling that she always seemed to carry.

Despite this good news, we were not quite out of the woods. If Stella were to remain on estrogen to protect her bones and alleviate other menopausal symptoms, she needed to take progesterone, too. We reintroduced it and found that now that she was taking the Zoloft, she tolerated it quite well. Her hormone-replacement needs well in hand, we turned our attention to the NURSE Program, which was to become an additional major support in her perimenopausal brain care.

With her depression resolved, Stella no longer craved sweets, which might have been due to the normalization of serotonin levels. She was able to maintain a healthful, low-fat diet. She began exploring physical activities and enrolled in a dance class. This weight-bearing exercise was an excellent way to strengthen her bones. Because she had a stressful job, we encouraged her to take a meditation class. With her renewed energy, Stella was also able to pursue a lifelong interest in art, which she had relegated to the back burner years earlier.

We would review Stella's progress over the next few years, watching her response to treatment to determine if and when we might discontinue the medication. The timing of this was unclear. In light of her long history of dysphoria, we suspected that Stella would relapse once off the antidepressant. She, of course, was in no hurry to discontinue the Zoloft. She was having too much fun.

Postpartum Depression Puts You at Risk During Menopause

If you've had a history of postpartum depression and have been well since, it is wise to be on the alert. Perimenopause can usher in a recurrence of the mood disturbance. That's what happened to our patient Ellena.

At forty-eight, Ellena noticed that her periods had become irregular—she never knew when she was going to menstruate, so she carried tampons in her bag so as not to be caught unprepared. She felt she could live with the night sweats and hot flushes, but slowly other uncomfortable feelings emerged. Some days her usual enthusiasm for life slipped. On other days time seemed to drag, and all she looked forward to was going to bed at night. This was completely out of character for her. She seemed edgier generally, from which a persistent anxiety arose. Her thoughts felt jumbled.

Had she ever felt like this in her life before? She thought back. There was something vaguely familiar about these peculiar symptoms.

Eventually even her bed offered no solace. Sleep eluded her, and she arose in the morning exhausted, anxious, and despairing. She was sure that these awful experiences were in some way related to her menopausal symptoms. I remember her desperate phone call one evening.

"There is something very wrong with me. I have been to so many doctors who can't figure it out. A friend of mine seems to think that you might have an answer."

Ellena had done well in her life. She was an accomplished cellist with an esteemed orchestra. Married in her early twenties, she had one daughter. Within a week of the birth of her daughter, she plunged into the abyss of a severe postpartum depression. Fortunately, she had been well cared for and had been treated with imipramine, an antidepressant available at that time. She responded to the medication, and the depression cleared. Eventually she stopped taking the drug. The depression didn't recur, although at times she had some premenstrual irritability.

Ellena's history told us that her brain-chemistry was exquisitely sensitive to hormonal shifts. Her postpartum depression gave us the clue to what was occurring now during perimenopause. The wild and unpredictable ebb and flow of estrogen and progesterone during this period confused her brain receptors and pathways. The end result was the reemergence of a depressive illness.

Ellena's perimenopausal mood changes were foreseeable. We treated her with an antidepressant, and her gynecologist prescribed hormone-replacement therapy. Collaboratively, we fine-tuned her dosages, and she is thriving again.

The Cafeteria Approach to Hormone Replacement

Hormone-replacement therapy (HRT) is a very personal choice that should be made only after careful consideration of the risks that pertain to you at this time in your life, along with your own family history and personal needs. For instance, although Stella tolerated the reintroduction of progesterone in her HRT regime, a number of women are unable to take this hormone in any form. As a rule we are cautious about the use of progesterone with women who have a history of mood problems, because of its capacity to worsen depression.

We encourage our patients to sample different kinds of progesterone, however, to determine if one will agree with their chemistry before giving up on its use altogether. A commonly prescribed form is medroxyprogesterone, also known as Provera.[1] If the smallest dose (2.5 milligrams) still produces problems in mood, we try a natural progesterone. It is available as a pill (in a micronized form, which means that the particles have been made small to enhance absorption) as well as skin and vaginal creams and suppositories. Micronized progesterone is now commercially available as Prometrium (100 milligrams). Another form of progesterone that may work is delivered by means of an intrauterine device that dispenses it directly onto the lining of the uterus. It remains in the uterus, and very little gets into the bloodstream or the brain.

If a patient has not yet started hormone replacement, we usually ask her to begin taking estrogen alone, at least for a couple of months, to ascertain its effectiveness in relieving her symptoms. If it is effective, only then do we cautiously add small amounts of progesterone. We prefer the micronized natural form that can be taken orally. This timetable helps us assess if the estrogen is effective in relieving symptoms and if the progesterone induces further mood disturbances. It also means that our patient doesn't go downhill over a lengthy period without anyone's realizing what's causing the problem, as happens so frequently.

Estrogens are available in many forms, too. Although there is no evidence at this time that one form is better than another, particularly within the brain, there are no long-term studies investigating the more recently introduced types, such as the estrogen patch or estrone replacement. As you may recall, estrone is the type of estrogen that is dominant after menopause.

Recently, pharmaceutical companies have been marketing low-dose estrogens that may not require added progesterone. These preparations may offer an important alternative to the millions of women who have difficulty tolerating progesterone, enabling them to take estrogen on its own and reap its benefits.

In preliminary studies low-dose estrogen appears to enhance bone structure, maintain the balance of HDLs to LDLs, and preserve estrogen's effect in dilating the blood-vessel walls. Moreover, it is likely to have a protective effect on memory and cognitive functions. It may also be a factor in slowing the processes that contribute to Alzheimer's disease later in life.

The lower dosage of estrogen varies among preparations. Premarin, a commonly prescribed form of estrogen, is available at 0.3 milligrams. Estrace, a natural estradiol, comes in 0.5-milligram tablets. Estratabs and some of the patch estrogens are available at dosages of 0.025 or 0.0375 milligrams. (See Appendix A for different estrogens.) Because you are not taking progesterone with this regime, your endometrium should be monitored for any overgrowth. This can be done by means of an endometrial biopsy once a year or transvaginal ultrasound twice a year. We recommend working with your care provider, asking plenty of questions, and being willing to try different preparations.

Alternatives to estrogen replacement have received a great deal of attention recently. These are called selective estrogen-receptor modulators (SERMs), and they affect some—but not all—of the same receptors that estrogen does. For instance, a SERM acts like estrogen in that it helps to prevent bone loss and can maintain the desired ratio of HDLs to LDLs, but it does not stimulate breast or endometrial tissue. Consequently, it has the potential to deter some of estrogen's effects that may lead to breast and uterine cancer. Evista (raloxifene) is in this new class of drugs. It is an alternative to estrogen for the prevention of bone loss in postmenopausal women and may also protect the heart.

Evista does occasionally have side effects, hot flashes being one. Additionally, some women have experienced nausea and vomiting while taking it. The bottom line is that there is no magic formula to offset all the hormonal changes you will experience during perimenopause or menopause. You need to be informed and talk with your health-care provider to determine the best treatment for you.

What Are the Risks?

Stella asked us what other choices she might have to protect her heart and bones if she elected not to take estrogen. She worried about the risks of breast cancer with long-term estrogen use. This is one of the biggest concerns women have about hormone-replacement therapy. Other women fail to pursue long-term use of HRT because they are not given adequate information about the pros and cons, or even why it has been prescribed. In fact, some surveys indicate that many women don't even fill the prescription.

At this time we don't have complete or final answers about the link between estrogen and breast cancer; opinions conflict. Some studies demonstrate a small increased risk of breast cancer with HRT, when women have used hormones for ten to fifteen years. That fact makes a case for judicious introduction and careful long-term follow-up. However, we also know that your risk of dying from a heart attack after menopause is significantly higher than your risk of dying from breast cancer. Because HRT offers greater protection against heart disease and osteoporosis, many health professionals believe that its benefits far outweigh its risks. But estrogen preparations may not be safe if you have a family history or if you have had breast or ovarian cancer (or other hormonally sensitive cancers), liver disease, gall-bladder disease, high blood pressure, or blood-clotting problems, or if you smoke. As you can see, this is an individual decision that you must make on the basis of your personal needs, particular risks, and family history. If you are healthy and carry no particular risks for heart disease and osteoporosis, you may do fine just using the NURSE program for menopause.

Stella had neither a history of breast cancer nor blood-clotting problems, and she did not smoke. Consequently, she had no primary reason to contradict her taking estrogen. Her history, however, did not exempt her from regular breast self-examination or yearly mammograms and Pap smears. Although no one had heart disease in her family, she seemed at greatest risk for osteoporosis because of her mother's condition. We suggested she take a baseline bone-density test to establish the condition of her bones, with follow-ups every two to three years thereafter. Estrogen replacement, calcium supplements, and weight-bearing exercise would also help keep her bones healthy.

Testosterone Replacement

Testosterone levels decrease after menopause, possibly contributing to loss of well-being and decreased libido. More and more these days there is a belief that testosterone may be an important addition to an HRT regimen. However, we have little information on dosages and levels that may be safe for women after menopause. There may also be added risks for breast cancer and elevated cholesterol. We advise a full discussion with your care provider of the risks and benefits of testosterone replacement.

Women who have had a hysterectomy and oophorectomy (removal of the uterus and ovaries, also known as "surgical menopause") experience a profound and acute loss of testosterone because of the loss of their ovaries. They often describe a much more tremendous and rapid decline in well-being than one would expect in the more gradual process of perimenopause/menopause. Some women also report significant loss of libido and profound depression. Although estrogen replacement is routine in these women, the effort to reclaim their well-being is often elusive, and their lives remain quite disrupted.

It is entirely likely that testosterone replacement is warranted in these cases but little research about testosterone replacement in such situations has been published. It is still unknown what role testosterone plays in women's sense of well-being. Much research is needed in this area.

The Worsening of an Already Present Depression

It's not unusual for women whose mood problems have been fairly well stabilized to find that their situation flies out of control or that they need to take higher doses of medication as they get older. Yet rarely does their clinician take into account the influence of perimenopause. Indeed, perimenopause can usher in a despairing voyage for some women.

Many find themselves on antidepressant treatment in their late thirties and forties. At forty-two, Dana had been treated for depression for a number of years. She had been fairly stable on a moderate dose of Prozac. Yet, seemingly out of the blue, she began to feel more despondent and anxious. Her insomnia returned.

Her doctor undertook all sorts of interventions. He increased her dose of Prozac, then switched her to other antidepressants, adding several together, to little avail. Nothing in her current family life seemed likely to contribute so intensely to the mood disturbance she was struggling with now.

When I saw Dana, I asked whether she had been experiencing hot flashes and night sweats.

"Why, yes," she said, "I've had them for a couple of years, but now they're getting worse. And since you mention it, my periods have become irregular. I skipped a few months a while back." These symptoms correlated with the onset of Dana's trouble in maintaining mood health. We felt sure that the change in her hormone status also contributed to her difficulties in finding a medication regimen that would stabilize her adequately.

There is some evidence that without adequate estrogen, antidepressant medications might not work as well. I believed that with the addition of estrogen, we might better influence the effectiveness of Dana's antidepressants. In her case we increased the dosage of the antidepressant, added estrogen, and later, when her mood had stabilized, added progesterone with success. The addition of estrogen clearly augmented the effectiveness of the Prozac, which by itself had been ineffective against the onset of her perimenopausal depressive symptoms.

The Depression Impostor at Perimenopause

Women who have mood-swing disorders can do particularly poorly during the early phases of perimenopause. In fact, even if they have been in treatment for a long time, they can enter a phase of destabilization at this time, yet reasons for their problems are rarely understood. Often as they try in vain to tell their clinicians how bad they actually feel, these care providers are unable to appreciate that something different is happening to their patients' mood state. Sometimes the caregivers even ignore patients when they say, "This feels hormonal." This lack of response often results in prolonged periods during which the affected women become increasingly distressed.

At forty-nine, Carrie reported an increasingly depressive mood to her therapist of twelve years, whom she had been seeing for family concerns as well as for her tendency to be impulsive and overly reactive to situations. Because Carrie had always been so functional and had tried to maintain her usual activities, her therapist was unable to appreciate that she was losing her ability to cope. Moreover, since she had never been diagnosed as having a bipolar disorder, Carrie was taking no mood-stabilizing medications.

Eventually Carrie reached such a depth of depression that she contacted her gynecologist. Believing Carrie to be experiencing early perimenopausal symptoms, given her shorter cycles and heavier periods of bleeding, he put her on a birth-control pill to regulate her cycles through this phase. After a week on the Pill she became unable to function. She couldn't get out of bed and became agitated and sleepless.

When she came to see me, the first thing I asked Carrie to do was to stop taking the birth-control pill. Until I knew more about the nature of her depression and the brain she had brought with her into this phase of life, I couldn't make further recommendations. Still, it was a safe bet that the progesterone in the Pill had acutely worsened her condition.

Looking at Carrie's genetic history, we found that her mother had violent mood swings and was an explosive person. Her father was an alcoholic. Clearly, she came to her life with a genetically loaded brain. She recalled that as an adolescent she had been quite depressed, but once she left her family's home she'd seemed to snap out of it, and her mood had changed to one of high energy. She became an overachiever and had periods of euphoria and tremendous stamina that she used to her advantage. She was continually promoted in her company. Premenstrually, she could rely on this extra energy burst, which would occur reliably within a day or two before her period.

During her pregnancy Carrie recalled feeling depressed. Her despair must have been quite profound, because she decided to have only one child as a result. Interestingly, she told no one about this. After the birth of her baby, she experienced a period of euphoria, which settled after a few months.

Carrie was fortunate that she had not developed ongoing depressive problems, although she had periods of anxiety and agitation, which she managed with meditation and other relaxation techniques. Now, however, within the perimenopausal hormone-shift period, something in her brain had changed. Unable to maintain its usual firing, it became subject to the influences of the hormonal fluctuations, and her usual coping strategies were being overpowered.

Since Carrie's new pattern of menstrual cycling (shorter periods, heavy bleeding, and sore, bloated breasts) indicated an excess of estrogen, she was not a good candidate for HRT at this particular time. It would further increase her already elevated levels of estrogen in this early phase of perimenopause. Interestingly, her pregnancy, a time of increased estrogen, was also correlated with a period of severe depression. I wondered whether those higher levels of estrogen had sensitized her brain.

I discussed with Carrie how her genetics, her baseline mood state, and the various junctures of her hormonal life were associated with her bipolar 2 disorder (see Chapter 4). She tended toward the energetic, slightly hypomanic end of the mood spectrum.

To begin treatment, we started Carrie on a mood-stabilizing agent, so that if we needed to add an antidepressant later, she would not swing into serious hypomania. Later we could consider estrogen replacement. I would help her evaluate what felt right for her, based on her lifestyle and family history of cancer, heart disease, osteoporosis, and Alzheimer's disease.

If you have bipolar disorder, you need to understand that normal hormonal fluctuations at this time can seriously impair your mood and mood stability. Furthermore, HRT may pose more problems: Progesterone may worsen a depressive mood, and estrogen can make you switch rapidly between mood states—a distressing situation.

Any hormonal-replacement treatments should be undertaken with the full knowledge of your psychiatrist, working in close collaboration with your gynecologist and with close attention to your moods. Start with estrogen alone at a low dose to assess if it causes you problems. Placing you on estrogen and progesterone together will confound any understanding of what may be disturbing your mood stability. If you find a type of estrogen that you tolerate well, cautiously add a low dose (100 milligrams) of progesterone.

A new patient recently called in great distress. She told us that she had had bipolar disorder since she was twenty. Now in her forties, she'd been given a progesterone-only birth-control pill because her periods had become heavy and irregular. Within a week of being on the Pill she became agitated, rageful, and suspicious of the people around her. She felt nonfunctional.

It was clear that the only recent change in her life was the introduction of the birth-control pill. We told her to stop the Pill immediately, and within one week her moods were regulated again. It may never be feasible for her to take progesterone.

Another middle-aged woman came to us complaining of the most severe PMDD she had ever experienced. She was thinking about resigning her job and moving out of her home because she was so impossible to live with. She complained of rage attacks, irritability, inability to sleep, agitation, uncontrollable crying, and depression. When we inquired further into her history, it became clear that she really had bipolar disorder and that the PMDD, from which she believed she had always suffered, had simply become predictably worse at perimenopause.

Among the interventions we made were a mood stabilizer and the NURSE Program. We also advised that she use progesterone only with great caution in any hormone-replacement regimen. We would deal with her hormone-replacement needs later, probably in the form of a low-dose estrogen, if she carried no risks for HRT in her menopausal years. Remember, with a mood-swing disorder it's important to introduce only one hormone at a time.

Every woman's situation is unique and must be evaluated based on her individual needs. If you have any mood history, bipolar or otherwise, you need to exercise caution in introducing HRT.

Estrogen and Memory

Recently I sat at my computer, staring at the screen; I couldn't take in and process the information that was there. I also noticed that I didn't remember what people had said to me a half hour earlier. I had to write everything down. It was a fairly frightening set of moments, particularly since we were in the middle of writing this book. This was no time to have memory disturbances!

Although I could have been tired, this felt different to me. I went to the laboratory and had some blood drawn. I found that even though I was still menstruating, albeit irregularly, my FSH was elevated to menopausal levels. I called my doctor and began taking estrogen. Within two weeks I started to feel better, and my thinking returned to normal. My memory improved, too. I had become my own case study in the effects of estrogen deficiency on memory.

Of course, I'm not the only one in this situation. Perimenopausal women often complain, "I just can't remember anything" or "My memory is like a sieve" or "I forget people's names." Or they may have to write down everything. "If I leave it to my memory," they gripe, "I'll just forget it." Other women bewail the fact that they are unable to retrieve words. The right one may be on the tip of the tongue, but they just can't get their brain to access it when they need it. Others lament, "I walk into a room and forget why I went there. I knew seconds ago, but suddenly it's gone."

How does estrogen attenuate memory and learning? In addition to its impact on mood, it can also affect your ability to learn new information adequately and recall it. It is involved in maintaining the specific cells in synapses—the intricate communication between nerve cells—in the hippocampus.

Furthermore, estrogen supports acetylcholine levels. Acetylcholine, a neurotransmitter found in the hippocampus and prefrontal cortex, is responsible for memory and those aspects of thought that relate to memory and retrieval of words. When estrogen is withdrawn in rats in experimental situations, acetylcholine levels decline in these brain areas and the rats' ability to recall learned behaviors degenerates.

This research on rats appears to apply to studies in women, demonstrating the beneficial effect of estrogen replacement on memory and other cognitive functions. For instance, Dr. Barbara Sherwin, a research psychologist at McGill University in Canada, has shown in a number of studies that women who are deficient in estrogen, either menopausally or after their ovaries have been surgically removed, experience a consistent decrease in their ability to recall recently learned material. This lessening in recall is confined to spoken material only and does not involve what they learned visually. Barbara Sherwin concludes that estrogen helps to maintain verbal memory and enhances the capacity for new learning in these women.

Moreover, a recent study evaluating sex differences in the aging brain by Dr. Declan Murphy at the National Institute of Mental Health demonstrated that women experience a more rapid decline in the structures essential for higher cognitive functioning. In particular, the hippocampus shrinks more substantially and more quickly in women between the ages of sixty and eighty-five than in men of the same age. The lack of estrogen may have something to do with this finding, but the researchers did not address this issue.

Other studies evaluating the effect of estrogen given to postmenopausal women have found mostly that the administration of estrogen enhances memory, learning, attention, and even IQ. For instance, Dr. Uriel Halbreich, a professor of psychiatry and gynecology at the State University of New York in Buffalo, has conducted numerous investigations into the effect of estrogen on the cognitive functioning of menopausal women. He has found that complex brain tasks such as recognition, interpretation, decision-making, eye-hand coordination, and some aspects of memory are markedly improved when women who were not receiving estrogen replacement begin taking the hormone. These results suggest that estrogen plays a role in helping maintain these functions at peak performance. When estrogen declines and remains at low levels, these functions can deteriorate.

It is possible that when the brain-ovary dialogue begins to fluctuate and slow, all these functions can be affected. Perimenopause (the period characterized by irregular hormonal variations) and menopause can prove to be a more difficult time for women as far as their memory goes.

When we affirm for women who report memory changes that they're not going mad, they are relieved. Often their doctors have told them "not to worry about it"—but this is not helpful when they are anxious that they're showing early symptoms of Alzheimer's—which they are not.

Alzheimer's Disease, Estrogen, and Menopause

Alzheimer's disease affects one in two women but only one in three men. Men retain their levels of testosterone well into the eighth decade, whereas women lose estrogen in their fifties. New understandings regarding Alzheimer's disease show that estrogen may play an important role in delaying the disease process in women. Estrogen may also be important in preventing the death of cells in crucial areas necessary for maintaining cognitive and memory functions.

Several preliminary studies suggest that the rate of Alzheimer's is one-third to one-half lower in women who have used estrogen compared to those who have never used it. Whether or not you have a family history of Alzheimer's disease, this is another important piece of information to help you decide if you should use estrogen-replacement therapy.

Use the NURSE Program for Perimenopausal Symptoms

We believe that if you proactively take care of yourself, you will enter perimenopause and menopause with part of the battle already won. Designing and implementing a perimenopausal NURSE Program is an important element of maintaining your mental and physical well-being. The following are some suggestions to tailor your NURSE Program to your own needs at the end of your reproductive cycle.

NOURISHMENT
Be sure that you:

- maintain a low-fat diet.
- have adequate calcium supplementation (see below).
- take a daily multivitamin that contains antioxidants. Antioxidants such as Vitamin C, Vitamin E, Vitamin B-complex, and selenium are substances that mop up harmful molecules called free radicals that can be damaging to cells. Vitamin E may alleviate hot flashes.
- eat foods rich in phytoestrogens, the naturally occurring estrogens in plant foods. Although there are still no controlled scientific studies on these products, they may help supply your brain with additional estrogen resources. Phytoestrogens also contain anticancer, antioxidant, antiviral, antibacterial, and anti-

fungal properties. Foods rich in phytoestrogens include yams, lentils, oat bran, tofu, and soy milk (or other soy-containing foods such as miso soup, cooked soy beans, soy "nuts," etc.).

- supplement your diet with alpha-omega-3 fatty acids (found in fish oil, flaxseed oil). Alpha-omega-3 fatty acids are an excellent source of phytoestrogens, in fact, more so than tofu.

UNDERSTANDING

Be sure that you understand the physiology of estrogen and neuro-transmitters. The decrease in your estrogen levels can affect the neurons, neurotransmitters, and limbic structures in your brain.

Use the Perimenopausal Rating Chart (in Appendix B) to help you rate the frequency and severity of perimenopausal symptoms you may be experiencing.

In addition, become informed on the pros and cons of hormone-replacement therapy (HRT) as an option for you. The decision to undertake HRT will be based on your family history, your symptoms, and your personal history.

Have regular physical examinations that include routine Pap smears, mammograms, bone-density scans, and cholesterol checks.

REST AND RELAXATION

Pay attention to your sleep patterns and rituals. Remember that your brain needs sleep to reregulate its biochemistry. If you begin to experience changes in your sleep patterns, think about what is going on. Are you experiencing increased stress in your life? Are your sleep patterns being disrupted by night sweats? Family issues?

Take naps if you're tired. You deserve to rest. Sometimes a ten-minute "power nap" can invigorate you for the rest of the day

SPIRITUALITY

Take time for yourself. Read that novel that's been lying on your bedside table. Keep a journal. This has been a powerful tool for many of our patients; it is a form of self-awareness.

Sign up for a yoga or meditation class or a stress-reduction program. Have a facial or a body massage—or maybe even both. Perhaps you've been thinking about going on a retreat or to a day spa—do it!

EXERCISE

Regular exercise is critical to your physical, mental, and spiritual health. Not only does exercise strengthen your bones and muscles, it can also reduce stress. Exercise also maintains your biological clock, aiding your sleep cycle. About twenty minutes of walking a day is an excellent choice. Weight-bearing exercise, such as walking, jogging, and weight-training, helps to strengthen bones. Swimming, on the other hand, will provide some cardiovascular benefits and will strengthen muscles and keep muscle tone but is less efficient in fortifying bones. Any form of aerobic activity, however, will protect your cardiovascular system.

Invite a friend. Sometimes it's easier to exercise with a buddy. Or listen to music. It helps to quicken the pace and can make the time pass more pleasantly.

Preventing Osteoporosis

For bone health it is important to supplement the amount of calcium you ingest during this vulnerable period. If you are taking estrogen replacement, you will need 1,000 milligrams of calcium a day. If you don't use estrogen, you would require a daily dose of 1,500 milligrams.

Take the calcium supplements in divided doses, because the body absorbs only about 500 milligrams at a time. Nutritionists recommend calcium citrate with Vitamin D or oyster-shell calcium, since these are the most easily absorbed. We also suggest chewing Tums tablets. Each tablet contains 500 milligrams of calcium, and Tums are much less expensive than calcium pills.

Of course, you can also derive calcium from the food you eat:

- Eight ounces of low-fat/nonfat yogurt provide 400 milligrams of calcium.
- An eight-ounce glass of low-fat or skim milk gives 350 milligrams.
- One ounce of Cheddar or Muenster cheese gives 200 milligrams.
- One cup of hard ice cream provides 150–250 milligrams. Soft-serve ice cream provides 300 or more milligrams.
- A cup of broccoli, soy beans, or turnip greens provides 100–200 milligrams.

After the travails of perimenopause, postmenopause can be a time of great energy and productivity in your life. Many women who have reached this milestone claim they have "never felt better." You may feel freer and better able to accomplish whatever you want at a moment's notice. In fact, the famed anthropologist Margaret Mead coined the phrase "postmenopausal zest" to characterize this period of renewed vigor.

By informing yourself about your potential for mood disruption and by designing and implementing your own perimenopausal NURSE Program, you, too, can enjoy this wonderful phase in your life.

EPILOGUE

TOWARD THE FUTURE: A HEALING JOURNEY

Whether the pattern is related to hormonal events or not, acknowledging that you are in need of help with an emotional illness is one of the first steps toward healing. Sadly, in our culture we still marginalize and deny these illnesses. You may worry that you will be considered weak or "crazy" if you admit to one and seek therapy. The stigma attached to mental disorders can interfere with your receiving adequate support and proper medical care.

But as the field of psychiatry is now showing, mental disturbances are often due to the brain's abnormal chemical functioning. They are not signs of personal weakness but are treatable brain diseases that warrant prompt attention.

Understanding this brain-mind-body connection can go a long way toward promoting healing. It removes the self-blame, shame, and stigma that so often accompany emotional illness and frees you to seek help.

Protect Yourself from Relapse

After an earthquake we bolt our homes to their foundations and reinforce masonry wherever possible. We pour additional concrete around bridge pilings and strengthen dams. We undertake these preventive measures because we care about our safety and we expect that more temblors may follow.

The same can be said of mood and anxiety disorders. Even if you are feeling well on or off maintenance medications, you must face the possibility that a mood or anxiety disorder can recur. Therefore, you'll want to do all you can to protect your brain from further episodes of chaos.

The NURSE Program includes all the elements of brain care that you'll need: nourishment (including medications as needed), understanding, relaxation, spirituality, and exercise. Based on the examples we've shared in this book, you can design and implement a plan that starts you down the road to authenticity and health. An important part of it includes valuing yourself in a loving way.

You may need to incorporate skills and strategies into your daily life that keep your brain biochemistry balanced. And you may need to develop new ways to integrate the changes that depression and anxiety already may have wrought in your biochemistry; the chemical underpinnings of the earthquake may have become a part of who you are. The NURSE Program coupled with psychotherapy can be very helpful in this regard.

Use Psychotherapy

An important step along the road to healing is understanding what precipitated the earthquake. What pressures affected you previously? If possible, try to reduce these as much as is reasonable in order to prevent a relapse.

We strongly recommend psychotherapy to help in this process of self-understanding and awareness. Therapy can provide the nurturing, reflective environment in which you can become more attuned to how you feel and how your behaviors relate to your feelings. It can also help you make sense of the changes in your life that the disorder has produced. You may assess its impact on your family as well as the factors that might have led to the episode. In therapy, you may also receive guidance to help you shape your future and counseling about how you can take better care of yourself.

There are many different types of therapy, including interpersonal, cognitive, and short-term. While these therapies are helpful, bear in mind that a short course of therapy may be ineffective for a long-term problem. You may need review and maintenance sessions at regular intervals. Remember, too, that in the same way that adverse events train your biology to respond negatively, psychotherapy promotes learning and insight, which has the capacity to enhance the *biology* of your mood pathways.

Therapy is an important adjunct to medical treatment. I recently had a surprising conversation with a well-known psychopharmacologist. Concerned about how long it took for antidepressants to kick in (up to eight weeks sometimes), he asked me how I manage the disease in the meantime. I replied, "That's not usually a problem, because I don't see my patients as a 'disease.' Besides, I usually rely on the relationship I establish with them through weekly meetings to support the healing and educational process." I sometimes wonder whether, in their zeal to prescribe medication, those in the field of psychopharmacology have forgotten the healing value of this relationship and that their patients still need to interact with them.

If, like so many people today, you simply receive medication without incorporating the other components of healing, you may run the risk of relapse. Here is another instance where you, as a whole person, must be considered. Most of the time you will be asked to stay on your medication for about a year. But what happens after you taper off? Do you just go on as before? The issue of preventing a relapse may never be raised—and that is wrong. It is our strong belief that if you are taking medication for your disorder, be sure that you are also in talk therapy with someone whom you trust. Both are necessary for your healing.

Accepting What You Can't Change

Many women find it difficult to accept that anxiety and depression can be long-term disorders that often worsen when their hormones shift. It is not unusual for us to discover that our patients are taking their medications only intermittently; they were curious about how they would do without them. Others stop their medications on their own and relapse several months later. They were testing whether we were telling them the truth. Some patients do this several times over; it's so difficult for them to accept the physiological disorder. Under these circumstances the healing journey is guaranteed to be bumpy, scary, and frustrating.

It is vital to recognize and accept that emotional disorders can be long-term problems. Think of it as living with an illness like diabetes, heart disease, or arthritis that flares up at intervals. Since the condition is ongoing, often there is no "cure." You learn to live alongside the disorder and find a way to accept it that doesn't victimize you. Psychotherapy can help in this process.

Protecting Our Children

As our patients recover, feel surer of themselves, and understand the disorders of depression and anxiety, they begin asking, "How can I prevent this from happening to my children?" This is a valid question. If you or a close family member has had a mood or anxiety disorder, it's possible that your children also will be vulnerable, and your daughters may be at particular risk. Consequently, you will want to arm them with the information and skills they'll need to care for themselves. Teaching them about their brains, how to manage the effects of stress, and how to recognize the early symptoms of depression can help circumvent future problems.

When I dropped my daughter Megan at college for her freshman year, my parting words to her were "Remember to take care of your brain."

She, of course, rolled her eyes and replied, "Mom, you've got to be the only mother in North America who sends her daughter off to college without crying about how sad she'll be!" Nevertheless, Megan knew what I meant and how important this was. She had heard about this vital aspect of caring for herself for a long time. Similarly, Jeanne has discussed moods, hormones, brain strain, and the components of brain health with her daughters.

We live with these vitally important concerns since we each have two daughters. As women's-health advocates, we worry how the mood disorders we have experienced might manifest in our girls. With an appreciation of the early emergence of mood disturbances and the brain's capacity to be loaded over time, we have raised our children with an awareness of how their brains interact with the world. We've been careful to teach them how to care for themselves.

The mother-daughter relationship can be an influential and intimate connection. If we, as mothers, become comfortable with who we are and with the vulnerabilities of our biochemistry, we can share that information with our daughters, watching and helping them become protective of themselves as they grow. This will enable them to be honest in their feelings and authentic in the world.

We have readily shared our strategies with our daughters, discussing with them what we have learned and how we have changed our own lives in response to our emerging knowledge. We validate what they feel and think so that they can have their own voices and develop relationships based on mutuality and respect. Jeanne's daughter Kate once remarked, "You know, Mom, if you're learning all this at forty-eight, and I'm learning it at twenty, my daughters may know all this by the time they're ten!" From the mouths of our daughters!

"What's going to happen to me when I have a baby, in light of what happened to you, Mom?" our daughters have asked us as they've grown older. We laugh and tell them that as long as we're both around, we'll take very good care of them. But they may well be at risk. Still, we'll make sure that they're well informed, and of course at any sign of problems, a treatment plan will be in place. In the meantime, we have taught them to stay in touch with their moods, brains, and hormones—and we hope that you and your daughters will, too!

Watch for Problems

Nurturing a child's mental and physical health begins at conception. If you or your partner have had a mood disorder, watch for signs of depression or anxiety in your children. Remember, depression need not start with mood disturbance, but with other symptoms such as problems sleeping, irritability, and fatigue. By the time a girl reaches puberty, she may be entering a risk period for depression.

One of my patients recently told me that her ten-year-old daughter was unable to fall asleep for a few hours and then awoke around 3:00 A.M., agitated and unable to go back to sleep. In light of her mother's and father's depressive disorders, it's likely that this young girl was showing early symptoms that might later unfold into depression.

I advocated immediate intervention, first with a behavioral approach (calming her before bedtime by avoiding boisterous games or TV shows and practicing quiet bedtime rituals), and if that didn't work, then medication. The alternative was to let this young girl's brain begin learning the depressive mode of functioning, which might guarantee a depressive earthquake a little later in her life.

Early education is imperative. By the time a girl reaches adolescence, many of her self-care habits are formed. She can enlarge her repertoire as she gains more cognitive and social knowledge. We have encouraged our daughters to learn and use the NURSE Program. You may find aspects of it helpful with your own children. As women and mothers, we do have the power to influence the next generation.

Using the NURSE *Program with Your Daughters*

Your child needs to take care of her brain. If she does, it will take care of her. The NURSE Program can help forestall future difficulties. Here are some suggestions about how you can apply it to your daughter's well-being.

NOURISHMENT

It's important for your daughter to nourish her mind, body, and soul. Like yours, her body needs a healthy balance of proteins, carbohydrates, fats, and fluids. Most people will tell you that they feel as though their body functions well when they make healthy food choices. You may have become more aware of the nutritional aspects of health during pregnancy or when your children were small, but there's no reason to stop there.

Mother-daughter outings can include visits with a nutritionist or enrolling in a nutritional workshop. Cooking together and discussing food preparation is another way to convey good nutritional thinking to the next generation.

Our daughters quickly imitate our behaviors, and in truth, we are often unaware of how much time they spend observing the way we function in the world. They are sensitive, attuned to their surroundings and to you in more ways than you may think. So when you pay attention to your food intake and attitudes, this will help your children, too.

Sadly, the pervasive cultural theme of "thin is in" can cause a young girl to diet excessively. If you nag your daughter about weight gain and body size, she may feel even more pressure to look like a supermodel. Nutrition and exercise are ongoing health issues, not part of a fad diet!

It's also important to nourish your child's mind. Encourage her to use the brain's cortex for the purpose for which it was designed. Keep your youngster's mind active through reading, problem-solving, critical thinking, negotiation, and communication. From a very early age, make reading to your child an important part of the day. Invite her to name, understand, and explain the pictures or concepts in books, on road signs, or at the grocery.

Another strategy that enhances cortical development is to respond to your child's questions by asking her what she thinks and feels rather than quickly supplying answers for her or telling her what she feels. This requires her to think and to name her emotions, enhancing her creativity, curiosity, and authenticity. It will also help you get to know who your child is in an intimate way. Reading the newspaper together and discussing the evening news are other "teachable moments" that can turn everyday life experiences into learning opportunities.

Brain nourishment may also come from medications. Preliminary research has begun to document that when a child shows signs of depression, intervention with psychiatric medications is far more effective than chalking up all behaviors as "just a phase" that will pass.

UNDERSTANDING

It's important for your daughters to know the information about neurochemistry and reproductive biochemistry we have presented. They need a good understanding of these magnificently complex aspects of their bodies' day-to-day functioning. They should be able to correctly name their genitals and reproductive organs as well as understand what is happening at a biochemical level during their menstrual cycle. Knowledge about their bodies will empower them.

Adolescents need to know that their monthly period is not just "something that happens so you can have a baby." Many teen pregnancies occur due to lack of information about fertility cycles and the physiological process of becoming pregnant. It is critical to talk with your daughters about sexuality, sensuality, and the risk of sexually transmitted diseases (particularly chlamydia, syphilis, gonorrhea, venereal warts, and HIV and AIDS). This will give them a sense of empowerment that may help them feel comfortable saying no if a disturbing or anxiety-provoking situation arises in a relationship.

The rate of depression begins to double for girls around adolescence—just when they're starting their menstrual cycles. This is an excellent time to continue the honest dialogue about how their bodies work and how their brain and body are interconnected.

If your daughter has a significant genetic history of mood and anxiety disorders, she may begin to experience some symptoms in her early adolescence. This is something to watch. In addition, she may not be a candidate for birth-control pills, Depo Provera, or Norplant. If she does try a biological contraceptive method, she must pay attention to any changes in her moods and work closely with her healthcare provider.

It's also important for your young daughter to have mentors and models. This may or may not be you. Some girls find mentors in other women, such as a teacher, a friend's mother, a Girl Scout leader, a coach, an aunt, or a grandmother. They can share their innermost thoughts and concerns with this person and not worry about being judged or negated.

Our work as mothers is to listen to our daughters and appreciate the reality of *their* experience. We must be careful not to project our beliefs and thoughts onto our girls at the expense of the expression of theirs.

REST AND RELAXATION

The brain needs sleep so it can reregulate its biochemical functions and be ready for a new day. A disruption in your daughter's sleep patterns is one of the first signs her brain gives that it's feeling strained. Disruption could mean that she wants to sleep all the time, that she wakes up in the middle of the night and can't get back to sleep, that she awakens earlier than normal without an alarm clock, or that she just can't get to sleep at all. If the sleep disruption occurs frequently and fatigue is getting in the way of daily living, something must be done to correct this dysregulation.

Early in our children's lives we focus on their sleep patterns and rituals, helping them to self-comfort and get to bed at the same time each night. Rituals may include taking a bath, putting on pajamas, brushing teeth, getting into bed, reading stories, talking about the day, saying prayers, and then falling asleep. It is the establishment and regularity of these regimes that help children gain a sense of competence and control.

As our children grow, it is time once again to remind them about sleep regularity—especially in adolescence. Some people recommend reading, the use of New Age or classical music, or white noise at bedtime to block out sounds of the night. Your children should avoid listening to a talk-radio or news station while they're failing asleep, as there is a potential to awaken with negative thoughts as a result of hearing the "news" of the day (which is usually unhappy) all night long.

It is not uncommon for young girls to experience sleep-pattern changes prior to their first periods, so be vigilant in your observation. Sleep disturbances can also be related to premenstrual hormonal changes, worries, stressors, interpersonal concerns, and the need to talk.

If you find that your adolescent is beginning to experience sleep disorders, it is important not just to ascribe it to her stage or age. Her brain is sending the message that it's unable to unwind and rest. This may be the time to enroll your child in a meditation or yoga course or to have the sleep disturbance evaluated. The brain needs to reset itself. If it doesn't get enough time to do that through sleep, mood and anxiety symptoms can result.

We also encourage the use of journal-keeping from a very early age. A diary can serve as part of your daughter's evening bedtime ritual, too. She can record her day's activities and write about feelings, relationships, thoughts, concerns, and private musings. A journal is a great way for her to listen to her inner voice. The exercise of writing can help your daughter become more conscious of what's going on in her mind.

SPIRITUALITY

Spirituality is a sense of self, balance, and connection with a higher power or being. The way you achieve spirituality is quite personal. Some find it within the context of their religious group. There they learn the guidelines, principles, and precepts of their faith. However, being part of a religious group and being spiritual can be two separate things. Indeed, spirituality can emanate from a personal philosophy of belief rather than affiliation with an organized religion.

Meditation, prayer, solitude, and mindfulness are all ways to incorporate spirituality into your life. If you or your daughter don't know how to practice relaxation breathing or mindfulness, many books and courses can teach you these easy techniques. For instance, simply sitting in a chair and being aware of your own breathing for fifteen minutes—just being present—is a form of relaxation.

This same kind of spiritual uplift may occur when you take a walk. Initially your mind may be spinning as you process the events of the day. But suddenly you find yourself noticing the flowers along the road or the clouds in the sky for the first time. Your breathing shifts, and your mind seems to clear. What a nice feeling. Your walk has made you more focused and centered.

You can use these techniques as part of an after-school ritual with your daughter as a way to influence her practice of meditation and mindfulness. Following her snack and a discussion of her day, ask her to lie on the floor alongside you and do your breathing exercises together. Consider signing her up for martial-arts courses that teach centering and self-control. Yoga is another practice that teaches centering and relaxation while strengthening the body. Sign up for a course together. When your child begins these self-care behaviors at an early age, it can set the stage for her to incorporate them into her life as she grows toward adulthood.

EXERCISE

Fifteen to twenty minutes of aerobic exercise can cause a surge in serotonin and endorphin levels that leaves your daughter with a sense of calm and well-being. Exercise can also help her focus on breathing and get in touch with her body's flexibility.

Many baby boomers were not raised on the concept of regular exercise for fitness and mental well-being. In fact, depending on your age, your school probably didn't offer sports (apart from intramural games or physical-education classes) in which girls could participate. Team sports were uncommon for girls in the 1950s, and exercise was often limited to ballet, gymnastics, tap, and jazz. But over the years girls' sports have become much more popular. Today there are girls' basketball, soccer, softball, baseball, hockey (field and ice), and la- crosse teams, to name a few.

Your exercise activities provide a great model for your daughter. She sees that they are important, especially if you share with her how you feel in response to them.

Exercise can also promote your relationship and communication with your daughter. Taking a walk, going for a bike ride, or playing a game of Frisbee, tennis, or catch—all of these are great ways to have uninterrupted one-on-one time together.

"Have You Taken Care of Your Brain Today?"

We hope that by providing you with basic information about how your brain and body work we have stimulated you to rethink aspects of your self-care. The key to brain health is knowing when and how you might be vulnerable and caring for your brain—your master com- puter—within the comprehensive NURSE framework. Each compo- nent of the NURSE Program provides a template for caring for yourself in a complete way. This goes a long way toward promoting mental and physical health.

Every woman is a unique person with distinct skills, experiences, coping strategies, and physiology. We hope that you are now able to assess your own situation. You have the power to understand your neurochemistry, and in that knowledge, you have the capacity to take care of your brain. As we often say, if you take care of your brain, it will take care of you. Indeed, this has become a mantra for us in our personal lives as well as in our practice. We feel so strongly about it that we have seriously considered creating a bumper sticker that asks, HAVE YOU TAKEN CARE OF YOUR BRAIN TODAY?

When you're struggling with an emotional earthquake, you may wonder if you will ever recover. "Will I ever feel normal again?" you may wonder. "Is there a light at the end of this horrible tunnel?" The "earthquake" may have changed your life—mental disorders are unlike any other experience.

Yet many women have told us that some years after their ordeal they look back on the earthquake as a gift. It caused them to regain power in their lives by learning how to care for themselves, by finding meaningful relationships, and by appreciating life in a way they never had before. Yes, you will recover, but you will have to work to achieve it. You and your family are worth it.

There is hope. There is life. You must do everything to find it.

Psychotropic Medications Currently Available

Drug Class/Generic Name	Trade Name
Antidepressants	
TriCyclic Antidepressants (TCA)	
Amitriptyline	Elavil, Endep
Amoxapine	Asendin
Clomipramine	Anafranil
Desipramine	Norpramin, Pertofrane
Doxepin	Adapin, Sinequan
Imipramine	Tofranil
Maprotiline	Ludiomil
Nortriptyline	Aventyl, Pamelor
Protriptyline	Vivactil
Trimipramine	Surmontil
Monoamine Oxidase Inhibitor (MAOIs)	
Phenelzine	Nardil
Tranylcypromine	Parnate

Selective Serotonin-Reuptake Inhibitors (SSRIs)

Fluoxetine	Prozac
Fluvoxamine	Luvox
Paroxetine	Paxil
Sertraline	Zoloft
Citalopram	Celexa

Selective Norepinephrine-Reuptake Blocker

Bupropion	Wellbutrin
	Wellbutrin SR

Serotonin- and Norepinephrine-Reuptake Blocker

Venlafaxine	Effexor
	Effexor XR

5HT2 Antagonist and Serotonin-Reuptake Blocker

Nefazodone	Serzone
Trazodone	Desyrel

Alpha-2, 5H2, 5HT3 Antagonist

Mirtazapine	Remeron

Antianxiety Agents
Benzodiazepines

Alprazolam	Xanax
Chlordiazepoxide	Librium
Clonazepam	Klonopin
Clorazepate	Tranxene
Diazepam	Valium
Estazolam	Prosom
Flurazepam	Dalmane
Lorazepam	Ativan
Oxazepam	Serax
Prazepam	Centrax
Quazepam	Doral
Temazepam	Restoril
Triazolam	Halcion
Zolpidem	Ambien

Serotonergic Antianxiety Agent

Buspirone	Buspar

Mood Stabilizers

Carbamazepine	Tegretol
Carbamazepine	XR Tegretol CR
Divalproex sodium	Depakote
Gabapentin	Neurontin
Lamotrigine	Lamictal
Lithium carbonate	Lithium
Lithium carbonate	Eskalith
Lithium citrate (elixir)	Cibalith-S
L-thyroxine	Synthroid
Nimodipine	Nimotop
Omega-3 fatty acids	Flaxseed oil or fish oil
Verapamil SR	Calan SR

Antipsychotic Drugs

Chlorpromazine	Thorazine
Chlorprothixene	Taractan
Fluphenazine	Prolixin
Haloperidol	Haldol
Loxapine	Loxitane
Mesoridazine	Serentil
Molindone	Moban
Perphenazine	Trilafon
Pimozide	Orap
Thioridazine	Mellaril
Thiothixine	Navane
Trifluoperazine	Stelazine

Atypical Antipsychotic Agents

Clozapine	Clozaril
Olanzapine	Zyprexa
Quetiapine	Seroquel
Risperidone	Risperdal

Charting Your Premenstrual or Perimenopausal Symptoms

Instructions for Premenstrual Daily Symptoms Chart:

Begin on the first day of your menstrual period, as Day 1. Mark each day you are menstruating with an M. Fill in the graph at the end of the day, recording your symptom severity according to the scale 0 to 3, with 0 representing no symptoms and 3 representing the worst you have ever experienced. If you have no symptoms, leave the square blank.

Note any specific stressful events that may have occurred during the day, any alcohol intake, and any medications you may be taking. If you should experience a symptom that is not already listed, please record it in the spaces provided.

Name																														
Day of cycle	1	2	3	4	5	6	7	8	9	10	11	12	13	14	15	16	17	18	19	20	21	22	23	24	25	26	27	28	29	30
Date																														
Menses																														
Symptoms																														
crying, tearful																														
anxiety, restlessness																														
sadness																														
overwhelmed by things																														
mood changeability																														
anger, rage attacks																														
irritability																														
overly sensitive																														
loss of interest																														
loss of enjoyment																														
feeling tired																														
feeling guilty																														
blaming self																														
disliking self																														
loss of libido																														
poor concentration																														
confusion																														
forgetfulness																														
social withdrawal																														
appetite: incr/decr																														
suicidal thoughts/plan																														
panic attacks																														
obsessional thoughts																														
compulsive behaviors																														
avoidant behavior																														
food cravings																														
sleep: incr/decr																														
nausea																														
abdominal bloating																														
hot flashes																														
clumsiness																														
breast swelling																														
abdominal cramps																														
headaches																														
increased energy																														
hyperactivity																														
talkative																														
start many projects																														
racing thoughts																														
buying sprees																														
elevated mood																														
euphoria																														
alcohol intake																														
medications																														
doses																														
other pertinent events																														

Scale: 1=mild symptoms, 2=moderate, 3=severe
If you do not have any symptoms, leave the box blank.

Illustration 12. Premenstrual Daily Symptoms Rating Chart

Instructions for Perimenopausal Symptom Chart:

Begin on the first day of your menstrual period, as Day 1. Fill in the graph at the end of the day, recording your symptom severity according to the scale 0 to 3, with 0 representing no symptoms and 3 representing the worst you have ever experienced. If you have no symptoms, leave the square blank.

Note any specific stressful events that may have occurred during the day, any alcohol intake, and any medications you may be taking. If you are taking estrogen and progesterone, record the pattern of replacement and dosage. If you should experience any symptom that is not already listed, please record it. Also record calcium intake.

If your cycle extends longer than the thirty days on the chart, go on to a new sheet and record the day, adding in 31, 32, 33, etc. If you experience any spotting or actual menstruation, use an S to record spotting and M for menses.

Activities of daily living (ADL) are the usual things that you do in the day, for example: bathing, shopping, calling people on the phone, cooking, dressing.

Name																														
Day of cycle	1	2	3	4	5	6	7	8	9	10	11	12	13	14	15	16	17	18	19	20	22	23	24	25	26	27	28	29	30
Date																														
Menses																														
Flow																														
Symptoms																														
hot flashes ?x day																														
breast changes																														
night sweats																														
interest in sex																														
burning on urinating																														
vaginal dryness																														
headaches																														
difficulty sleeping																														
increased sleep																														
feeling tired																														
not feeling well																														
diffic make decision																														
feeling emotional																														
sadness																														
feeling low																														
loss of interest																														
overwhelmed																														
loss of enjoyment																														
feeling a failure																														
blaming self																														
looking unattractive																														
crying, tearful																														
feeling guilty																														
hopeless, worthless																														
hard to do ADL																														
restlessness																														
anger, irritability																														
increased tension																														
anxiety																														
agitation																														
isolating self																														
suicidal thoughts																														
poor concentration																														
forgetfulness																														
word finding difficulty																														
not thinking clearly																														
hard to take in info																														
difficulty organizing																														
incr/dcre appetite																														
elevated mood																														
feeling wonderful																														
talkative																														
racing thoughts																														
buying sprees																														
increased energy																														
estrogen dose																														
progesterone dose																														
other meds																														
calcium intake																														

Scale: 1=mild symptoms, 2=moderate, 3=severe
If you do not have any symptoms, leave the box blank.

Illustration 13. Perimenopausal Daily Symptoms Rating Chart

Estrogen and Progesterone Preparations

There are many estrogen preparations on the market, some new and some old. More are becoming available every day. Although the table beginning on page 308 lists some of the preparations you may encounter, it is important for you to have some general information about these preparations and which questions to ask your doctor so you can feel comfortable about what is prescribed for you.

In their natural state, estrogen and progesterone are unstable and poorly absorbed orally, so pharmaceutical companies have developed ways to maximize their stability and absorption rates. Any type of estrogen, even those coming from a natural source such as yams, must be modified in the lab to maximize these properties.

You can take estrogen orally, vaginally, or through the skin. It can be surgically inserted beneath the skin or delivered via a device inserted into the uterus.

Some women prefer the estrogen they are taking to be derived from "nature" rather than synthesized in a laboratory. However, even if a drug is marketed as "natural" because it is made from plant sources, it will still have been modified. Indeed, the newer preparations derived from the plant source are still altered and refined in the laboratory for better stability and absorption.

Rather, you should focus on whether the form and dose of estrogen achieves the desired preventive measures in the bones, heart, and blood fats and does not produce adverse side effects for you. Currently the estrogen used in most of the studies is Premarin, the oldest and most commonly prescribed form of estrogen in hormone-replacement therapy. The active estrogen ingredients in this preparation are *equilins,* or horse estrogens. They are removed from the urine of pregnant mares and include a number of different estrogens. Newer preparations have been approved for menopausal use, but no one preparation has been shown to be superior to another.

Estrogen preparations may be unsafe if you have a family history of or have had breast or ovarian cancer (or other hormone-sensitive cancers), liver disease, gallbladder disease, blood-clotting problems, or high blood pressure, or if you smoke. In these situations, discuss alternatives with your doctor (see the NURSE Program in Chapter 18).

It is preferable that you not have undesirable side effects such as bloating, breast tenderness and swelling, weight gain, nausea, or any blood-clotting problems or abnormal vaginal bleeding. Mood changes in either direction (depression or unwarranted elation) are also unwelcome.

You and your doctor may embark on one type of dosing regime, find that it does not work for you, and then seek out another. This is quite common. Don't give up, but rather work with your doctor to achieve what is comfortable for you.

Progesterone is given in different combinations with estrogen to protect the lining of the uterus. One way is to take it continuously with estrogen, so that after a while no further menstrual bleeding occurs. In the beginning you may experience irregular bleeding. These bleeds must be evaluated, because the cause of any irregular bleeding should be determined. However, many postmenopausal women tolerate the combined daily dosing well. You can also take progesterone between days one and twelve of the cycle or add it between days fifteen and twenty-five. These regimens give rise to withdrawal bleeds and a monthly period. Another way of adding progesterone is to do it continuously with estrogen for twenty-five days with a five- to six-day break, during which bleeding may occur. The HRT (hormone-replacement therapy) is then resumed on day thirty-two of the cycle.

Remember that progesterone can induce irritability, mood changes, and depression. Check with your doctor about the best dosages for you and how best to balance the progesterone with the estrogen you take.

Use of testosterone preparations is not widespread at the moment, though there is interest in adding this to hormone-replacement regimens. Since using testosterone over long periods in postmenopausal women is not well studied, you should check with your doctor about the advisability of using these preparations in your particular case.

In some situations estrogens have been mixed with progesterones, and in others with testosterone. In a short time there will no doubt be preparations available that combine all three.

ESTROGEN PREPARATIONS

Brand Name	Dosages	Type of Estrogen	Manufacturer
Premarin	0.3 mg	conjugated equine estrogens	Wyeth-Ayerst
	0.625 mg	made from pregnant mares' urine	
	0.9 mg		
	1.25 mg		
	2.5 mg		

Premarin also comes combined with testosterone.

Estrace	0.5 mg	micronized estradiol	Mead Johnson
	1.0 mg	metabolized to estrone	
	2.0 mg		
Estratabs	0.3 mg	esterified estrogens—mostly estrone	Solvay
	0.625 mg		
	2.5 mg		

Estratabs are also mixed with testosterone and marketed as Estratest regular, with 1.25 mg of estrogen and 2.5 mg of testosterone, and Estratest HS (half strength), with 0.625 mg of estrogen and 1.25 mg of testosterone.

Ogen	0.625 mg	estropipate— an estrone	Abbott
	1.25 mg		

| Ortho-est | 0.625 mg | estropipate | 1.25 mg |
| | | Ortho | |

All of these preparations, except those with testosterone, are available as vaginal creams.

Estrogen Patch Preparations—delivered through the skin

Climara	0.5 mg	estradiol	Berlex
	1.0,g		
Estraderm	0.05 mg	estradiol	Ciba-Geigy
	0.1 mg		
Fempatch	0.025 mg	estradiol	Parke-Davis
Vivelle	0.0375 mg	estradiol	Ciba-Giegy
	0.05 mg		
	0.075 mg		
	0.1 mg		

PROGESTERONE PREPARATIONS

Aygestin	5 mg	norethindrone	Wyeth Ayerst
Cycrin	2.5 mg	medroxyproges-terone	Wyeth-Ayerst
	5 mg		10 mg
	5 mg		
	10 mg		
Megace	2.5 mg	megesterol	Bristol-Myers
	20 mg		
Norfluate	5 mg	norethindrone	Parke-Davis
Prometrium	100 mg	micronized progesterone (natural)	Solvay
Provera	2.5 mg	medroxyproges-terone	Upjohn

ESTROGEN-PROGESTERONE COMBINATIONS

| Premphase | Same doses as Prempro but the progesterone part is included only in the last two weeks | Wyeth-Ayerst |

| Prempro | 0.625 mg estrogen + 5 mg or 2.5 mg medroxyprogesterone | | Wyeth-Ayerst |
| | Both hormones taken through the month | | |

Testosterone Preparations—oral

| Android-10 | Methyltestos-terone | | ICN |
| Halotestin | fluoxymester-one | | Upjohn |

Injection

| Delatestryl | testosterone | enanthate | Upjohn |
| Depotestos-terone | testosterone | cypionate | Gynex |

Notes

Chapter 2. The Invisible Woman

1. R.E. Kendell, J. C. Chalmers, and C. Platz. 1987. Epidemiology of puerperal psychosis. *British Journal of Psychaitry* 150:662–673.

2. B.L. Parry. 1989. Reproductive factors affecting the course of affective illness in women. *Psychiatric Clinics of North America* 12, 1:207–217. K.A. Yonkers. 1997. The association between premenstrual dysphoric disorder and other mood disorders. *Journal of Clinical Psychiatry* 58, suppl. 15:19–25. J.A. Hamilton, M. Grant, and M.F. Jensvold. *Sex and the treatment of depression, when does it matter?* in M.F. Jensvold, U. Halbreich, and J.A. Hamilton, eds. 1996. *Psychopharmacology and women.* Washington, D.C.: American Psychiatric Press, pp. 241–257.

3. E. Leibenluft. 1997. Issues in the treatment of women with bipolar illness. *Journal of Clinical Psychiatry* 58, suppl. 15:5–11.

4. E. Leibenluft, P.L. Fiero, and D.R. Rubinow. 1994. Effects of the menstrual cycle on dependent variable in mood disorder research. *Archives of General Psychiatry* 51:761–781.

5. Personal communication from Selwyn Oskowitz, M.D.

6. P.E. Greenberg et al. 1993. The economic burden of depression. *Journal of Clinical Psychiatry* 54, 11:405–418.

7. Kolata, Gina. 1997. Which comes first: depression or heart disease? *New York Times*, January 14.

8. At the Howard Mahoney Neuroscience Forum, Boston, Massachusetts, October 1996.

9. Michael O'Hara, Ph.D., a researcher at the University of Iowa, has shown that 10 percent of women will have an episode of depression during their pregnancies. M.W. O'Hara et al. 1990. Controlled prospective study of mood disorders: compar-

ison of childbearing and nonchildbearing women. *Journal of Abnormal Psychology* 99, 1:3–15. Also, Channi Kumar, a professor at the Institute of Psychiatry in London, in Kumar, R., and K.M. Robson. 1984. A prospective study of emotional disorders in childbearing women. *British Journal of Psychiatry* 144:35–47.

10. J. Harasty et al. 1997. Language associated cortical regions are proportionally larger in the female brain. *Archives of Neurology* 54, 2:171–176.

Chapter 3. Your Brain: The Cornerstone of Your Emotional Health

1. W.C. Drevets et al. 1992. A functional anatomical study of unipolar depression. *Journal of Neuroscience* 12:3628–3641.

2. P. McLean, 1993. Perspectives on the cingulate cortex in the limbic system, in *The Neurobiology of the Cingulate Cortex,* ed. Brent A. Vogt and Michael Gabriel, published by Birkenhauser.

3. Confirming earlier research conducted by a colleague, in J.S. Stamm. 1955. The function of the median cerebral cortex in maternal behavior in rats. *Journal of Comparative Physiology and Psychology* 45:347–356.

4. W.C. Drevets et al. 1997. Subgenual prefrontal cortex abnormalities in mood disorders. *Nature* 386:824–827.

5. Small building-block proteins form one type, of which *glutamate* is a major stimulator of nerve activities. The other class of messengers, which themselves affect many mood and behavior states, are the peptide hormones, of which there are hundreds.

6. Insufficient norepinephrine, which regulates alertness, may also contribute to the lethargy associated with depression.

7. This is due to the electrical charge in the calcium, potassium, and chlorine ions in the nerve's membrane.

8. Serotonin and the limbic brain mobilize a peptide hormone called *cortisol-releasing factor* (CRF). The secretion of CRF activates an important circuit of the body's stress response called the *hypothalamus-pituitary-adrenal circuit* (HPA).

9. Under conditions of acute loss or prolonged trauma, stress-specific proteins called *transcriptional factors* are coaxed into activity. These can induce a series of longer-acting, critical changes to occur in the neurotransmitter cells that influence mood stability by altering a part of the genes of the cell. This regulation of gene expression (transcription) by social factors explains how the environment can alter brain functioning and thus behavior. When the elevated rates of firing of the cells in these pathways persist, as happens during periods of prolonged stress, the transcriptional proteins spur changes within the genes of the cell. With repeated negative events over time, these alterations can eventually change how the genes respond, so that they learn to function as if stress were present all the time.

The entire pathway will now function in an altered, dysregulated state. Indeed, this chemically dysregulated state may become the new norm, possibly contributing to the chronic nature of depressive illness.

Note: Genes have two functions. One is stable, responsible for providing copies of each gene to successive generations. This is called the *template function.* The other function is transcriptional, which is responsive to changes in the environment. This is the function that alters as a result of continued stress. Psychotherapy and drug therapy may induce important positive changes in the neuronal pathways, indicating how important these interventions are in the long-lasting effects of treatment.

Chapter 4. "What I'm Feeling Has a Name?" Mental Illnesses Affected by Hormones

1. *ESM-IV Diagnostic and Statistical Manual of Mental Disorders.* 1994. 4th ed Washington, D.C.: American Psychiatric Association.

2. H.S. Akiskal. 1996. The prevalent clinical spectrum of bipolar disorder: beyond DSM-IV. *Journal of Clinical Psychopharmacology 16,* suppl. 1: 4S-14S.

Chapter 5. Demystifying the Menstrual Cycle

1. This cluster of nerve cells is called the *arcuate nucleus,* just in case you are on *Jeopardy!* and you choose a question on neurochemistry!

2. The hypothalamus is located in the limbic brain.

3. This rise of estrogen must be above 200 picograms for at least fifty hours to "switch" on the luteinizing hormone (LH). A picogram is the unit used to measure estrogen in the blood. Estrogen levels range from the lowest point at menstruation of 30–50 picograms to a peak range of 100–400 picograms at ovulation and then around 200–300 picograms before the premenstrual drop.

4. That is, levels greater than 2 nanograms, the measurement for progesterone in the blood.

5. Endorphins are peptides that are secreted in the limbic brain.

Chapter 6. Putting It All Together

1. R.M. Post. 1992. Transduction of psychosocial stress into neurobiology of recurrent affective disorder. *American Journal of Psychiatry* 149:999–1010.

Chapter 8. PMDD Is a Biochemical Problem, Not an Emotional One

1. Some people rely on oil of evening primrose for fatty acids. But oil of evening primrose contains alpha-omega-6 and -9. This may be insufficient to combat the worst PMDD symptoms.

2. In our practice, it is routine to get a baseline set of blood levels. We do a complete blood count and blood chemistry to ascertain liver and kidney functions, as well as thyroid and prolactin screening.

3. The generic names are sertraline, fluvoxamine, and paroxetine.

4. The generic name is venlafaxine.

5. I. Wikender. 1998. Citalopram in premenstrual dysphoria is intermittent treatment more effective than continuous medication throughout the menstrual cycle? *Journal of Clinical Psychopharmacology* 18. Citalopram is the generic name.

6. These medications are Danazol, Lupron, and Synnarel.

Chapter 9. The Mimics of PMDD

1. 900 milligrams.

2. She had a level drawn on day three and on day twenty of her menstrual cycle. Kelly's level in the first half of the cycle was 0.8, and in the luteal phase it had dropped to 0.5. The normal lithium level is 0.7 to 1.2 milliequivalents.

3. 150–300 milligrams.

Chapter 10. "How Did This Happen?" Depression in Pregnancy

1. In his 1984 paper in the *British Journal of Psychiatry*. Supporting Kumar's statistics are the findings by Dr. Michael O'Hara, a research psychologist at the University of Iowa. He showed in his 1986 *Archives of General Psychiatry* article that 8 to 10 percent of the pregnant women he studied demonstrated evidence of depressive disturbance.

2. During the critical first trimester, vital structures of the heart, brain, and spinal cord are forming, and the embryo is most vulnerable to the influence of substances that can produce birth defects. This is why we must be so careful about exposure to medication or potentially toxic environments during this time. It's not always easy. Most women discover that they are pregnant only when they miss their period—that means they are already four to five weeks along. Whatever medication a woman was taking will already have had access to the tiny embryo.

3. We know that when cortisol-releasing factor (CRF), which is responsible for elevating cortisol levels, is injected into the brain, it produces symptoms similar to depression, namely, decreased appetite and libido, disrupted sleep, and anxiety. So it is possible that both cortisol and CRF are involved in how depressive symptoms occur.

4. One study carries a startling title: "Production of Fetal Asphyxia by Maternal Psychological Stress." This investigation, carried out by Ronald Myers at the National Institutes of Health, was published in the *Pavlovian Journal of Biological Science* 12 (1977):51–52.

5. Another series of experiments, 1977. The influence of maternal stress on the fetus. *American Journal of Obstetrics and Gynecology* 131:286–290 confirms these findings.

6. He published these results in July 1993. Psychological distress in pregnancy and preterm delivery: association between prenatal stress and infant birth weight and gestational age at birth. *British Medical Journal* 307:234–238.

7. It repeated Hedegaard's results, published in 1993 by Pathik Wadhwa, a physician researcher at the University of California, Irvine. Also Rachel Copper, a science researcher at the National Institute for Child Health and Human Development, published in R.L. Copper et al. 1995. The preterm prediction study: maternal stress is associated with spontaneous preterm birth at less than 35 weeks gestation. *American Journal of Obstetrics and Gynecology* 175:1286–1292.

8. C. Chambers. 1993. C.D. Chambers et al. 1996. Birth outcomes in pregnant women taking fluoxetine. *New England Journal of Medicine* 335:1010–1015.
I. Nulman, 1996. I. Nulman, and G. Koren. 1996. The safety of fluoxetine during pregnancy and lactation. *Teratology* 53:304–308.
G. Koren, A. Pastuszak, and S. Ito. 1998. Drugs in pregnancy. *New England Journal of Medicine* 338:1128–1137.

9. Dr. Gideon Koren, who leads a world-renowned research group at the Motherisk Program in Toronto. Also, Christina Chambers. 1996. Birth outcomes in pregnant women taking fluoxetine. *The New England Journal of Medicine* 335:1010–1015. This study has been criticized by many researchers for its method and interpretation of results. Dr. Elisabeth Roberts states clearly in her editorial in the same journal that many of the women who went into premature labor were taking other medications.

10. In a group of 267 women, information was gathered about the outcomes of the use of these medications during pregnancy. In March 1998, a study, again conducted by Dr. Koren's group, Pregnancy outcome following maternal use of new selective serotonin reuptake inhibitors. *Journal of the American Medical Association* 279:609–610, could not substantiate any ill effects on the babies or pregnancies in the women.

11. D.G. Dutton and S.K. Golant. 1995. *The batterer: a psychological profile.* New York: Basic Books. Also, the U.S. Bureau of Justice reports that male partners seriously assault over two million women in a one-year period. A 1986 publication.

12. In D.E. Stewart. 1994. Incidence of postpartum abuse in women with a history of abuse during pregnancy. *Canadian Medical Association Journal* 151, 11: 1601–1604.

Chapter 11. "Is It Safe for Me to Get Pregnant?" Bipolar Disorder and Pregnancy

1. Five-milligram dose.
2. Ebstein's anomaly.
3. Dr. Cohen published the results of a reevaluation of the statistics and the extent of the risk in L.S. Cohen et al. 1994. A reevaluation of risk of in utero exposure to lithium. *Journal of the American Medical Association* 271:146–150: correction 271: 1485.
4. Dr. Morgens Schou examined sixty children in Sweden. In Schou, M. 1976. What happened to the lithium babies? A follow-up study of children born without malformations. *Acta Psychiatrica Scandanavica* 54:193–197.
5. Heather was taking 1,200 milligrams per day and doing well.
6. For Heather, this meant decreasing her daily dose of lithium to 900 milligrams.

Chapter 12. Anxiety Disorders in Pregnancy

1. Dr. Donald Klein, a psychiatrist-researcher and world authority on anxiety disorders at Columbia University, found a similar result in his study of pregnant women. D.F. Klein. 1994. Pregnancy and panic disorder. *Journal of Clinical Psychiatry* 55: 293–294.
2. She responded to a dose of 0.5 milligrams, three times a day.
3. V.C. Hendrick and L.L. Altshuler. 1997. Management of breakthrough panic symptoms during pregnancy. *Journal of Clinical Psychopharmacology* 17:228–229.
4. 20 milligrams.
5. 0.5 milligrams.

Chapter 13. Postpartum Depression: There Is a Light at the End of the Painful Journey

1. R.E. Kendell, J.C. Chalmers, and C. Platz. (1987). Epidemiology of puerperal psychosis. *British Journal of Psychiatry* 150:662–673.
2. At the International Meeting of the Marce Society, Iowa City, Iowa, June 1998.
3. K. Wisner. 1994. Prevention of postpartum major depression. *Hospital and Community Psychiatry* 45:1191.

4. Z.N. Stowe et al. 1997. Sertraline and desmethylsertraline in human breast milk and nursing infants. *American Journal of Psychiatry* 154:1255–1260.

5. Between 1 and 3 nanograms per milliliter.

Chapter 16. Avoidable Tragedies: Postpartum Psychosis

1. The postpartum period is a time of increased risk for the development of blood clots anyway, and we don't want to heighten the dangers. A blood clot that travels to the brain can cause a stroke. If a clot from one of the veins in the leg breaks off and lodges in the lung, it can cause serious lung problems, since a portion of the lung tissue dies.

Chapter 17. Menopause: The Dialogue Ceases

1. An FSH level over 40 IU per milliliter in the absence of several periods generally indicates a menopausal state.

2. In a 1997 Gallup poll, 46 percent of women surveyed thought that breast cancer accounted for the greatest number of deaths in women, and only 4 percent knew that heart disease was actually the more serious problem.

Chapter 18. Menopause, Moods, and Memory

1. This is given in 2.5-, 5-, or 10-milligram dosages.

A SELECTED BIBLIOGRAPHY

Bipolar Disorders

Akiskal, H.S. 1996. The prevalent clinical spectrum of bipolar disorder: beyond DSM-IV. *Journal of Clinical Psychopharmacology* 16. Suppl. 1:4S–14S.

Akiskal, H.S. 1997. Exploring the richness of Bipolar II Disorder. Bipolar Disorders Letter. *Psychiatric Times.* Suppl. 1:4.

Baldessarini, R.J.; Tondo, L.; Faedda, G.L.; Suppes, T.A.; Floris, G.; and Rudas, N. 1996. Effects of the rate of discontinuing lithium maintenance treatment. *The Journal of Clinical Psychiatry* 57:441–448.

Blehar, M.C.; DePaulo, J.R.; Gershon, E.S.; Reich,T.; Simpson, S.G.; and Nurnberger, J.I. 1998. Women with bipolar disorder: findings from the NIMH Genetics Initiative Sample. *Psychopharmacology Bulletin* 34:239–243.

Cohen, L.S.; Sichel, D.A.; Robertson, L.M.; Heckscher, B.; and Rosenbaum, J.F. 1995. Postpartum prophylaxis for women with bipolar disorder. *American Journal of Psychiatry* 152:1641–1645.

Faedda, G.L.; Tondo, L.; Baldessarini, R.J.; Suppes, T.; and Tohen, M. 1993. Outcome after rapid vs. gradual discontinuation of lithium treatment in bipolar disorders. *Archives of General Psychiatry* 50:448–455.

Fatemi, S.H.; Rappaport, D.J.; Calabrese, J.R.; and Thuras, P. 1997. Lamotrigine in rapid-cycling bipolar disorder. *The Journal of Clinical Psychiatry* 58:522–527.

Frances, A. J.; Kahn, D.A.; Carpenter, D.; Docherty, J.P.; and Donovan, S.L. 1998. The expert consensus guidelines for treating depression in bipolar disorder. *The Journal of Clinical Psychiatry* 59. Suppl. 4:73–79.

Leibenluft, E. 1997. Issues in the treatment of women with bipolar illness. *The Journal of Clinical Psychiatry* 58. Suppl. 15:5–11.

Rosenblatt, J.E.; and Rosenblatt, N.C., eds. 1998. Update on treatment of bipolar depression. Part II of an interview with Paul E. Keck. *Currents in Affective Illness: Literature Review and Commentary* 17:5–11.

Brain Biochemistry

Brown, J.R.; Ye, H.; Bronson, R.T.; Dikkes, P.; and Greenberg, M.E. 1996. A defect in nurturing in mice lacking the immediate early gene *fosB*. *Cell* 86:297–309.

Drevets, W.C.; Price, J.L.; Simpson, J.R.; Todd, R.D.; Reich, T.; and Raichel, M.E. 1997. Subgenual prefrontal cortex abnormalities in mood disorders. *Nature* 386: 824–827.

Duman, R.S.; Heninger, G.R.; and Nestler, E.J. 1997. A molecular and cellular theory of depression. *Archives of General Psychiatry* 54:597–606.

Fink, G.; Sumner, B.E.; Rosie, R.; Grace, O.; and Quinn, J.P. 1996. Estrogen control of central neurotransmission: effect on mood, mental state and memory. *Cellular & Molecular Neurobiology* 16:325–344.

Marangell, L.B.; George, M.S.; Callahan, A.M.; Ketter, T.A.; Pazzaglia, P.J.; L'Herrou, T.A.; Leverich, G.S.; and Post, R. M. 1997. Effects of intrathecal thyrotropin-releasing hormone (protirelin) in refractory depressed patients. *Archives of General Psychiatry* 54:214–222.

Nemeroff, C.B. 1989. Clinical significance of psychoneuronendocrinology in psychiatry: focus on the thyroid and adrenal. *The Journal of Clinical Psychiatry* 50. Suppl. 5:13–20.

Reiman, E.M.; Lane, R.D.; Ahearn, G.L.; Schwartz, G.E.; Davidson, R.J.; Friston, K.J.; Yun, L.S.; and Chen, K. 1997. Neuroanatomical correlates of externally and internally generated human emotion. *American Journal of Psychiatry* 154:918–925.

Restak, R.M. 1989. The brain, depression, and the immune system. *The Journal of Clinical Psychiatry* 50. Suppl. 5:23–25.

Slotnick, B.M. 1967. Disturbances of maternal behavior in rats following lesions of the cingulate cortex. *Behavior* 24:204–236.

Spring, B.; Chiodo, J.; Harden, M.; Bourgeois, M.J.; Mason, J.D.; and Lutherer, L. 1989. Psychobiological effects of carbohydrates. *The Journal of Clinical Psychiatry* 50. Suppl. 5:27–33.

Stahl, S.M. 1997. Apoptosis: neuronal death by design. *The Journal of Clinical Psychiatry* 58: 183–184.

Stamm, J.S. 1955. The function of the median cerebral cortex in maternal behavior in rats. *Journal of Comprehensive Physiology Psychology* 55:347–356.

Stein, M. 1989. Stress, depression, and the immune system. *The Journal of Clinical Psychiatry* 50. Suppl. 5:35–40.

Weiss, J.M.; Sundar, S.K.; Becker, K.J.; and Cierpial, M.A. 1989. Behavioral and neural influences on cellular immune responses: effects of stress and Interleukin-1. *The Journal of Clinical Psychiatry* 50. Suppl. 5:43–53.

Depression

Akiskal, H.S. 1989. New insights into the nature and heterogeneity of mood disorders. *The Journal of Clinical Psychiatry* 50. Suppl. 5:6–10.

Akiskal, H.S. 1996. The new anatomy of melancholy: who gets depressed and why. *Medical Advances—Health in Mind & Body* 1:9–10.

Almeida, D.M.; and Kessler, R.C. 1998. Everyday stressors and gender differences in daily distress. *Journal of Perspectives in Social Psychology* 75:670–680.

American Psychiatric Association. 1993. American Psychiatric Association practice guidelines for major depressive disorder in adults. *American Journal of Psychiatry* 150. Suppl. 4:1–26.

American Psychiatric Association. 1995. Practice guidelines for psychiatric evaluation of adults: American Psychiatric Association. *American Journal of Psychiatry* 152. Suppl. 11:63–80.

Beeber, L.S. 1996. Pattern integrations in young depressed women: Part 1. *Archives in Psychiatric Nursing* 10:151–156.

Beeber, L.S.; and Caldwell, C.L. 1996. Pattern integrations in young depressed women: Part II. *Archives of Psychiatric Nursing* 10:157–164.

Bifulco, A.; Brown, G.W.; Moran, P.; Ball, C.; and Campbell, C. 1998. Predicting depression in women: the role of past and present vulnerability. *Psychological Medicine* 28:39–50.

Dowling, C. 1993. *You mean I don't have to feel this way? New help for depression, anxiety, and addiction.* New York: Bantam Books.

George, M.S.; Guidottik, A.; Rubinow, D.; Pan, B.; Mikalauskas, K.; and Post, R.M. 1994. CSF neuroactive steroids in affective disorders: pregnenolone, progesterone, and DBI. *Biological Psychiatry* 35:775–780.

Greenberg, P.E.; Stiglin, L.E.; Finkelstein, S.N.; and Berndt, E.R. 1993. The economic burden of depression. *Journal of Clinical Psychiatry* 54:405–418

Hauenstein, E.J. 1996. A nursing practice paradigm for depressed rural women: theoretical basis. *Archives in Psychiatric Nursing* 10:283–292.

Judd, J.L.; Akiskal, H.S.; and Paulus, M.P. 1997. The role and clinical significance of subsyndromal depressive symptoms (SSD) in unipolar major depressive disorder. *Journal of Affective Disorders* 45:5–18.

Kandel, E.R. 1998. A new intellectual framework for psychiatry. *American Journal of Psychiatry* 155:457–469.

Kendler, K.S.; Kessler, R.C.; Walters, E.E.; MacLean, C.; Neale, M.C.; Heath, A.C.; and Eaves, L.J. 1995. Stressful life events, genetic liability, and onset of an episode of major depression in women. *American Journal of Psychiatry* 152:833–842.

Kendler, K.S.; Gallagher, T.J.; Abelson, J.M.; and Kessler, R.C.1996. Lifetime prevalence, demographic risk factors, and diagnostic validity of nonaffective psychosis as assessed in a U.S. community sample. *Archives of General Psychiatry* 53:1022–1031.

Kendler, K.S. 1993. Prediction of major depression in women. *American Journal of Psychiatry* 150:1139–1148.

Kendler, K.S.; and Gardner, C.O. Jr. 1998. Boundaries of major depression: an evaluation of DSM-IV criteria. *American Journal of Psychiatry* 155:172–177.

Kessler, R.C.; and Walters, E.E. 1998. Epidemiology of DSM-III-R major depression and minor depression among adolescents and young adults in the National Comorbidity Survey. *Depression and Anxiety* 7:3–14.

Kessler, R.C.; Nelson, C.B.; McGonagle, K.A.; Liu, J.; Swartz, M.; and Blazer, D.G. 1996. Comorbidity of DSM-III-R major depressive disorder in the general population: results from the U.S. National Comorbidity Survey. *British Journal of Psychiatry* Suppl. June:17–30

Kessler, R.C.; McGonagle, K.A.; Zhao, S.; Nelson, C.B.; Hughes, M.; Eshleman, S.; Wittchen, H.U.; and Kendler, K.S. 1994. Lifetime and 12-month prevalence of DSM-IVR psychiatric disorders in the United States. Results from the National Comorbidity Survey. *Archives of General Psychiatry* 51:8–19.

Llewellyn, A.M.; Stowe, Z.N.; and Nemeroff, C.B. 1997. Depression during pregnancy and the puerperium. *The Journal of Clinical Psychiatry* 58. Suppl. 15:26–32.

McGrath, E.; Keita, G.P.; Strickland, B.R.; and Russo, N.F., eds. 1990. *Women and depression: risk factors and treatment issues.* Washington, D.C.: American Psychological Association.

Mueller, T.I.; Keller, M.B.; Leon, A.C.; Solomon, D.A.; Shea, M.T.; Coryell, W.; and Endicott, J. 1996. Naturalistic recovery after five years of unremitting Major Depressive Disorder. *Archives of General Psychiatry* 53:794.

Pardes, H. 1998. Depression and health-care policy. *Journal of Gender-Specific Medicine* 1:443–447.

Randel, E.R. 1998. A new intellectual framework for psychiatry. *American Journal of Psychiatry* 155:457–469.

Rothschild, A.J. 1992. Advances in the management of depression: implications for the obstetrician/gynecologist. *American Journal of Obstetrics and Gynecology* 173:659–666.

Schreiber, R. 1996. Understanding and helping depressed women. *Archives of Psychiatric Nursing* 10:165–175.

Solomon, A. 1998. Anatomy of melancholy. *The New Yorker* January 12:46–61.

Stahl, S.M. 1998. Augmentation of antidepressants by estrogen. *Psychopharmacology Bulletin* 34:319–321.

Stahl, S.M. 1998. Neuropharmacology of obesity: my receptors made me eat it. *The Journal of Clinical Psychiatry* 59:447–448.

Steer, R.A.; Scholl, T.O.; Hediger, M.L.; and Frisher, R.L. 1992. *Journal of Clinical Epidemiology* 45:1093–1099.

Wagner, K.D. 1996. Major depression and anxiety disorders associated with Norplant. *The Journal of Clinical Psychiatry* 57:152–157.

Weissman, M.M.; Gammon, G.D.; Merikangas, K.R.; Warner, V.; Prusoff, B.A.; and Sholomskas, D. 1987. Children of depressed parents. *Archives of General Psychiatry* 44:847–853.

Weissman, M.M.; and Klerman, G.I. 1977. Sex differences and the epidemiology of depression. *Archives of General Psychiatry* 34:98–100.

Weissman, M.M.; Bland, R.; Joyce, P.R.; Newman, S.; Wells, J.E.; and Wittchen, H.U. 1993. Sex differences in the rates of depression: cross national perspectives. *Journal of Affective Disorders* 29:77–84.

Weissman, M.M.; and Olfson, M. 1995. Depression in women: implications for health-care research. *Science* 269:799–801.

Whiffen, V.E.; and Gotlib, I.H. 1993. Comparison of postpartum and nonpostpartum depression: clinical presentation. *Journal of Consulting and Clinical Psychology* 61:485–494.

Yonkers, K.A.; and Chantilis, S.J. 1995. Recognition of depression in obstetric/gynecology practices. *American Journal of Obstetrics & Gynecology* 173:632–638.

Eating Disorders

Becker, A.E.; Grinspoon, S.K.; Klibanski, A.; and Herzog, D.B. 1999. Eating disorders. *New England Journal of Medicine* 340:1092–1098.

Becker, A.E.; Hamburg, P.; and Herzog, D.B. 1998. The role of psychopharmacologic management in the treatment of eating disorders. *Psychiatric Clinics of North America: Annual of Drug Therapy* 5:17–51.

Kaye, W.H.; Berrettini, W.H.; Gwirtsman, H.E.; Gold, P.W.; George, D.T.; Jimerson, D.C.; and Ebert, M.J. 1989. Contribution of CNS neuropeptide (NPY, CRH, and beta-endorphin) alterations to psychophysiological abnormalities in anorexia nervosa. *Psychopharmacology Bulletin* 25:433–438.

Exercise

Aganoff, J.A.; and Boyle, G.J. 1994. Aerobic exercise, mood states, and menstrual cycle symptoms. *Journal of Psychosomatic Research* 38:183–192.

Drinkwater, B.L. 1990. Physical exercise and bone health. *Journal of American Medical Women's Association* May/June:91–97.

Dua, J.; and Hargreaves, L. 1992. Effect of aerobic exercise on negative affect, positive affect, stress, and depression. *Perceptual Motor Skills* 75:355–361.

Goldfarb, A.H.; Hatfield, B.D.; Armstrong, D.; and Potts, J. 1990. Plasma beta-endorphin concentration: response to intensity and duration of exercise. *Medical Science of Sports and Exercise* 22:241–244.

McMurray, R.G.; Forsythe, W.A.; Mar, M.H.; and Hardy, C.J. 1987. Exercise intensity-related responses of beta-endorphin and catecholamines. *Medical Science Sports Exercise* 19:570–574.

Steege, J.F.; and Blumenthal, J.A. 1993. The effects of aerobic exercise on premenstrual symptoms in middle-aged women: a preliminary study. *Journal of Psychosomatic Research* 37:127–133.

Steptoe, A.; Kimbell, J.; and Basford, P. 1998. Exercise and the experience of appraisal of daily stressors: a naturalistic study. *Journal of Behavioral Medicine* 21:363–374.

Gender Differences

Allen, L.A.; Richey, M.F.; Chai, Y.M.; and Gorski, R.A. 1991. Sex differences in the corpus callosum of the living human being. *Journal of Neuroscience* 11:933–942.

Allen, L.; and Gorski, R.A. 1992. Sexual orientation and the size of the anterior commissure in the human brain. *Proceedings of National Academy of Science USA* 89:7199–7202.

Andreason, P.J.; Zametkin, A.J.; Guo, A.C.; Baldwin, P.; and Cohen, R.M. 1994. Gender-related differences in regional cerebral glucose metabolism in normal volunteers. *Psychiatry Research* 51:175–183.

Baxter, L.R. Jr.; Mazziotta, J.C.; Phelps, M.E.; Selin, C.E.; Guze, B.H.; and Fairbanks, L. 1987. Cerebral glucose metabolic rates in normal human females versus normal males. *Psychiatry Research* 21:237–245.

Berg, M.J. 1998. Drugs, vitamins, and gender. *Journal of Gender-Specific Medicine* 1:10–11.

Blehar, M.C.; and Oren, D.A. 1997. Gender differences in depression. *Medscape Women's Health* 2.

Blehar, M.C.; DePaulo, J.R. Jr.; Gershon, E.S.; Reich, T.; Simpson, S.G.; and Nurnberger, J.I. Jr. 1998. Women with bipolar disorder: findings from the NIMH Genetics Initiative Sample. *Psychopharmacology Bulletin* 34:239–243.

Carlsson, M.; and Carlsson, A. 1988. A regional study of sex differences in rat brain serotonin. *Progress in Neuropsycholopharmacological Biological Psychiatry* 12:53–61.

Ditkoff, E.C.; Crary, W.G.; Cristo, M.; and Lobo, R.A. 1991. Estrogen improves psychological function in asymptomatic postmenopausal women. *Obstetrics and Gynecology* 78:991–995.

Downey, J.I. 1996. Recognizing the range of mood disorders in women. *Medscape Women's Health* 1.

Gelenberg, A.J. 1998. Sex hormones and sexual desire. *Biological Therapies in Psychiatry Newsletter* 21:1–2.

George, M.S.; Wassermann, E.M.; Williams, W.A.; Steppel, J.; Pascual-Leone, A.; Basser, P.; Hallett, M.; and Post, R.M. 1996. Changes in mood and hormone levels after rapid-rate transcranial magnetic stimulation (rTMS) of the prefrontal cortex. *Journal of Neuropsychiatry & Clinical Neuroscience* 8:172–180.

George, M.S.; Ketter, T.A.; Parekh, P.I.; Herscovitch, P.; and Post, R.M. 1996. Gender differences in regional cerebral blood flow during transient self-induced sadness or happiness. *Biological Psychiatry* 40:859–871.

George, M.S.; Ketter, T.A.; Gill, D.S.; Haxby, J.V.; Ungerleider, L.G.; Herscovitch, P.; and Post, R.M. 1993. Brain regions involved in recognizing facial emotion or identity: an oxygen-15 PET study. *Journal of Neuropsychiatry & Clinical Neuroscience* 5:384–394.

Gur, R.C.; Gur, R.E.; Obrist, W.D.; Hungerbuhler, J.P.; Younkin, D.; Rosen, A.D.; Skolnick, B.E.; and Reivich, M. 1982. Sex and handedness differences in cerebral blood flow during rest and cognitive activity. *Science* 217:659–661.

Gur, R.C.; Mozley, L.H.; Mozley, P.D.; Resnick, S.M.; Karp, J.S.; Alavi, A.; Arnold, S.E.; and Gur, R.E. 1995. Sex differences in regional cerebral glucose metabolism during a resting state. *Science* 267:528–531.

Gur, R.E.; and Gur, R.C. 1990. Gender differences in regional cerebral blood flow. *Schizophrenia Bulletin* 16:247–254.

Gur, R.C.; Skolnick, B.E.; and Gur, R.E. 1994. Effects of emotional discrimination tasks on cerebral blood flow: regional activation and its relation to performance. *Brain Cognition* 25:271–286.

Halbreich, U.; Lemus, C.Z.; Lieberman, J.A.; Parry, B.; and Schiavi, R.C. 1990. Gonadal hormones, sex and behavior. *Psychopharmacology Bulletin* 26:297–301.

Hamilton, J.A.; Grant, M.; and Jensvold, M.F. 1996. Sex and the treatment of depression, when does it matter? Chapter in Jensvold, M.F.; Halbreich, U.; and Hamilton, J.A.; eds. 1996. *Psychopharmacology and Women*. Washington, D.C.: American Psychiatric Press.

Harasty, J.; Double, K.L.; Halliday, G.M.; Kril, J.J.; and McRitchie, D.A. 1997. Language-associated cortical regions are proportionally larger in the female brain. *Archives of Neurology* 54:171–176.

Jaeger, J.J.; Lockwood, A.H.; Van Valin, R.D. Jr.; Kemmerer, D.L.; Murphy, B.W.;

and Wack, D.S. 1998. Sex differences in brain regions activated by grammatical and reading tasks. *Neuroreport* 9:2803–2807.

Jensvold, M.R.; Halbreich, U.; and Hamilton, J.A. 1996. *Psychopharmacology and women: sex, gender, and hormones.* Washington, D.C.: American Psychiatric Press.

Kendell, D.; Stancel, G.; and Enna, S. 1982. The influence of sex hormones, on antidepressant-induced alteration in neurotransmitter receptor binding. *Journal of Neuroscience* 2:354–360.

Kessler, R.C.; and McLeod, J.D. 1984. Sex differences in vulnerability to undesirable life events. *Sociological Review* 49:620–631.

Klaiber, E.L.; Kobayahi,Y.; Broverman, D.M.; and Hall, F. 1971. Plasma monoamine oxidase activity in regularly menstruating women and in amenorrheic women receiving cyclic treatment with estrogens and a progestin. *Journal of Clinical Endocrinology and Metabolism* 33:630–638.

Klaiber, E.L.; Broverman, D.M.; Vogel, W.; Kobayashi,Y.; and Moriarty, D. 1972. Effects of estrogen therapy on plasma MAO activity and EEG driving responses of depressed women. *American Journal of Psychiatry* 128:1492–1498.

Klaiber, E.L.; Broverman, D.M.; Vogel, W.; Kobayashi, Y.; and Moriarity, D. 1979. Estrogen therapy for severe persistent depression in women. *Archives of General Psychiatry* 36:550–554.

Klein, D.F. 1993. False suffocation alarms, spontaneous panics, and related conditions: an integrated hypothesis. *Archives of General Psychiatry* 50:306–317.

Kornstein, S.G. 1997. Gender differences in depression: implications for treatment. *The Journal of Clinical Psychiatry* 58. Suppl. 15:12–18.

Majewska, M.D. 1992. Neurosteroids: endogenous modulators of the GABA-A receptor: mechanism of action and physiological significance. *Progress in Neurobiology* 38:379–395.

Majewska, M.D.; and Schwartz, R.D. 1987. Pregnenolone-sulfate: an endogenous antagonist of the y-aminobutyric acid receptor complex in the brain? *Brain Research* 404:355–360.

Majewska, M.D.; Ford-Rice, F.; and Falkay, G. 1989. Pregnancy-induced alterations of GABAa receptor sensitivity in the maternal brain: an antecedent of postpartum blues? *Brain Research* 482:397–401.

Majewska, M.D.; Demirgoren, S.; and Spivak, C.H. 1990. Neurosteroid dehydroepiandrosteroine sulfate in an allosteric antagonist of the GABA a receptor. *Brain Research* 526:143–146.

Mercurio, M.G. 1998. Gender and dermatology. *Journal of Gender-Specific Medicine* 1:16–20.

Merikangas, K.R.; Weissman, M.M.; and Pauls, D.L. 1985. Genetic factors in the sex ratio of major depression. *Psychological Medicine* 15:63–69.

Mustard, C.A.; Kaufert, P.; Kozyrskyj, A.; and Mayer, T. 1998. Sex differences in the use of health care services. *The New England Journal of Medicine* 338:1678–1683.

Steiner, M. 1992. Female-specific mood disorders. *Clinical Obstetrics and Gynecology* 35:599–611.

Sun, L. 1998. Gender differences in pain sensitivity and responses to analgesia. *Journal of Gender-Specific Medicine* 1:28–30.

Tamminga, C.A. 1996. Gender and schizophrenia. *The Journal of Clinical Psychiatry* 58. Suppl. 15:33–37.

Warnock, J.K.; Bundren, J.C.; and Morris, D.W. 1997. Female hypoactive sexual desire disorder due to androgen deficiency: clinical and psychometric issues. *Psychopharmacology Bulletin* 33:761–766.

Young, E.A. 1998. Sex differences and the HPA axis: implications for psychiatric disease. *Journal of Gender-Specific Medicine* 1:21–27.

Hormones

Chakravorty, S.G.; and Halbreich, U. 1997. The influence of estrogen on monoamine oxidase activity. *Psychopharmacology Bulletin* 32:229–233.

Cohen, L.S. and Rosenbaum, J.F. 1994. Hormonal therapies for psychiatric symptoms in women: possibilities and cautions. *Harvard Review of Psychiatry* 1:353–355.

Coplan, J.D.; Pine, D.S.; Papp, L.A.; and Gorman, J.A. 1997. A view of noradrenergic hypothalamic-pituitary-adrenal axis and extrahypothalamic corticotrophin-releasing factor function in anxiety and affective disorders: the reduced growth hormone response to clonidine. *Psychopharmacology Bulletin* 33:193–204.

Demitrack, M.A.; Lesem, M.O.; Brandt, H.A.; Pigott, T.A.; Jimerson, D.C.; Altemus, M.; and Gold, P.N. 1989. Neurohypophyseal dysfunction: implications for the pathophysiology of eating disorders. *Psychopharmacology Bulletin* 25:439–443.

Dorn, L.D.; and Chrousos, G.P. 1997. The neurobiology of stress: understanding regulation of affect during female biological transitions. *Seminars in Reproductive Endocrinology* 15:19–35.

Freeman, E.W.; Sondheimer, S.J.; and Rickels, K. 1997. Gonadotropin-releasing hormone agonist in the treatment of premenstrual symptoms with and without ongoing dysphoria: a controlled study. *Psychopharmacology Bulletin* 33:303–309.

Freeman, E.W.; Purdy, R.H.; Rickels, K.; and Paul, S.M. 1993. Anxiolytic metabolites of progesterone: correlation with mood and performance following oral progesterone administration to healthy female volunteers. *Clinical Neuroendocrinology* 58:478–484.

Grodstein, F.; Stampfer, M.J.; Colditz, G.A.; Willett, W.C.; Manson, J.E.; Joffee, M.; Rosner, B.; Fuchs, C.; Hankinson, S.E.; Hunter, D.J.; Hennekens, C.H.; and Speizer, F.E. 1997. Postmenopausal hormone therapy and mortality. *The New England Journal of Medicine* 336:1769–1775.

Halbreich, U. 1990. Gonadal hormones and antihormones, serotonin and mood. *Psychopharmacology Bulletin* 26:291–295.

Halbreich, U. 1997. Hormonal interventions with psychopharmacological potential: an overview. *Psychopharmacology Bulletin* 33:281–286.

Halbreich, U.; Lemus, C.Z.; Lieberman, J.A.; Parry, B.; and Schiavi, R.C. 1990. Gonadal hormones, sex and behavior. *Psychopharmacology Bulletin* 26:297–301.

Heim, C.; Owens, M.J.; Plotsky, P.M.; and Nemeroff, C.B. 1997. 1. Endocrine factors in the pathophysiology of mental disorders. *Psychopharmacology Bulletin* 33:185–192.

Hendrick, V.; Altshuler, L.L.; and Suri, R. 1998. Hormonal changes in the postpartum and implications for postpartum depression. *Psychosomatics* 39:93–101.

Khanna, S.; Ammini, A.; Saxena, S.; and Mohan, D. 1988. Hypopituitarism presenting as delirium. *International Journal of Psychiatry in Medicine* 18:89–92.

Klaiber, E.; Broverman, D.M.; Vogel, W.; Peterson, L.G.; and Snyder, M.B. 1996. Individual differences in changes in mood and platelet monamine oxidase (MAO) during hormonal replacement therapy in menopausal women. *Psychoneuroendocrinology* 7:575– 592.

Lindamer, L.A.; Lohr, J.B.; Harris, M.J.; and Jeste, D.V. 1997. Gender, estrogen, and schizophrenia. *Psychopharmacology Bulletin* 33:221–228.

Love, S.M.; and Lindsey, K. 1997. *Dr. Susan Love's Hormone Book.* New York: Random House.

McEwen, B.S. 1998. Multiple ovarian hormone effects on brain structure and function. *Journal of Gender-Specific Medicine* 1:33–41.

Magiakou, M.A.; Mastorakos, G.; Webster, E.; and Chrousos. G.P. 1997. The hypothalamic-pituitary-adrenal axis and the female reproductive system. *Annals of New York Academic Science* 816:42–56.

Meyers, B.S.; and Moline, M.L. 1997. The role of estrogen in late-life depression: opportunities and barriers to research. *Psychopharmacology Bulletin* 33:289–291.

Morrison, M.F. 1997. Androgens in the elderly: will androgen replacement therapy improve mood, cognition, and quality of life in aging men and women. *Psychopharmacology Bulletin* 33:293–296.

Ober, K.P. 1990. Case report: postpartum hypopituitarism with preservation of the pituitary-ovarian axis. *American Journal of Medical Science* 299:257–259.

Oppenheim, G. 1983. Estrogen in the treatment of depression: neuropharmacological mechanisms. *Biological Psychiatry* 18:721–725.

Pearlstein, T.B. 1995. Hormones and depression: what are the facts about premenstrual syndrome, menopause, and hormonal replacement therapy? *American Journal of Obstetrics and Gynecology* 173:646–653.

Warnock, J.K.; and Bundren, J.C. 1997. Anxiety and mood disorders associated with gonadotropin-releasing hormone agonist therapy. *Psychopharmacology Bulletin* 33:311–316.

World Health Organization. 1981. Temporal relationships between ovulation and defined changes in the concentration of plasma estradiol-17b, luteinizing hormone, follicle-stimulating hormone, and progesterone, I: probit analysis. *American Journal of Obstetrics and Gynecology* 138:383–390.

Medications: Breast-feeding

Altshuler, L.L.; Burt, V.K.; McMullen, M.; and Hendrick, V. 1995. Breast-feeding and sertraline: a 24-hour analysis. *The Journal of Clinical Psychiatry* 56:243–245.

Epperson, C.N.; Anderson, G.M.; and McDougle, C.J. 1997. Sertraline and breast-feeding. *The New England Journal of Medicine* (correspondence) 336:1189–1190.

Goldberg, H.L.; and Nissim, R. 1994. Psychotropic drugs in pregnancy and lactation. *International Journal of Psychiatry of Medicine* 24:129–149.

Goodnick, P.J. 1994. Pharmacokinetics optimization of therapy with newer antidepressants: a review. *Clinical Pharmacokinetics* 27:307–330.

Hale, T.W. 1998. *Medications and Mother's Milk.* 7th Edition. Amarillo, TX: Pharmasoft Medical Publishing.

Hatzopoulos, F.K.; and Nissim, R. 1994. Antidepressant use during breast-feeding. *Journal of Human Lactation* 139:139–141.

Isenberg, K.E. 1990. Excretion of bupropion in breast milk. *The Journal of Clinical Psychiatry* 51:169.

Lester, B.M.; Cucca, J.; Andreozzi, L.; Flanagan, P.; and Oh, W. 1993. Possible association between fluoxetine hydorchloride and colic in an infant. *Journal of the American Academy of Child & Adolescent Psychiatry* 32:1253–1255.

Mammen, O.K.; Perel, J.M.; Rudolph, G.; Foglia, J.P.; and Wheeler, S.B. 1997. Sertraline and norsertraline levels in three breast-fed infants. *The Journal of Clinical Psychiatry* 58:100–103.

Miseri, S.; and Sivertz, K. 1991. Tricyclic drugs in pregnancy and lactation: a preliminary report. *International Journal of Psychiatry in Medicine* 21:157–171.

Nulman, I.; and Koren, G. 1996. The safety of fluoxetine during pregnancy and lactation. *Teratology* 53:304–308.

Pons, G.; Rey, E.; and Matheson, I. 1994. Excretion of psychoactive drugs into breast milk. Pharmacokinetic principles and recommendations: a review. *Clinical Pharmacokinetics* 27:270–289.

Schimmell, M.S.; Katz, E.Z.; Shaag, Y.; Pastuszak, A.; and Koren, G. 1991. Toxic neonatal effects following maternal clomipramine therapy. *Journal of Toxicology-Clinical Toxicology* 29:479–484.

Sovner, R. and Orsulak, P.J. 1979. Excretion of Imipramine and Desipramine in human breast milk. *American Journal of Psychiatry* 136:451–452.

Spencer, M.J. 1993. Fluoxetine hydrochloride (Prozac) toxicity in a neonate. *Pediatrics* 92:721– 722.

Spigset, O. and Hagg. S. 1998. Excretion of psychotropic drugs into breast milk: Pharmacokinetic overview and therapeutic implications. *CNS Drugs* 9:111–134.

Spigset, O.; Carleborg, L.; Ohman, R.; and Norstrom, A. 1997. Excretion of Citalopram in breast milk. *British Journal of Pharmacology* 44:295–298.

Stowe, Z.N.; Owens, M.J.; Landry, J.C.; Kilts, C.D.; Ely, T.; Llewellyn, A.; and Nemeroff, C.B. 1997. Sertraline and desmethylsertraline in human breast milk and nursing infants. *American Journal of Psychiatry* 154:1255–1260.

Taddio, A.; Ito, S.; and Koren, G. 1996. Excretion of fluoxetine and its metabolite, norfluoxetine, in human breast milk. *Journal of Clinical Pharmacology* 36:42–47.

Wisner, K.L.; and Perel, J.M. 1998. Serum levels of valproate and carbamazepine in breast-feeding mother-infant pairs. *Journal of Clinical Psychopharmacology* 18:167–169.

Wisner, K.L.; Perel, J.M.; and Findling, R.L. 1996. Antidepressant treatment during breast-feeding. *American Journal of Psychiatry* 153:1132–1137.

Wisner, K.L.; Perel, J.M.; Peindl, K.S.; Findling, R.L.; and Hanusa, B.H. 1997. Effects of the postpartum period on nortriptyline pharmacokinetics. *Psychopharmacology Bulletin* 33:243–248.

Wisner, K.L.; Perel, J.M.; Findling, R.L.; and Hinne, R.L. 1997. Nortriptyline and its hydroxymetabolites in breast-feeding mothers and newborns. *Psychopharmacology Bulletin* 33:249–251.

Medications: Pregnancy and Postpartum

Altshuler, L.L.; Cohen, L.; Szuba, M.P.; Burt, V.K.; Gillin, M.; and Mentz, J. 1996. Pharmacologic management of psychiatric illness during pregnancy: dilemmas and guidelines. *American Journal of Psychiatry* 153:592–606.

Bergman, U.; Rosa, F.W.; Baum, C.; Wiholm, B.E.; and Faich, G.A. 1992. Effects of exposure to benzodiazepine during fetal life. *The Lancet* 340:694–696.

Chambers, C.D.; Johnson, K.A.; Dick, L.M.; Felix, R.J.; and Jones, K.L. 1996. Birth outcomes in pregnant women taking fluoxetine. *The New England Journal of Medicine* 335:1010–1015

Cohen, L.S.; and Rosenbaum, J.F. 1997. Birth outcomes in pregnant women taking fluoxetine. Letter to the Editor. *The New England Journal of Medicine* 33:872.

Cohen, L.; and Rosenbaum, J.F. 1998. Psychotropic drug use during pregnancy: weighing the risks. *Journal of Clinical Psychiatry* 59. Suppl. 2:18–28.

Delgado-Escueta, A.V.; and Janz, D. 1992. Consensus guidelines: preconception counseling, management, and care of the pregnant woman with epilepsy. *Neurology* 42. Suppl. 5:149–160.

Gelenberg, A.J. (1998). Citalopram (Celexa): SSRI#5. *Biological Therapies in Psychiatry: Newsletter* 2:1–2.

Glod, C.A. 1996. Recent advances in the pharmacology of major depression. *Archives of Psychiatric Nursing* 10:355–364.

Goldstein, D.J.; Sundell, K.L.; and Corbin, L.A. 1997. Birth outcomes in pregnant women taking fluoxetine. Letters to the Editor. *The New England Journal of Medicine* 336:873.

Grant, I. 1996. Where now SSRIs? Reflections on Prozac's tenth birthday. *Medical Advances—Health in Mind & Body* 1:1–5.

Greenberg, P.E.; Stiglin, L.E.; Finkelstein, S.N.; and Berndt, E.R. 1993. The economic burden of depression in 1990. *Journal of Clinical Psychiatry* 54:405–418.

Greenberg, P.E.; Stiglin, L.E.; Finkelstein, S.N.; and Berndt, E.R. 1993. Depression: a neglected mental illness. *Journal of Clinical Psychiatry* 54:419–424.

Hiilesmaa, V.K. 1992. Pregnancy and birth in women with epilepsy. *Neurology* 42. Suppl. 5:8–11.

Jensvold, M.F.; Halbreich, U.; and Hamilton, J.A. 1996. *Psychopharmacology and women: sex, gender, and hormones.* Washington, D.C.: American Psychiatric Press.

Jones, K.L.; Johnson, K.A.; and Chambers, C.D. 1997. Birth outcomes in pregnant women taking fluoxetine. Letters to the Editor. *The New England Journal of Medicine* 336:873.

Koren, G.; Pastuszak, A.; and Ito, S. 1998. Drugs in pregnancy. *The New England Journal of Medicine* 338:1128–1137.

Kulin, N.A.; Pastuszak, A.; Sage, S.R.; Schick-Boschetto, B.; Spivey, G.; Feldkemp, M.; Ormond, K.; Matsui, D.; Stein-Schechman, A.K.; Cook, L.; Brochu, J.; Rieder, M.; and Koren, G. 1998. Pregnancy outcome following maternal use of new selective serotonin reuptake inhibitors. *Journal of the American Medical Association* 279:609–610.

Leavitt, A.M.; Yerby, M.S.; Robinson, N.; Sells, C.J.; and Erickson, D.M. 1992. Epilepsy in pregnancy: developmental outcome of offspring at 12 months. *Neurology* 42. Suppl. 5:141–143.

Manford, M.S.; and Patton, J.H. 1993. In utero exposure to Fluoxetine HCL increases hematoma frequency at birth. *Pharmacology, Biochemistry and Behavior* 45: 959–962.

Nulman, I.; and Koren, G. 1996. The safety of fluoxetine during pregnancy and lactation. *Teratology* 53:304–308.

Nulman, I.; Rovet, J.; Stewart, D.E; Wolpin, J.; Gardner, H.A.; Theis, J.G.W.; Kulin, N.; and Koren, G. 1997. Neurodevelopment of children exposed in utero to antidepressant drugs. *The New England Journal of Medicine* 336:258–262.

Santiago, J.M. 1994. Commentary: the costs of treating depression. *The Journal of Clinical Psychiatry* 54:425–426.

Scolnik, D.; Nulman, I.; Rovet, J.; Gladstone, D.; Czuenta, D.; Gardner, H.A.; Gladstone, R.; Ashby, P.; Weksberg, R.; and Einarson, T. 1994. Neurodevelopment of children exposed in utero to phenytoin and carbamazepine monotherapy. *Journal of the American Medical Association* 271:767–770.

Sitland-Marken, P.A.; Rickman, L.A.; Wells, B.G.; and Mabie, W.C. 1989. Pharmacologic management of acute mania in pregnancy. *Journal of Clinical Psychopharmacology* 9:78–87.

St. Clair, S.M.; and Schirmer, R.G. 1992. First-trimester exposure to Alprazolam. *Obstetrics and Gynecology* 80:843–846.

Tanganelli, P.; and Regesta, G. 1992. Epilepsy, pregnancy, and major birth anomalies: an Italian prospective, controlled study. *Neurology* 42. Suppl. 5:89–93.

Wegner, C.; and Nau, H. 1992. Alteration of embryonic folate metabolism by valproic acid during organogenesis. *Neurology* 42. Suppl. 5:17–24.

Wisner, K.L.; Perel, J.M.; and Wheeler, S.M. 1993. Tricyclic dose requirements across pregnancy. *American Journal of Psychiatry* 150:1541–1542.

Yerby, M.S.; Friel, P.N.; and McCormick, K. 1992. Antiepileptic drug disposition during pregnancy. *Neurology* 42. Suppl. 5:12–16.

Menopause

Abraham, G.E. 1993. The chemical, biochemical, physiological and clinical basis for the use of natural steroid hormones during the postmenopause. *Physician Information Manual.* Lakewood, CO: Belmar Pharmacy.

Albery, N. 1997. Politics of menopause: my body, my life, my choice. Chapter in Wren, B.G., ed. 1997. *Progress in the Management of the Menapause.* New York: The Parthenon Publishing Group.

Avis, N.E.; and McKinlay, S.M. 1995. The Massachusetts Women's Health Study: An epidemiologic investigation of the menopause. *Journal of American Medical Women's Association* 50:45–48.

Balfour, J.A.; and McTavish, D. 1992. Transdermal Estradiol. A review of its pharmacological profile and therapeutic potential in the prevention of postmenopausal osteoporosis. *Drugs & Aging* 2:487–507.

Birge, S.J. 1997. The role of estrogen in the treatment of Alzheimer's disease. *Neurology* 48. Suppl. 7:S36–S41.

Borton, J.C. 1992. *Drawing from the women's well: reflections on the life passage of menopause.* San Diego, CA: LuraMedia.

Buckler, H.M.; and Robertson, W.R. 1997. Androgen production over the female life span. Chapter in Wren, B.G., ed. 1997. *Progress in the Management of the Menopause*. New York: The Parthenon Publishing Group.

Cooke, D. 1985. Psychosocial vulnerability to life events during the climacteric. *British Journal of Psychiatry* 147:71–75.

de Lignieres, B. 1997. Hormone-replacement therapy in women over 60: management of compliance. Chapter in Wren, B.G., ed. 1997. *Progress in the Management of the Menopause*. New York: The Parthenon Publishing Group.

Ditkoff, E.C.; Crary, W.G.; Cristo, M.; and Lobo, R.A. 1991. Estrogen improves psychological factors in asymptomatic postmenopausal women. *Obstetrics and Gynecology* 78:991–995.

Erikson, E.F. 1997. Clinical aspects of estrogens and osteoporosis. Chapter in Wren, B.G., ed. 1997. *Progress in the Management of the Menopause*. New York: The Parthenon Publishing Group.

Foidart, J.M.; Desreux, J.; Beliard, A.; Delvigne, A.C.; Denoo, X.; Colin, C.; Fournier, S.; and de Lignieres, B. 1997. Hormone-replacement therapy in women over 60: managment of cancer risks. Chapter in Wren, B.G., ed. 1997. *Progress in the Management of the Menopause*. New York: The Parthenon Publishing Group.

Gorodeski, G.I. 1997. Mechanism of action for estrogen in cardioprotection. Chapter in Wren, B.G., ed. 1997. *Progress in the Management of the Menopause*. New York: The Parthenon Publishing Group.

Graziottin, A. 1997. Hormones and libido. Chapter in Wren, B.G., ed. 1997. *Progress in the Management of the Menopause*. New York: The Parthenon Publishing Goup.

Greenwood, S. 1992. *Menopause naturally: preparing for the second half of life*. Volcano, CA: Volcano Press.

Grimwade, J.C.; Farrell, E.A.; and Murkies, A.L. 1997. Ultrasound and the endometrium in postmenopausal women. Chapter in Wren, B.G., ed. 1997. *Progress in the Management of the Menopause*. New York: The Parthenon Publishing Group.

Grodstein, F.; Stampfer, M.J.; Colditz, G.A.; Willett, W.C.; Manson, J.E.; Joffe, M.; Rosner, B.; Fuchs, C.; Hankinson, S.E.; Hunter, D.J.; Hennekens, C.H.; and Speizer, F.E. 1997. Postmenopausal hormone therapy and mortality. *The New England Journal of Medicine* 336:1769–1775.

Halbreich, U. 1997. Role of estrogen in postmenopausal depression. *Neurology* 48. Suppl. 7:S16–S20.

Henderson, V.W. 1997. Estrogens and dementia: a clinical and epidemiological update. Chapter in Wren, B.G., ed. 1997. *Progress in the Management of the Menopause*. New York: The Parthenon Publishing Group.

Henderson, V.W. 1997. The epidemiology of estrogen replacement therapy and Alzheimer's disease. *Neurology* 48. Suppl. 7:S27–S35.

Horrigan, B.J. 1996. *Red Moon Passage: The power and wisdom of menopause*. New York: Three Rivers Press.

Hughes, C.L.; Cline, J.M.; Williams, J.K.; Anthony, M.S.; Wagner, J.D.; and Clarkson, T.B. 1997. Dietary soy phytoestrogens and the health of menopausal women: overview and evidence of cardioprotection from studies in non-human primates. Chapter in Wren, B.G., ed. 1997. *Progress in the Management of the Menopause*. New York: The Parthenon Publishing Group.

Jordan, V.C.; MacGregor, J.I.; and Tonetti, D.A. 1997. Selective estrogen receptor modulators as a new postmenopausal prevention-maintenance therapy. Chapter in

Wren, B.G., ed. 1997. *Progress in the Management of the Menopause*. New York: The Parthenon Publishing Group.

Kindig, S.; and Sanford, D.G. 1998. *Midlife and menopause: celebrating women's health*. Washington, D.C.: Association of Women's Health, Obstetric and Neonatal Nurses.

Knight, D.C.; and Eden, A.A. 1996. Review of the clinical effects of phytoestrogens. *Obstetric and Gynecology* 87:897–904.

LeBoeuf, F.J.; and Carter, S.G. 1996. Discomforts of the perimenopause; *Journal of Obstetric, Gynecologic and Neonatal Nursing* 25:173–180.

Liberman, U.A.; Weiss, S.R.; Broll, J.; Minne, H.W.; Quan, H.; Bell, N.H.; Rodriguez-Portales, J.; Downs, R.W. Jr.; Dequeker, J.; and Farvus. M. 1995. Effect of oral aldendronate on bone mineral density and the incidence of fractures in postmenopausal osteoporosis. *The New England Journal of Medicine* 333:1437–1443.

McEwen, B.S.; Alves, S.E.; Bulloch, K.; and Weiland, N.G. 1997. Ovarian steroids and the brain: implications for cognition and aging. *Neurology* 48. Suppl. 17:S8–S15.

Moore, A.A.; and Noonan, M.D. 1996. A nurse's guide to hormone-replacement therapy. *Journal of Obstetric, Gynecologic, and Neonatal Nursing* 25:24–31.

Mosekilde, L.; and Thomsen, J.S. 1997. Bone structure and function in relation to aging and the menopause. Chapter in Wren, B.G., ed. 1997. *Progress in the Management of the Menopause*. New York: The Parthenon Publishing Group.

Palinkas, L.A.; and Barrett-Connor, E. 1992. Estrogen use and depressive symptoms in postmenopausal women. *Obstetrics and Gynecology* 80:30–36.

Pickar, J.H. 1997. Clinical implications for the endometrium of hormone-replacement therapy. Chapter in Wren, B.G., ed. 1997. *Progress in the Management of the Menopause*. New York: The Parthenon Publishing Group.

Prior, J.C. 1994. One voice on menopause. *Journal of the American Medical Women's Association* 49:27–29.

Punyahotra, S.; and Limpaphayom, K. 1997. An Asian perspective of menopause. Chapter in Wren, B.G., ed. 1997. *Progress in the Management of the Menopause*. New York: The Parthenon Publishing Group.

Resnick, S.M.; Maki, P.M.; Golski, S.; Kraut, M.A.; and Zonderman, A.B. 1998. Effects of estrogen replacement therapy on PET cerebral blood flow and neuro-psychological performance. *Human Behavior* 34:171–182.

Santoro, N. et al. 1996. Hyperestrogenism in the perimenopause. *Journal of Clinical Endocrinology and Metabolism* 81:1495–1501.

Schiff, I.; and Parson, A.B. 1996. *Menopause*. New York: Random House.

Sheehy, G. 1992. *The silent passage: menopause*. New York: Random House.

Sherwin, B.B. 1996. Hormones, mood, and cognitive functioning in postmenopausal women. *Obstetrics and Gynecology* 87:20S–26S.

Sherwin, B.B. 1997. Estrogen effects on cognition in menopausal women. *Neurology* 48. Suppl. 7:S21–S26.

Sherwin, B.B. 1997. The use of androgens in the postmenopause: evidence from clinical studies. Chapter in Wren, B.G., ed. 1997. *Progress in the Management of the Menopause*. New York: The Parthenon Publishing Group.

Stefanick, M.L.; Mackey, S.; Sheehan, M.; Ellsworth, N.; Haskell, W.L.; and Wood,

P.D. 1998. Effects of diet and exercise in men and postmenopausal women with low levels of HDL cholesterol and high levels of LDL cholesterol. *The New England Journal of Medicine* 339:12–20.

Stewart, D.E.; Boydell, K.; Derzko, C.; and Marshall, V. 1992. Psychologic distress during the menopausal years in women attending a menopause clinic. *International Journal of Psychiatry in Medicine* 22:213–220.

Stewart, D.E.; and Boydell, K.M. 1993. Psychologic distress during menopause: associations across the reproductive life cycle. *International Journal of Psychiatry and Medicine* 162.

Tailor, D. and Sumrall, A.C. 1991. *Women of the 14th Moon: writings on menopause*. Freedom, CA: The Crossing Press.

Wallis, C. 1995. The estrogen dilemma. *Time* June 26:46–53.

Wren, B.G., ed. 1997. *Progress in the Management of the Menopause*. New York: The Parthenon Publishing Group.

Menstruation

Endicott, J. 1993. The menstrual cycle and mood disorders. *Journal of Affective Disorders* 29:193–200.

Leibenluft, E.; Fiero, P.L.; and Rubinow, D.R. 1994. Effects of the menstrual cycle on dependent variables in mood disorder research. *Archives of General Psychiatry* 51:761– 781.

Tailor, D. 1988. *Red Flower: rethinking menstruation*. Freedom, CA: The Crossing Path.

Wagner, K.D. 1996. Major depression and anxiety disorders associated with Norplant. *The Journal of Clinical Psychiatry*. 57:152–157.

Mind and Body

Borysenko, J. 1987. *Minding the body, mending the mind*. New York: Bantam Books.

Breathnach, S.B. 1995. *Simple Abundance: a daybook of comfort and joy*. New York: Warner Books.

Goleman, D.; and Gurin, J. 1993. *Mind-body medicine: how to use your mind for better health*. Yonkers, New York: Consumer Report Books.

Hamer, D.; and Copeland, P. 1998. *Living with our genes: Why they matter more than you think*. Garden City, NY: Doubleday.

Kabat-Zinn, J. 1990. *Full catastrophe living*. New York: Delacorte.

Kabat-Zinn, J. 1992. Effectiveness of meditation-based stress reduction program in treatment of anxiety disorders. *American Journal of Psychiatry* 149:7.

Maton, K.I. 1989. The stress-buffering role of spiritual support: cross-sectional and prospective investigations. *Journal for the Scientific Study of Religion* 28:310–323.

Omega-3 Fatty Acids

Mes, M.; Smith, R.; Christophe, A.; Cosyns, P.; Desnyder, R.; and Meltzer, H. 1996. Fatty acid composition in major depression: decreased omega-3 fractions in cholesteryl esters and increased C20: 4 omega-6/C20:5 omega-3 ration in cholesteryl esters and phospholipids. *Journal of Affective Disorders* 38:35–46.

Peet, M.; Murphy, B.; Shay, J.; and Horrobin, D. 1998. Depletion of omega-3 fatty acid levels in red blood cell membranes of depressive patients. *Biological Psychiatry* 43:315–319.

Severus, W.E.; Ahrens, B; and Stoll, AL. 1999. Omega-3 fatty acids—the missing link? *Archives of General Psychiatry* 56:380–381,

Panic Disorder

Beck, C.T. 1996. A concept analysis of panic. *Archives of Psychiatric Nursing* 10: 265–275.

Beck, C.T. 1998. Postpartum onset of panic disorder. *Image: Journal of Nursing Scholarship* 30:131–135.

Carr, D.B.; and Sheehan, D.V. 1984. Panic attack: a new biological model. *The Journal of Clinical Psychiatry* 45:323–330.

Cohen, L.S.; Rosenbaum, J.F.; and Heller, V.L. 1989. Panic attack associated with placental abruption: a case report. *The Journal of Clinical Psychiatry* 50:266–268.

Cohen, L.S.; Sichel, D.A.; Dimmock, J.A.; and Rosenbaum, J.F. 1994. Impact of pregnancy on panic disorder: a case study. *The Journal of Clinical Psychiatry* 55: 284–288.

Cohen, L.S.; Sichel, D.A.; Dimmock, J.A.; and Rosenbaum, J.F. 1994. Postpartum course in women with preexisting panic disorder. *The Journal of Clinical Psychiatry* 55:289–292.

Cowley, D.S.; and Arana, G.W. 1990. The diagnostic utility of lactate sensitivity in panic disorder. *Archives in General Psychiatry* 47:277–284.

Cowley, D.S.; Dager, S.R.; and Dunner, D.L. 1986. Lactate-induced panic in primary affective disorder. *American Journal of Psychiatry* 143:646–648.

Facchinetti, F.; Romano, G.; Fava, M.; and Genazzani, A.R. 1992. Lactate infusion induces panic attacks in patients with premenstrual syndrome. *Psychosomatic Medicine* 54:288–96.

Hendrick, V.C.; and Altshuler, L. 1997. Management of breakthrough panic disorder symptoms during pregnancy. *Journal of Clinical Psychopharmacology* 17:228–229.

Klein, D.F. 1994. Commentary: pregnancy and panic disorder. *The Journal of Clinical Psychiatry* 55:293–294.

Koenigsberg, H.W.; Pollak, C.P.; Fine, J.; and Kakuma, T. 1992. Lactate sensitivity in sleeping panic disorder patients and healthy controls. *Biological Psychiatry* 32: 539–542.

Liebowitz, M.R.; Fyer, A.J.; Gorman, J.M.; Dillon, D.; Appleby, I.L.; Levy, G.; Anderson, S.; Levitt, M.; Palij, M.; Davies, S.O.; and Klein, D.F. 1984. Lactate provocation of panic attacks. *Archives of General Psychiatry* 41:764–770.

Morishima, H.O.; Pedersen, H.; and Finoher, M. 1978. The influence of maternal stress on the fetus. *American Journal of Obsetetrics and Gynecology* 131:286–290.

Myers, R.E. 1977. Production of fetal asphyxia by maternal psychological stress. *Pavlov Journal of Biological Science* 12:51–62.

Sandberg, D.; Endicott, J.; Harrison, W.; Nee, J.; and Gorman, J. 1993. Sodium lactate infusion in late luteal phase dysphoric disorder. *Psychiatry Research* 46: 79–88.

Villeponteaux, V.; Lydiard, B.; Laraia, M.; et al 1992. The effects of pregnancy on preexisting panic disorder. *The Journal of Clinical Psychiarty* 53:201–205.

Physiology

Angier, N. 1999 *Woman: an intimate geography*. Boston: Houghton Mufflin Company.

Pert, C.B. 1997. *Molecules of emotion: why you feel the way you feel*. New York: Scribner.

Raey, J.J.; and Johnson, C. 1997. *Shadow syndromes*. New York: Pantheon Books.

Speroff, L.; Glass, R.H.; and Kase, N.G. 1989. *Clinical gynecologic endocrinology and infertility*. Baltimore: Williams & Wilkins.

Pregnancy

Chelmow, D.; and Halfin, V.P. 1997. Pregnancy complicated by obsessive-compulsive disorder. *Journal of Maternal and Fetal Medicine* 6:31–34.

Coverdale, J.H.; McCullough, L.B.; Chervenak, F.A.; Bayer, T.; and Weeks, S. 1997. Clinical implications of respect for anatomy in the psychiatric treatment of pregnant patients with depression. *Psychiatric Services* 48:209–212.

Diket, A.L.; and Nolan. T.E. 1997. Anxiety and depression: diagnosis and treatment during depression. *Obstetrics and Gynecological Clinics of North America* 24:535–558.

Driscoll, J.W.; and Sozanski, G.K. 1990. Care of the pregnant woman with a pre-existing mental illness. Chapter in *NAACOG's Clinical Issues in Perinatal and Womens' Health Nursing*. Vol. 1 Philadelphia: Lippincott.

Hedegaard, M.; and Henriken, T. 1993. Psychological distress in pregnancy and preterm delivery. *British Medical Journal* 307:234–238.

Llewellyn, A.M.; Stowe, Z.N.; and Nemeroff, C.B. 1997. Depression during pregnancy and the puerperium. *The Journal of Clinical Psychiatry* 58. Suppl. 15:26–32.

Northcott, C.J.; and Stein, M.B. 1994. Panic disorder in pregnancy. *The Journal of Clinical Psychiatry* 55:539–542.

Oretti, R.G.; Hunter, C.; Lazarus, J.H.; Parkes, A.B.; and Harris, B. 1997. Antenatal depression and thyroid antibodies. *Biological Psychiatry* 41:1143–1146.

Spinelli, M.G. 1997. Interpersonal psychotherapy for depressed antepartum women: a pilot study. *American Journal of Psychiatry* 154:1028–1030.

Teixeira, J.M.A.; Fisk, N.M.; and Glover, V. 1999. Association between maternal anxiety in pregnancy and increased uterine artery resistance index: cohort-based study. *British Medical Journal* 18:153–157.

Viguera, A.C.; and Cohen, L.S. 1998. The course and management of bipolar disorder during pregnancy. *Psychopharmacology Bulletin* 34:339–345.

Wadhwa, P. 1993. Association between prenatal stress and infant birth weight and gestational age at birth. *American Journal of Obstetrics & Gynecology* 169:858–865.

Premenstrual Dysphoric Disorder (Premenstrual Syndrome)

Altshuler, L.L.; Hendrick, V.; and Parry, B. 1995. Pharmacological management of premenstrual disorder. *Harvard Review of Psychiatry* 2:233–245.

Bancroft, J. 1993. The premenstrual syndrome: a reappraisal of concept and the evidence. *Psycological Medicine.* Suppl. 24:1–47.

Berga, S.L. 1998. Understanding premenstrual syndrome. *Lancet* 351:465–466.

Brown, W.A. 1996. PMS: a quiet breakthrough. *Psychiatric Annal* 26:569–570.

Dalton, K. 1987. *The premenstrual syndrome.* New York: Fawson Associates.

Freeman, E.W.; Sondheimer, S.J.; Rickels, K.; and Alpert, J. 1993. Gonadotropin-releasing hormone agonist in treatment of premenstrual symptoms with and without comorbidity of depression: a pilot study. *The Journal of Clinical Psychiatry* 54: 192–195.

Freeman, E.W.; Rickels, K.; Sondheimer, S.J.; and Wittmaack, F.M. 1996. Sertraline versus desipramine in the treatment of premenstural syndrome: an open-label trial. *The Journal of Clinical Psychiatry* 57:7–11

Freeman, E.W.; and Halbreich, U. 1998. Premenstrual syndromes. *Psychopharmacology Bulletin* 34:291–295.

Freeman, E.W.; Rickels, K.; and Sondheimer, S.R. 1990. Ineffectiveness of progesterone suppository treatment for premenstrual syndrome. *Journal of the American Medical Association* 264:349.

Gallo, M.A.; and Smith, S.S. 1993. Progesterone withdrawal decreases latency to and increases duration of electrified prod burial: a possible rate model of PMS anxiety. *Pharmacology Biochemistry and Behavior* 46:897–904.

Gelenberg, A.J. 1995. Psychotropic drugs for premenstrual dysphoria. *Biological Therapies in Psychiatry: Newsletter* 18:1–2.

Gelenberg, A.J. 1997. Treating PMS. *Biological Therapies in Psychiatry: Newsletter.* January:1.

Gelenberg, A.J. 1998. Sertraline for PMDD. *Biological Therapies in Psychiatry: Newsletter* 21:1–2.

Gold, J.H. 1985. *The psychiatric implications of menstruation.*Washington, D.C.: American Psychiatric Press.

Halbreich, U. 1996. Reflections on the cause of premenstrual syndrome. *Psychiatric Annals* 26:581–585.

Halbreich, U.; Endicott, J.; and Nee, J. 1983. Premenstrual depressive changes. *Archives of General Psychiatry* 40:535–542.

Halbreich, U.; and Tworek, H. 1993. Altered serotonergic activity in women with dysphoric premenstrual syndromes. *International Journal of Psychiatry in Medicine* 23:1–27.

Harrison, M. 1985. *Self-help for premenstrual syndrome.* New York: Random House.

Harrison, W.M.; Rabkin, J.G.; and Endicott, J. 1985. Psychiatric evaluation of premenstrual changes. *Psychosomatics* 26:789–799.

Levitte, S.S. 1997. Treatment of premenstrual exacerbation of schizophrenia. *Psychosomatics* 38:582–584.

Misri, S.; and Susak, L. 1991. Premenstrual syndrome: fact and fiction. *The Canadian Journal of Ob/Gyn & Women's Health Care* 3:201–205.

Mortola, J.F. 1992. Assessment and management of premenstrual syndrome. *Current Opinion in Obstetrics and Gynecology* 4:877–885.

Mortola, J.F. 1998. Premenstrual syndrome—pathophysiologic considerations. *The New England Journal of Medicine* 338:256–257.

Pearlstein, T. 1996. Nonpharmacologic treatment of premenstrual syndrome. *Psychiatric Annals* 26:590–594

Price, W.A.; and Giannini, A.J. 1985. Premenstrual tension syndrome. *Resident & Staff Physician* 31:34–38.

Roca, C.A.; Schmidt, P.J.; Bloch, M.; and Rubinow, D.R. 1996. Implications of endocrine studies of premenstrual syndrome. *Psychiatric Annals* 26:576–580.

Rubinow, D.R.; and Schmidt, P.J. 1995. The treatment of premenstrual syndrome—forward into the past. *The New England Journal of Medicine* 332:1574–1575

Rubinow, D.R. 1992. The premenstrual syndrome. *Journal of the American Medical Association* 268:1908–1912.

Sampson, G.A.; and Jenner, F.A. 1977. Studies of daily recordings from the Moos Menstrual Distress Questionaire. *British Journal of Psychiatry* 130:265–271.

Schmidt, P.J.; Nieman, K.L.; Danaceau, M.A.; and Rubinow, D.R. 1998. Differential behavioral of gonadal steroids in women with and in those without premenstral syndrome. *The New England Journal of Medicine* 338:209–216.

Shangold, G.A. 1993. The premenstrual syndrome: theories of etiology with relevance to the therapeutic use of GnRH agonists. *Seminars in Reproductive Endocrinology* 11:172–186.

Smith, S.; and Schiff, I. eds. 1993.. *Modern management of premenstrual syndrome.*New York: Norton Medical Books.

Sondheimer, S.J.; Freeman, E.W.; Scharlop, B.; and Rickels, K. 1985. Hormonal changes in premenstrual syndrome. *Psychosomatics* 26:803–810.

Steiner, M.; and Wilkins, A. 1996. Diagnosis and assessment of premenstrual dysphoria. *Psychiatric Annals* 26:571–575.

Steiner, M.; Korzekwa, M.; Lamont, J.; and Wilkins, A. 1997. Intermittent fluoxetine dosing in the treatment of women with premenstural dysphoria. *Psychopharmacology Bulletin* 33:771–774.

Steiner, M.; Steinberg, S.; Stewart, D.; Carter, D.; Berger, C.; Reid, R.; Grover, D.; and Streiner, D. 1995. Fluoxetine in the treatment of premenstrual dysphoria. *The New England Journal of Medicine* 332:1529–1534.

Sugawara, M.; Toda, M.A.; Shima, S.; Mukai, T.; Sakakura, K.; and Kitamura, T. 1997. Premenstrual mood changes and maternal mental health in pregnancy and the postpartum period. *The Journal of Clinical Psychology* 53:225–232

Taylor, D.L. 1994. Evaluating therapeutic change in symptom severity at the level of the individual woman experiencing severe PMS. *Image: Journal of Nursing Scholarship* 26:25–33.

Wikender, I.; Sunblad, C.; Andersch, B.; Dagnell, I.; Zylberstein, D.; Bengtsson, F.; and Ericksson, E. 1998. Citalopram in premenstrual dysphoria: is intermittent treatment during luteal phases more effective than continuous medication throughout the menstrual cycle? *The Journal of Clinical Psychopharmacology.* 18:390–398.

Yonkers, K.A. 1996. The association between premenstural dysphoric disorder and other mood disorders. *The Journal of Clinical Psychiatry* 58. Suppl. 15:16–25.

Yonkers, K.A.; and Brown, W.A. 1996. Pharmacologic treatments of premenstrual dysphoric disorder. *Psychiatric Annals* 26:586–589.

Yonkers, K.A.; and White, K. 1992. Premenstrual exacerbation of depression: one process or two? *The Journal of Clinical Psychiatry* 53:289–292.

Postpartum Mood and Anxiety Disorders

Affonso, D.D. 1992. Postpartum Depression: a nursing perspective on women's health and behaviors. *Image: Journal of Nursing Scholarship* 24:215–221.

Ahokas, A.J.; Turtianinen, S.; and Aito, M. 1998. Sublingual estrogen treatment for postnatal depression. *Lancet* 351:109.

Albright, A. 1993. Postpartum Depression: an overview. *Journal of Counseling & Development* 71:316–320.

Altshuler, L.L.; Hendrick, V.; and Cohen, L.S. 1998. Course of mood and anxiety disorders during pregnancy and the postpartum period. *The Journal of Clinical Psychiatry* 59. Suppl. 2:29–33.

Amino, N.; Mori, H.; Iwatani, I.; Tanizawa, O.; Kawashima, M.; Tsuge, I.; Ibaragi, K.; Kamahara, Y.P.; and Miyal, K. 1996. High prevalence of transient post-partum thyrotoxicosis and hypothyroidism. *The New England Journal of Medicine* 306: 849–851.

Appleby, L.; Gregoire, A.; Platz, C.; Prince, M.; and Kumar, R. 1994. Screening women for high risk of postnatal depression. *Journal of Psychosomatic Research* 38:439–445.

Austin, M.P.V. 1992. Puerperal affective psychosis: is there a case for lithium prophylaxis? *British Journal of Psychiatry* 161:692–694.

Barnett, B. 1991. *Coping with postnatal depression.* Melbourne, Australia: Lothian Books.

Beck, C.T. 1992. The lived experience of postpartum depression: a phenomenological study. *Nursing Research* 41:166–170.

Beck, C.T. 1993. Teetering on the edge: a substantive theory of postpartum depression. *Nursing Research* 42:42–48.

Beck, C.T. 1995. Screening methods for postpartum depression. *Journal of Obstetric, Gynecologic, and Neonatal Nursing* 24: 308–312.

Beck, C.T. 1995. The effects of postpartum depression on maternal-infant interaction: a meta-analysis. *Nursing Research* 44:298–304.

Beck, C.T. 1996. A meta-analysis of the relationship between postpartum depression and infant temperment. *Nursing Research* 44:225–230.

Beck, C.T. 1996 Postpartum depressed mothers' experiences interacting with their children. *Nursing Research* 45:98–104

Beck, C.T. 1998. The effects of postpartum depression on child development: a meta-analysis. *Archives of Psychiatric Nursing* 12:12–20.

Beck, C.T. 1998. Postpartum onset of panic disorder. *Image: Journal of Nursing Scholarship* 30:131–135.

Bernazzani, O.; Saucier, J.F.; David, H.; and Borgeat, F. 1997. Psychosocial predictors of depressive symptomatology level in postpartum women. *Journal of Affective Disorders* 46:39–49.

Bing, E.; and Colman, L. 1994. Shades of Blue. *Childbirth Instuctor Magazine.* Autumn:35–41.

Brockington, I.F.; Cernik, K.F.; Schofield, E.M.; Downing, A.R.; Francis, A.F.; and Keelan, C. 1981. Puerperal psychosis. *Archives of General Psychiatry* 38:829–833.

Burak, C.S.; and Remington, M.G. 1994. *The cradle will fall.* New York: Donald I. Fine, Inc.

Cohen, L.S. 1997. Currents Interview: update on postpartum psychiatric disorders: an interview with Lee S. Cohen, M.D. *Currents in Affective Illness* 16:5–12.

Cooper, P.J.; and Murray, L. 1995. Course and recurrence of postnatal depression. Evidence for the specificity of the diagnostic concept. *British Journal of Psychiatry* 166:191–195.

Cox, J.L.; Holden, J.M.; and Sagovsky, R. 1987. Detection of postnatal depression. Development of the 10-item Edinburgh Postnatal Depression Scale. *The British Journal of Psychiatry* 150:782–786.

Cox, J.L.; Murray, D.; and Chapman, G. 1993. A controlled study of the onset, duration and prevalence of postnatal depression. *British Journal of Psychiatry* 163: 27–31.

Cramer, B. 1993. Are postpartum depressions a mother-infant relationship disorder? *Infant Mental-health* 14:283–297.

Dalton, K. 1980. *Depression after childbirth.* New York: Oxford University Press.

Dix, C. 1985. *The new mother syndrome.* Garden City, NY: Doubleday.

Driscoll, J.W. 1990. Maternal parenthood and the grief process. *Journal of Perinatal and Neonatal Nursing* 4:1–10.

Driscoll, J.W. 1992. Postpartum depression. Chapter in Angelini, D.J.; and Whelan Knapp, C., eds. 1992. *Case Studies in Perinatal Nursing.* Gathersburg, MD: Aspen Publications.

Dunnewold, A.; and Sanford, D.G. 1994. *Postpartum survival guide.* Oakland, CA: New Harbinger Publications.

Fossey, L.; Papiernik, E.; and Bydlowski, M. 1997. Postpartum blues: a clinical syndrome and predictor of postnatal depression? *Journal of Psychosomatic Obstetrics and Gynecology* 18:17–21.

Fowles, E.R. 1998. The relationship between maternal role attainment and postpartum depression. *Health Care of Women International* 19:83–94.

Gregoire, A.J.; Kumar, R.; Henderson, A.F.; and Studd, J.W.W. 1996. Transdermal estrogen for treatment of severe postnatal depression. *Lancet* 347:930–933.

Gruen, D.S. 1990. Postpartum depression: a debilitating yet often unassessed problem. *Health and Social Work* 15:261–269.

Gruen, D.S. 1993. A group psychotherapy approach to postpartum depression. *International Journal of Group Psychotherapy* 43:191–203.

Hamilton, J.A.; and Harberger, P.N. 1992. *Postpartum Psychiatric Illness: a picture puzzle.* Philadelphia: University of Pennsylvania Press.

Handley, S.L.; Dunn, T.L.; Baker, J.M.; Cockshott, C.; and Gould, S. 1977. Mood changes in the puerperium and plasma tryptophan and cortisol concentrations. *British Medical Journal* 2:18–20.

Harris, B. 1993. A hormonal component to postnatal depression. *British Journal of Psychiatry* 163:403–405.

Hay, D.F.; and Kumar, R. 1995. Interpreting the effects of mothers' postnatal depression on children's intelligence: a critique and re-analysis. *Child Psychiatry & Human Development* 25:165–181.

Henderson, A.F.; Gregoire, A.J.P.; Kumar, R.C.; and Studd, J.W.W. 1991. Treatment of severe postnatal depression with oestradiol skin patches. Letter. *The Lancet* 338:816–817.

Hobfoll, S.E.; Ritter, C.; Lavin, J.; Hulsizer, M.R.; and Cameron, R.P. 1995. Depression prevalence and incidence among inner-city pregnant and postpartum women. *Journal of Consulting & Clinical Psychology* 63:445–453.

Kendell, R.E.; Chalmers, J.C.; and Platz, C. 1987. Epidemiology of puerperal psychosis. *British Journal of Psychiatry* 150:662–673.

Kirschenbaum, S. 1995. More than blue. *Mothering* Spring:73–79.

Klaiber, E.L.; Broverman, D.M.; Vogel, W.; and Kobayashi, Y. 1979. Estrogen therapy for severe persistent depression in women. *Archives of General Psychiatry* 36:742–747.

Kleiman, K.R.; and Raskin, V.D. 1994. *This isn't what I expected. Recognizing and recovering from depression and anxiety after childbirth*. New York: Bantam Books.

Kumar, R.C. 1997. "Anybody's child": severe disorders in mother-to-infant bonding. *British Journal of Psychiatry* 171:175–181.

Kumar, R.; and Robson, K. 1984. A prospective study of emotional disorders in childbearing women. *British Journal of Psychiatry* 144:45–37.

McIntosh, J. 1993. Postpartum depression: women's help-seeking behaviour and perceptions of cause. *Journal of Advanced Nursing* 18:178–184.

Madsen, L. 1994. *Rebounding from childbirth*. Westport, CT: Bergin & Garvey.

Mallett, P.; Andrew, M.; Hunter, C.; Smith, J.; Richards, C.; Othman, S.; Lazarus, J.; and Harris, B. 1995. Cognitive function, thyroid status and postpartum depression. *Acta Psychiatry Scandanavica* 91:243–246.

Mayberry, L.J.; and Affonso, D.D. 1993. Infant temperment and postpartum depression: a review. *Health Care of Women International* 14:201–211.

Meakin, C.; Brockington, I.F.; Lynch, S.E.; and Jones, J.R. 1995. Dopamine supersensitivity and hormonal status in puerperal psychosis. *British Journal of Psychiatry* 166:73–79.

Midmer, D.; Wilson, L.; and Cummings, S. 1995. A randomized, controlled trial of the influence of prenatal parenting education on postpartum anxiety and marital adjustment. *Family Medicine* 27:200–205.

Milgrom, J.; Westley, D.T.; and McCloud, P.I. 1995. Do infants of depressed mothers cry more than other infants? *Journal of Paediatrics & Child Health* 31:218–221.

Misri, S. 1995. *Shouldn't I be happy? Emotional problems of pregnant and postpartum women*. New York: The Free Press.

Murray, L. 1991. The impact of postnatal depression on infant development. *The Journal of Clinical Psychology and Psychiatry* 3:543–561.

Nonacs, R. et al. 1998. Postpartum mood disorders: diagnosis and treatment guidelines. *The Journal of Clinical Psychiatry* 59 Suppl. 2:29–33.

O'Hara, M.W. 1994. *Postpartum Depression: Causes and Consequences*. New York: Springer Verlag.

O'Hara, M.W.; and Swain, A.M. 1996. Rates and risk of postpartum depression- a meta-analysis. *International Review of Psychiatry* 8:37–54.

O'Hara, M.W. and Engeldinger, J. 1989. Postpartum mood disorders: detection and prevention. *The Female Patient* 14:19–27.

Pacific Postpartum Support Society. 1987. *Post partum depression and anxiety: a self-help guide for mothers.* Vancouver, British Columbia: Pacific Postpartum Support Society.

Pajer, K. 1995. New strategies in the treatment of depression in women. [Review] *The Journal of Clinical Psychiatry* 56. Suppl. 2:30–37.

Pariser, S.F.; Nasrallah, H.A.; and Gardner, D.K. 1997. Postpartum mood disorders: clinical perspectives. *Journal of Women's Health* 6:421–434.

Parry, B.L. 1989. Reproductive factors affecting the course of affective illness in women. *Psychiatric Clinics of North America* 12:207–219.

Placksin, S. 1994. *Mothering the new mother: your postpartum resource companion.* New York: Newmarket Press.

Pop, V.J.; de Rooy, H.A.; Vader, H.; van der Heide, D.; and vander von Son, M.M. 1993. Microsomal antibodies during gestation in relation to postpartum thyroid dysfunction and depression. *Acat Endocrinology (Copenhagen)* 129:26–30.

Purdy, D.; and Frank, E. 1993. Should postpartum depression be given a more prominent place in the DSM-IV? *Depression* 1:59–70.

Rees, B.l. 1995. Effect of relaxation with guided imagery on anxiety, depression, and self-esteem in primiparas. *Journal of Holistic Nursing* 13:255–267.

Roan, S.L. 1997. *Postpartum depression: every woman's guide to diagnosis, treatment, & prevention.* Holbrook, MA: Adams Media Corporation.

Robinson, G.E. 1994. Postpartum psychiatric disorders. *Contemporary OB/GYN* April:11–19.

Rubinow, D.R.; Schmidt, P.J.; and Roca, C.A. 1998. Hormone measures in reproductive endocrine-related mood disorders: diagnositic issues. *Psychopharmacology Bulletin* 34:289–290.

Ross, S.; Jennings, K.D.; and Popper, S.D. 1993. Identifying maternal depression in an early intervention setting. *Infants and Young Children* 5:12–21.

Sichel, D.A. 1992. Psychiatric Issues of the Postpartum Period: an interview with Deborah A. Sichel, M.D. *Currents in Affective Illness* 11:5–12.

Sichel, D.A.; Cohen, L.S.; Rosenbaum, J.F.; and Driscoll, J.W. 1993. Postpartum onset of obsessive-compulsive disorder. *Psychosomatics* 34:277–279.

Sichel, D.A.; Cohen, L.S.; Ammock, J.A.; and Rosenbaum, J.F. 1993. Postpartum obsessive compulsive disorder: a case series. *The Journal of Clinical Psychiatry* 54:156–159.

Sichel, D.A.; Cohen, L.S.; Robertson, L.M.; Ruttenberg, A.; and Rosenbaum, J.F. 1995. Prophylactic estrogen in recurrent postpartum affective disorder. *Biological Psychiatry* 38:814–818.

Stamp, G.E.; Williams, A.S.; and Crowther, C.A. 1996. Predicting postnatal depression among pregnant women. *Birth* 23:218–223.

Stamp, G.E.; Williams, A.S.; and Crowther, C.A. 1995. Evaluation of antenatal and postnatal support to overcome postnatal depression: a randomized controlled study. *Birth* 22:138–143.

Steiner, M. 1990. Postpartum psychiatric disorders. *Canadian Journal of Psychiatry* 35:89–95.

Susman, V.L.; and Katz, J.L. 1988. Weaning and depression: another postpartum complication. *American Journal of Psychiatry* 145:498–501.

Taylor, V. 1996. *Rock-a-by baby: feminism, self-help, and postpartum depression.* New York: Routledge.

Ugarriza, D.N. 1992. Postpartum affective disorders: incidence and treatment. *Journal of Psychosocial Nursing* 30:29–32.

Videbech, P.; and Gouliaev, G. 1995. First admission with puerperal psychosis: 7–14 years of follow-up. *Acat Psychiatrica Scandinavica* 91:167–173.

Weick, A.; Kumar, R.; Hirst, A.D.; Marks, M.N.; Campbell, I.C.; and Checkley, S.A. 1991. Increased sensitivity of dopamine receptors and recurrence of affective psychosis after childbirth. *British Medical Journal* 303:613–616.

Weinberg, M.K.; and Tronick, E.Z. 1998. The impact of maternal psychiatric illness on infant development. *Journal of Clinical Psychiatry* 59. Suppl. 2:53.

West, M.G. 1992. *If only I were a better mother.* Walpole, NH: Stillpoint Publishing.

Whiffen, V.E. 1992. Is postpartum depression a distinct diagnosis? *Clinical Psychological Review* 12:485–508.

Williams, K.E.; and Koren, L.M. 1997. Obsessive-compulsive disorder in pregnancy, the puerperium, and the premenstruum. *The Journal of Clinical Psychiatry* 58:330–334.

Winnicott, D.W. 1958. *Collected papers: through paediatrics to psychoanalysis.* New York: Basic Books.

Winnicott, C.; Shepherd, R.; and Davis, M., eds. 1987. Winnicott, D.W. *Babies and their mothers.* Reading, MA: Addison-Wesley Publishing Company, Inc.

Winnicott, C.; Bollas, C.; Davis, M.; and Shepherd, R. 1993. *Talking to parents: D.W. Winnicott.* Reading, MA: Addison-Wesley Publishing Company, Inc.

Wisner, K.L.; Peindl, K.; and Hanusa, B.H. 1993. Relationship of psychiatric illness to childbearing status: a hospital-based epidemiologic study. *Journal of Affective Disorders* 28:39–50.

Wisner, K.L.; and Wheeler, S.B. 1994. Prevention of recurrent postpartum major depression. *Hosptial and Community Psychiatry* 45:1191–1196.

Wisner, K.L.; Peindl, K.S.; and Hanusa, B.H. 1995. Psychiatric episodes in women with young children. *Journal of Affective Disorders* 34:1–11.

Wisner, K.L.; and Stowe, Z. 1997. Psychobiology of postpartum mood disorders. *Seminars in Reproductive Endocrinology* 15:77–89.

Wisner, K.L.; Perel, J.M.; Peindl, K.S.; Findling, R.L.; and Hanusa, B.H. 1997. Effects of the postpartum period on nortriptyline pharmacokinetics. *Psychopharmacology Bulletin* 33:243–248.

Wisner, K.L.; Peindl, K.S.; and Hanusa, B.H. 1996. Effects of childbearing on the natural history of panic disorder with comorbid mood disorder. *Journal of Affective Disorders* 41:173–180.

Post-Traumatic Stress Disorder

Ballard, C.G.; Stanley, A.K.; and Brockington, I.F. 1995. Post-traumatic strss disorder (PTSD) after childbirth. *British Journal of Psychiatry* 166:525–528.

Friedman, M.J. 1988 Toward rational pharmacology for PTSD. *American Journal of Psychiatry* 145:281–285.

Goldbeck-Wood, S. 1996. Post-traumatic stress disorder may follow childbirth. *British Medical Journal* 313:774.

Kessler, R.C.; Sonnega, A.; Bromet, E.; Hughes, M.; and Nelson, C. 1995. Post-traumatic stress disorder in the national comorbidity survey. *Archives of General Psychiatry* 52:1048–1060.

Reynolds, J.L. 1997. Post-traumatic stress disorder after childbirth: the phenomenon of traumatic birth. *Canadian Medical Asssociation Journal* 156:831–835.

Rhodes, N.; and Hutchinson, S. 1994. Labor experiences of childhood sexual abuse survivors. *Birth* 21:213–220.

Van der Kolk, B.; and Saporta J. 1993. Biological responses to psychic trauma. In Wilson, J.; and Raphael, B., eds. 1993. *International Handbook of Traumatic Stress Syndrome*. New York: Plenum Press.

Solomon, S.D.; Gerrity, E.T.; and Muff, A.M. 1992. Efficacy of treatments for post-traumatic stress disorder: an empirical review. *Journal of the American Medical Association* 268:633–638.

Stress

Copper, R.L.; Goldenberg, R.L.; Das, A.; Elder, N.; Swain, M.; Norman, G.; Ramsey, R.; Cotroneo, P.; Collins, B.A.; Johnson, F.; Jones, P.; Meier, A.; and the National Institute of Child Health and Human Development Maternal-Fetal Medicine Units Network. 1996. The preterm prediction study: maternal stress is associated with spontaneous preterm birth at less than thirty-five weeks' gestation. *American Journal of Obstetrics and Gynecology* 175:1286–1292.

Dolan, R.J.; Calloway, S.P.; Fonagy, P.; et al. 1985. Life events, depression and the hypothalamic pituitary adrenal axis. *British Journal of Psychiatry* 147:429–433.

Dorn, L.D.; and Chrousos, G.P. 1997. The neurobiology of stress: understanding regulation of affect during female biological transitions. *Seminars in Reproductive Endocrinology* 15:19–35.

Jaffe, R.; Jauniaux, E.; and Hustin, J. 1997. Maternal circulation in the first-trimester human placenta—myth or reality? *American Journal of Obstetrics and Gynecology* 176:695–705.

Lewinsohn, P.M.; Hoberman, H.M.; and Rosenbaum, M. 1988. A prospective study of risk factors in unipolar depression. *Journal of Abnormal Psychology* 97:251–264.

Lloyd, C. 1980. Life events and depressive disorder reviewed. *Archives of General Psychiatry* 37:529–535.

McEwen, B.S. 1995. Stressful experience, brain, and emotions: developmental, genetic, and hormonal influences. Chapter in Gazzaniga, M.S., ed. 1995. *The Cognitive Neurosciences*. Cambridge, MA: The MIT Press.

McEwen, B.S. 1998. Protective and damaging effects of stress mediators. *The New England Journal of Medicine* 338:171–179.

McEwen, B.S.; and Stellar, E. 1993. Stress and the individual: mechanisms leading to disease. *Archives of Internal Medicine* 153:2093–2101.

Myers, R.E. 1977. Production of fetal asphyxia by maternal psychological stress. *Pavlovian Journal of Biological Science* 12:51–52.

Paykel, E.S. 1978. Contribution of life events to causation of psychiatric illness. *Psychological Medicine* 8:245–253.

Post, R.M. 1992. Tranduction of psychosocial stress into neurobiology of recurrent affective disorder. *American Journal of Psychiatry* 149:999–1010.

Shrout, P.E.; Link, B.G.; Dohrenwend, B.P.; Skodol, A.E.; Stueve, A.; and Mirotznik, J. 1989. Characterizing life events as risk factors for depression: the role of fateful loss events. *Journal of Abnormal Psychology* 98:460–467.

Thyroid

Kaptein, E.M. 1996. Thyroid testing. *Medical Advances–Health in Mind & Body* 1: 8.

Oreti, R.G.; Hunter, C.; Lazarus, J.H.; Parkes, A.B.; and Harris, B 1997. Antenatal depression and thyroid antibodies. *Biological Psychiatry* 41:1143–1146.

Prange, A.J. 1996. Thyroid disorders related to depression. *Medical Advances–Health in Mind & Body* 18.

Tremont, G.; and Stern, R.A. 1997. Use of thyroid hormone to diminish the cognitive side effects of psychiatric treatment. *Psychopharmacology Bulletin* 33:273–280.

Women's Issues

Baron-Faust, R. 1997. *Mental wellness for women.* New York: William Morrow & Company, Inc.

Belenky, M.F.; Clinchy, B.M.; Goldberger, N.R.; and Tarule, J.M. 1986. *Women's ways of knowing: the development of self, voice, and mind.* New York: Basic Books, Inc.

Borysenko, J. 1996. *A woman's book of life: the biology, psychology, and spirituality of the feminine life cycle.* New York: Riverhead Books.

Colditz, G.A.; Manson, J.E.; and Hankinson, S.E. 1997. The Nurses' Health Study: 20-year contribution to the understanding of health among women. *Journal of Women's Health* 6.

Foley, D.; and Nechas, E. 1993. *Women's encyclopedia of health and emotional healing.* Emmaus, PA: Rodale Press.

Gilligan, C. 1982. *In a different voice.* Cambridge, MA: Harvard University Press.

Gilligan, C.; Ward, J.V.; and Taylor, J.M., eds. 1988. *Mapping the moral domain.* Cambridge, MA: Harvard University Press.

Halbreich, U. 1998. Future directions for studies of women's mental health. *Psychopharmacology Bulletin* 34:327–328.

Hancock, E. 1989. *The girl within: recapture the childhood self, the key to female identity.* New York: E.P. Dutton.

Jordan, J.V.; Kaplan, A.G.; Miller, J.B.; Stiver, I.P.; and Surrey, J.L. 1991. *Women's growth in connection: writings from the Stone Center.* New York: Guilford Press.

Leibenluft, E.; Fiero, P.L.; and Rubinow, D.R. 1994. Effects of the menstrual cycle on dependent variables in mood disorder research. *Archives of General Psychiatry* 51:761–781.

Miller, J.B. 1986. *Toward a new psychology of women.* 2d Edition. Boston: Beacon Press.

Mirkin, M.P. 1994. *Women in context: toward a feminist reconstruction of psychotherapy.* New York: The Guilford Press.

Northrup, C. 1994. *Women's bodies, women's wisdom: creating physical and emotional health and healing.* New York: Bantam Books.

Parry, B.L. 1996. Women and depression. *Medical Advances–Health in Mind & Body* 1:1–2.

Speroff, L., ed. 1996. Oral contraceptives and breast cancer. *OB/GYN Clinical Alert* 13:25–28.

Stewart, D. E.; and Stotland, N.L., eds. 1993. *Psychological aspects of women's health care.* Washington, D.C.: American Psychiatric Press.

Swedo, S.; and Leonard, H. 1996. *It's not all in your head.* San Francisco: HarperSanFrancisco.

INDEX